FOREWORD

Little need be said by way of foreword to this work. The demand that is daily multiplying from the students of medicine and the profession at large is sufficient evidence that the book is one which should be republished.

The plan on which the book rests covers the questions and answers relating to the field of clinical work, and the book with many improvements and additions as made has been so neatly arranged that it can be claimed to be an indispensable guide for beginners and practitioners alike. It became a question whether the book should be republished in two volumes, one covering the questions, the other the answers. In the belief, however, that in a work in which numerous cross-references are unavoidable, it has been decided to keep it as a single volume.

It is hoped that the book will be widely welcome and will prove helpful in the field of practical solution for the complicated problems of clinical diagnosis.

Cordial thanks are extended to Messrs. Boericke & Tafel, Philadelphia, U.S.A., for giving us the privilege of being the publishers of this novel book in India.

A HANDBOOK FOR VIVA-VOCE

A Syllabus of Diagnosis

(with Practice of Medicine & Surgery Covered in Depth)

WILLIAM F. BAKER, A.M., M.D.

CLINICAL INSTRUCTOR OF MEDICINE IN THE
HAHNEMANN MEDICAL COLLEGE
OF PHILADELPHIA, PA.

FIRST INDIAN EDITION
(Thoroughly Revised & Augmented)

B. Jain Publishers (P) Ltd.
An ISO 9001 : 2000 Certified Company
USA—EUROPE—INDIA

A HANDBOOK FOR VIVA-VOCE

4th Impression: 2009

All rights reserved. No part of this book may be reproduced, stored in a retrieval system or transmitted, in any form or by any means, mechanical, photocopying, recording or otherwise, without any prior written permission of the publisher.

© with the Publisher

Published by Kuldeep Jain for
B. JAIN PUBLISHERS (P) LTD.
An ISO 9001 : 2000 Certified Company
1921/10, Chuna Mandi, Paharganj, New Delhi 110 055 (INDIA)
Tel.: 91-11-2358 0800, 2358 1100, 2358 1300, 2358 3100
Fax: 91-11-2358 0471 • *Email:* info@bjain.com
Website: **www.bjainbooks.com**

Printed in India by
J.J. Offset Printers

ISBN: 978-81-319-0834-1

PREFACE

In presenting a syllabus of such an ever widening field of medical science as diagnosis, the writer feels that he is supplying a need not only of the student undertaking the subject for the first time, but also of the advanced student in the research connected with his clinical work. It seems to have been the complaint of students in general that they "hardly know where to begin the study of such a large subject." In order that the book may be of particular service to Hahnemann College student, the same plan of arrangement is carried out as is found in that excellent work of Dr. Clarence Bartlett on the subject.

The questions are taken direct from the teachings of Profs. Bertlett, and Snader, and with their consent published after being reviewed by them.

The questions on Physical Diagnosis are the first series Dr Snader has compiled for publication.

1425 Spruce St., Phila.,
    U. S. A.

CONTENTS

CHAPTER		PAGE
I.	EXAMINATION OF THE PATIENTS	1
II.	TEMPERATURE *including* SUB-NORMAL TEMPERATURE, RIGORS and SWEAT	4
III.	THE PULSE *including* PHLEBITIS, AND VENOUS PULSATIONS	26
IV.	RESPIRATION	41
V.	THE DIGESTIVE TRACT LIPS—MOUTH—GUMS—TEETH—TONGUE—LINGUAL TONSIL—SALIVA—OFFENSIVE BREATH—FAUCES—PHARYNX—TONSILS—ŒSOPHAGUS—STOMACH—INTESTINES—RECTUM.	47
VI.	THE DIGESTIVE TRACT (*continued*) LIVER—GALL-BLADDER—BILE-DUCTS	114
VII.	THE DIGESTIVE TRACT (*continued*) SPLEEN	120
VIII.	THE DIGESTIVE TRACT (*continued*) PANCREAS	121
IX.	THE RESPIRATORY ORGANS NOSE—PHYSICAL DIAGNOSIS—CHEST	124
X.	THE RESPIRATORY ORGANS (*continued*) LARYNX	147

CONTENTS

CHAPTER		PAGE
XI.	THE RESPIRATORY ORGANS (*continued*) GENERAL DISEASES	160
XII.	THE RESPIRATORY ORGANS (*continued*) LUNGS—TRACHEA—BRONCHI	175
XIII.	THE CIRCULATORY SYSTEM THE HEART	184
XIV.	THE URINE	200
XV.	THE KIDNEYS	218
XVI.	THE BLOOD	225
XVII.	THE EXTERNAL SURFACE ALTERATIONS in SIZE *and* SHAPE	238
XVIII.	THE NERVOUS SYSTEM	258
XIX.	THE CEREBRAL LOCALIZATION	307
XX.	THE SPINAL LOCALIZATION	318
XXI.	THE EYE	327
XXII.	THE EAR	350
XXIII.	THE X-RAY DIAGNOSIS	367
	THE INDEX	376

A SYLLABUS OF DIAGNOSIS

CHAPTER I.

EXAMINATION OF THE PATIENTS.

1. **Outline one practical way of Questioning the Patients.**

    When visiting a patient for the first time a physician should begin with some commonplace words and try to become familiar with the patient and extract from him indirectly every possible information of his sufferings.

    When conducting subsequent examinations, after putting some general questions, such as, how the patient is progressing and such others, he should enquire specifically as to the condition of each of the symptoms noted on previous visits.

2. **Why is it necessary that a Physician should keep Accurate and Systematic Records?**

    They cultivate proper methods of clinical works and make the recorder a finished clinician. They enable the physician to consult the past history of the patient and formulate his method of treatment and also present them as finished scientific treatises to his colleagues and followers.

3. **Name the principal Subjects of Enquiry in medical cases.**

    The principal subjects of enquiry are—
    (i) The GENERAL HISTORY of the patient, by *interrogation*.

(ii) If the DISORDER relates to one or more special physiological systems—by *interrogation*.
(iii) The GENERAL CONDITION of the patient—by *observation* or *investigation*.
(iv) The CONDITION of the system most affected and finally of each of the other affected systems—by *examination*.

4. What constitutes a Physical Examination?

Examination of the corporal symptoms of a disease in a patient by *investigation* of his general state, and of the organ most affected, and finally each of the other special systems by *inspection, palpation, percussion, auscultation*, etc.

5. What do you understand by the term Symptom: Sign?

By SYMPTOM, we understand the change or phase which occurs in the body or its functions, either subjective or objective, synchronously with a disease or indicating a disease and serves to point out its nature and origin. *It is perceived only by the patient.*

By SIGN, we understand any diagnostic or indicative symptom—an objective evidence of a disease, *appreciable by some one other than the patient.*

6. In general what do Physical Signs represent?

They represent the purely local evidences of a disease, afforded by the direct examination of the organs involved.

7. Give an instance in which the Family History plays an important part in the diagnosis.

In the diagnosis of congenital Syphilis a through study of the family history for several generations, as to the occurrence of a previous affection, plays an important part.

8. Give an example of a Congenital Defect.

Malformations—Atelocheilia, Ateloprosopia.

9. Name some diseases peculiar to children.

Scarlatina. Measles. Mumps. Whooping-Cough, etc.

10. Give an example where Age plays a part in diagnosis.

Convulsions.

11. Give an example where Sex plays a part in diagnosis.

Nervous diseases.

12. Give an example where Occupation plays a part in diagnosis.

Indigestion.

13. Give an example where Habits play a part in diagnosis.

In a case of nervous prostration.

14. Give an example where Environment plays a part in diagnosis.

In a doubtful Small Pox case.

15. Give an example where History of Preceding Disease plays a part in diagnosis.

In a chonic disease.

16. How may physical conditions be recorded in a record?

Physical conditions may be recorded in printed or rubber-stamped diagrams, outlining the different sections of the human body, which can be had from the noted chemists. In it the various lesions can be noted specifically, and placed on the same sheets as the balance of the records.

CHAPTER II.

TEMPERATURE

1. What is the only accurate way for determining the Bodily Temperature?

By observation of the same, with a good clinical *thermometer*, allowing sufficient time to obtain a correct reading.

2. What are the necessary factors in order that the observation with the Thermometer should be accurate?

(i) *Accuracy* of the instrument. (ii) Allowance of *sufficient time*. (iii) *Proper placing*—avoiding the seat of the local disease as the place of observation.

3. How long should a Thermometer be kept in situ when taking the Temperature?

An ordinary one—for 5 minutes. Rapidly-acting thermometers—double the time instructed in the instrument.

* 4. How does the Age of the Thermometer affect its Reading?

After an year or so, the instrument records about a degree above the correct temperature.

5. How do local diseases influence the reading of the Thermometer?

In the seat of local diseases the heat is much higher than the general temperature of the body.

6. What places are available for Thermometric observations?

The mouth. The axilla. The rectum. The vagina. The folds of the groins.

7. What precautions are to be adopted when taking Temperature Observations in the Mouth?

The bulb should be placed well beneath the tongue and completely covered by that organ. The thermometer should be thoroughly disinfected after use.

8. What precautions are to be observed when taking Axillary Temperature?

The bulb should be placed in the thoroughly dried axillary folds, not too deep as to protrude posteriorly. The muscles must be thoroughly relaxed.

9. What precautions are to be adopted when taking Temperature Observations in the Rectum and Vagina?

The bulb should be inserted about 2 inches in the verge of the anus or vagina.

10. In what class of cases would you use the Rectum or Vagina for taking Temperature?

In *comatose* and *convulsive* patients.

11. Under what circumstances is the taking of the Mouth Temperature inadmissible?

After partaking of any kind of food or when the patient suffers from stomatitis or dental diseases.

* **12. What are the relative differences of Temperatures taken in the Mouth, Axilla and Rectum?**

In the mouth about ½ a degree higher than those taken in the axilla; in the rectum and vagina half a degree higher than those of the mouth.

13. How frequently should Temperature Observations be taken?

Depends upon the nature of the case; generally 4 times a day.

* **14. Name the Physiological Influences causing variations in the Temperature.**

Taking of food; exercise; atmospheric heat; age; time of the day; and mental excitement.

15. What means have we for keeping an accurate Record of Temperature Observations?

Printed temperature charts.

✶ 16. How do you convert degrees Centigrade into degrees Fahrenheit and vice versa?

To convert degrees Centigrade into degrees Fahrenheit muliply the number by 9, divide by 5, and add 32.

In the reverse case, substract the number by 32, multiply by 5 and then divide by 9.

✶ 17. How does taking of Food influence Temperature?

Frequently, the temperature rises about half a degree after taking a full meal.

18. How does Exercise influence Temperature?

Exercise of a violent nature raises the temperature.

✶ 19. How does the Age of the Patient influence Temperature?

The temperature during infancy is slightly higher than the normal, but lower in advanced life. The temperature of the new-born infants varies from 99°F to 99.7°F. In persons past middle-life, it may be as low as 96°F. without being suggestive of illness.

20. How does Time of the Day influence Temperature?

The maximum temperature is attained in the afernoon or early evening; the minimum between midnight and early morning. In persons, who work at night and sleep during the day, these variations are reversed.

21. What is Fever?

Fever is a disordered state of the body marked by an elevation of temperature, attended with quick pulse indicating inrecased katabolism or tissue-waste and diminished secretion. Usually it is accompanied by thirst, loss of appetite and restlessness.

22. Define Slight Fever.

A febrile condition whose temperature varies from 99.5°F. to 101°F.

23. Define Moderate Fever.

Moderate fever is one whose temperature varies from 101°F. to 103°F.

24. Define High Fever.

A high fever is one whose temperature varies from 103°F. to 105.5°F.

25. Define Hyperpyrexia.

A hyperpyrexia is one whose temperature rises above 105.5°F.

26. What is the relative prognostic value of high temperature in Typhoid Fever and Pneumonia?

In TYPHOID FEVER, high temperature is looked upon with increasing gravity—much depending upon the duration of the pyrexia. If of short duration, say an hour or so, it does not signify much; when *lasting for days it is very serious*, but if unattended with nervous symptoms or rapid pulse (over 120 beat per minute), it need not be regarded with much alarm.

In PNEUMONIA, high temperature is one of the constant features of typical cases. It is *not so damaging* as that of Typhoid Fever because it is of short duration in Pneumonia.

*27. What is indicated by a fresh accession of fever after the temperature has fallen to the normal?

Indicates the advent of some complications.

*28. What is the indication afforded by fall of temperature without improvement in the associated symptoms?

Indicates the decline of vital powers with deficient heat production in the body. It is an evidence of collapse.

It also indicates the perforation of a hollow organ and the advent of hæmorrhage.

29. What are the general Pathological Factors producing fever?

(i) Infection of the blood by micro-organisms. (ii) The disturbances of the thermotaxic or the central heat-regulating mechanism. (iii) Peripheral nerve irritation.

✗ 30. In studying a case of fever to what points in the course of the disease should you pay attention?

In the initial stage—nature of the onset, whether gradual or rapid, the presence or absence of rigors, and the premonitory and associated symptoms.

The *fastigium* requires a study of its duration, the daily fluctuations of temperature and the character of the associated symptoms.

The *Stage of decline* demands a study of the fall of temperature whether lyterian or critical, if critical, the character of the symptoms associated with it.

Note.—Every case of fever must be studied according to the phenomena depicted in the individual stages, together with all associated symptoms.

31. What is Defervescence?

The stage of the fever when the temperature falls. With the abatement of the associated symptoms it is favourable, without which it is critical suggesting failing of vital powers.

32. What is Defervescence by Crisis?

When the fall of temperature is rapid it is called defervescence by *crisis*.

33. What is Defervescence by Lysis?

When the fall of temperature is gradual it is called defervescence by *lysis*. It is characterized by evening exacerbations and morning remissions.

34. Into what varieties may we divide fevers according to their temperature curves?

Continued. Remittent. Intermittent. Relapsing.

35. What is Continued Fever?

The fever in which the rise of temperature is slow and continuous.

36. What is Remittent Fever?

A paroxysmal fever in which the temperature remains persistently above the normal, with a wide diurnal variation amounting to 2 or more degrees is called a Remittent Fever.

37. What is Intermittent Fever?

The fever in which the symptoms intermit, with intermediate periods of freedom from febrile attack, is called an Intermittent Fever.

38. Name some Continued Fevers.

Simple Continued Fever, Typhoid Fever, Typhus Fevers, Pneumonic Fevers, Erysipelas, Small Pox, etc.

39. Name some disease which may present either continued, remittent or intermittent temperature-curves.

Typhoid Fever, Tuberculosis, Influenza, Malaria.

40. What is the special character of the mode of onset of the fever in Scarlatina?

As a rule, *sudden*, with disproportionately high pulse rate.

41. What relation does the fever of Scarlatina have to the time of appearance of the eruption?

The relation is definite and distinctive. The eruption appears on the day following the advent of fever.

42. What is the usual cause of suddenly appearing fever without apparent physical or other signs of local disease in infants?

Gastro-intestinal disorder (Acute Gastric Catarrh).

43. What are the usual symptoms associated with fever?

Increased frequency of pulse and respiration; alteration in pulse-tensions, and more or less disturbance of the secretory functions.

44. Describe the typical temperature-curve of Typhoid Fever.

The typical temperature-curve portrays a gradual rise of the curve for the first 5 or 6 days, rising about 2°F. in the evening and falling about 1°F. in the morning daily, *in a step-like manner*, to the highest point, travels in the same line with slight daily variations for a week or more, and then inclines downwards by steps, as it rose gradually, until it reaches the normal point in the 21st day or later.

45. Describe some of the departures from the typical temperature-curve observed in Typhoid Fever.

When the disease sets in with a chill, or in children with a convulsion, the temperature rises at once to 103°F. or 104°F.

Sometimes, a drop of over 6°F. follows an intestinal hæmorrhage or perforation.

Sometimes during the Anæmia which follows a severe hæmorrhage from the bowels there are remarkable oscillations in the temperature.

In some cases, there is a higher fever in the morning than in the afternoon or evening.

46. What is suggested by the sudden fall of the temperature in the course of Typhoid Fever?

A suggestion for *alertness*. If associated with the cardinal symptoms, it is suggestive of intestinal hæmorrhage or perforation.

47. Describe the usual mode of onset of the fever in Croupous Pneumonia.

The fever begins *with the very inception* of the disorder. The height of the fever may be 104° to 106°F. and is attained almost at once, sometimes within 12 hours.

48. Describe some of the temperature symptoms of Tuberculosis.

In the *initial stage*, the morning temperature varies from 97° to 97.5°F., while the evening temperature from 99° to 100.5°F.; in more severe cases it may reach 103° to 104°F. As a rule the maximum is attained between 2 and 6 P.M., while the minimum between 2 and 6 A.M.

In *advanced cases*, the tempeature usually attains a fairly high level and oscillates between 101° to 104°F. or more. The temperature begins to rise in the afternoon reaching the maximum between 8 and 10 P.M.—sometimes well into the night, which offers an unfavourable prognosis.

49. Describe the febrile curve of Small Pox.

There is an initial rise in the curve, often to a high point (103° to 105°) which falls on the 2nd or 3rd day, almost to the normal point and remaining slightly above the normal until the 8th or 9th day, it again rises to as high or higher point than in the beginning. With slight variations till the 14th day, it inclines downwards gradually day by day, till it reaches the normal point in about 7 to 10 days.

50. Describe the temperature-curve of Septicæmia.

The tempeature curve in Septicæmia rises moderately at first and then more or less rapidly, being characterized by irregular remissions and exacerbations, even intermissions.

51. Mention some fevers with sudden onset.

Scarlet Fever, Pneumonic Fevers, Malarial Fevers, Inflammatory Fevers, Typhus Fever, Fevers of Erysipelas, Measles, Variola, and fevers of the gastro-intestinal disorders.

52. Mention some fevers of gradual onset.

Typhoid Fever, Influenza, etc.

53. Give the usual concomitant symptoms of fever.

Exhaustion, emaciation, disturbances of the nervous system and indigestion.

54. Give some nervous symptoms of fever.

Restlessness, sleeplessness, headache, delirium, apathy and coma.

55. Outline what is meant by the term Simple Continued Fever.

A continued fever which is not associated with symptoms other than those of the febrile process especially, and have not its origin in any known specific infection or local pathological process.

56. What is the value of persistent high fever in Typhoid?

See Ans. to Q. 26.

57. How may an Intestinal Perforation be suggested from the temperature-curve?

Sudden abnormal drop of temperature in the curve during the course of Typhoid Fever suggests an intestinal perforation. See also answer to Q. 46 above.

58. Describe the temperature-curve of Measles.

The temperature-curve of Measles begins either with an initial rise to 101°F. or thereabout in the 1st day, falling promptly to a little above the normal and remaining at the same position for the next 2 days with evening rises (very little) and morning falls, it rises again to a very high point (which may be as high as 106°F) on *the 4th day* with the appearance of rashes. It remains at the maximum point until the time the eruptions begin to fade, which is not longer than 2 days—usually one, when it slopes gradually to the normal point, within a period of 24 to 36 hours.

59. What is the character of the fever usually associated with Vaccination?

Though the temperature may rise as high as 104.5°F. it subsides within 48 hours. The symptoms associated are trivial.

60. Describe the fever of Erysipelas.

It is characterized by a severe chill, followed by a rapid rise in the temperature—which may be upto

104°F. or higher. It follows a continuous course without marked remissions for 4 or 5 days, after which it becomes intermittent and later usually irregular. Defervescence by crisis or lysis, usually the former.

61. Describe the fever of the Acute Miliary Tuberculosis.

No settled type. Generally sometime after the infection an irregular fever appears. It increases rapidly with evening exacerbations and morning remissions. The pulse *exceedingly rapid*. It is associated with *profuse* and *exhausting perspiration*. The temperature disturbance is of highest importance from both diagnostic and prognostic standpoint.

62. When do the temperature-curves of Septiæmia resemble those of Tuberculosis?

When Septicæmias develop without any local site of infection their temperature-curves resemble those of Tuberculosis.

63. What can you say of the activity of the Pathological process as related to the fever in Tuberculosis?

The activity of the fever suggests the activity of the pathological process. They are directly proportionate. When the cavities are blocked and their secretions retained, the temperature rises promptly and falls as the cavities are emptied.

64. How would you differentiate the fever of Miliary Tuberculosis from that of Typhoid Fever?

Disproportionately rapid pulse in Tuberculous fever from the beginning, differentiates it with Typhoid Fever, whose pulse-beat is proportionate to the temperature present. The former is associated with profuse and exhausting sweat.

65. What variety of Tuberculosis is usually characterized by a high Remittent Fever?

Caseous Tuberculosis.

66. In what form of Tuberculosis, (a) the temperature is characterized by great variety of range ; (b) is there almost a complete absence of fever ?

(a) Chronic Fibro-caseous Tuberculosis.
(b) Fibroid Tuberculosis.

67. Name two general characteristics of Malarial Fevers.

Periodicity & intermittence.

68. Mention the varieties of Malarial fevers as to recurrence of the paroxysms.

(1) Quotidian, (2) Tertian and (3) Quartan.

69. Describe the fever of Dengue.

Sudden onset, high temperature, rapid or gradual, may rise upto 105°F. or more. Fever continues at its maximum from 3 to 5 days, after which it begins to subside gradually, reaching the normal within 12 to 36 hours. Associated with most severe pain in the joints and muscles. Full and bounding pulse.

70. Describe the temperature-curve of Cerebro-spinal Meningitis.

It has no definite temperature curve. An ordinary case presents a curve with a gradual rise upto 102°F. from the 1st or the 2nd day of attack for a week or 10 days with morning falls and evening rises. Defervescence by lysis.

71. Describe the fever of Influenza.

The fever is of no settled type. May be continued or remittent or intermittent with sudden or gradual onset. Generally there is a rapid rise of temperature (upto 104°F. or more). When uncomplicated, the height of the fever is reached on the day of attack or at the latest, at the end of the 2nd day, and as a rule, disappears within 3 or 4 days, in advance of the symptoms associated with it.

72. Describe what is meant by Relapsing Fever.

A specific infectious disease, a mild form of

epidemic malignant remittent fever, caused by the Spirochætes, and characterized by terminating suddenly within a week, only to return after a like period of a febrile state. It is also called the Famine Fever.

73. Describe the course of the fever in Yellow Fever.

Sudden onset with chilly feeling in the morning and rapid rise of temperature of any degree upto 106°F. It remains the same till the morning of the 2nd day and keeps on going with slight diurnal variation till the 3rd day, after which it falls by lysis. In fatal cases, continuous, the temperature becoming higher.

74. Describe the course of the fever in Miliary Fever.

High temperature from the beginning, which may rise upto 104°F. In mild cases a slight fever.

75. Name the varieties of Septic Fevers.

Sapræmia. Toxæmia. Septicæmia. Pyæmia.

76. Describe the fevers of Septicæmia and Pyæmia.

The *fevers of Septicæmia* run a very irregular course. It comes with a chill or chilliness with moderate rise in temperature, more or less rapid, marked by irregular daily remissions and exacerbations, even intermissions. In fatal case, the fever runs high till the end and may be complicated with a typhoid state.

The *fevers of Pyæmia* may be remittent or intermittent with sudden onset, following a severe chill. Rapid rise of temperature to 103° or 104°F., followed by a profuse sweat. Temperature irregular, varies from hour to hour. When intermittent, it simulates Malaria, but is marked by the irregularity of its return with chills and sweat. The course of the fever may prolong for a long time irregularly.

77. Give the characteristics of the fever in Malta Fever.

Irregular temperature of a variable length of a distinctly remittent character. Liable to a series of relapses.

78. Tell the course of the fever in infantile indigestion.

Sudden onset with a rise in temperature without any objective signs of local disease. Similar to the fever of Scarlatina (vide Q. 40) but without the disproportionately high pulse-rate of the latter. It may run a continued or remittent course, of long or short duration.

79. Mention the characteristics of the fevers of the Morphia Habitutes.

The fever is intermittent and apt to be accompanied with neuralgic pains and intense prostration. Quinine has no effect over it—a dose of Morphia relieves it quickly.

80. Describe the fever of Syphilis.

In the initial stage, the fever is usually slight, sometimes sharp and remittent and is accompanied with a malaise.

At the time of the secondary outbreaks, the fever may be slight or intense and very variable in character; ordinarily it ranges between 101° and 102°F., the evening temperature being one degree higher than the morning, continuing throughout the night regularly. In exceptional cases the temperature ranges from 104° to 106°F. and may be confused with Rheumatic fever and Typhoid Fevers.

The fevers of the *tertiary stage* are persistently high.

81. Describe the fever associated with the Anæmias.

The fevers associated with the Anæmias have no special characteristic except that their temperature-curves are marked by *irregularities*.

In *Chlorosis* and *Secondary Anæmia*, the fever is slight. In *Pernicious Anæmia*, moderate. In *Lukœmia*, moderate—seldom rises above 102°F., exceptionally it may be as high as 104°F. In Acute *Lymphatic Lukœmia* the fever is usually high—may run a continuous course simulating Typhoid Fever. In *Lymphadenoma* the fever presents different types; in the initial stage—moderate fever with somewhat irregular course ; towards the terminal stage the temperature becomes decidedly irregular with higher intensity exhibiting remarkable daily remissions and intermissions ; during the progress of the disease it may assume the type of a Relapsing Fever with high temperature of a steady rise and gradual fall. In *Purpura Rheumatica* and *Purpura Hæmorrhagica* the fever is moderate.

82. What are the characteristics of the fever of Cholera Infantum ?

The temperature is unusually high with coolness of the surface of the body ; the variance of the axillary temperature with that of the rectum, is greater than usual.

83. When is fever present in Appendicitis ?

The fever of a moderate intensity (100° to 102°F.) is always present *in the early stage*, which continues if the case goes on to the formation of a local abscess.

84. Describe the phenomena of Heat-stroke or Thermic Fever.

The *heat-stroke* is a state of *nervous exhaustion* caused by exposure to intense heat. It begins with a staggering gait, pallid face, a small and soft pulse, enfeebled respiration developing into a syncope or profound prostration. Muscular spasms are frequent. Severe cases end in deep coma and finally death due to heart failure. The attack is preceded by giddiness and vertigo or headache.

The *Thermic fever* originating from the same cause as the Heat-stroke comes on suddenly with a malaise, giddiness, vertigo, headache, photophobia, sometimes vomiting, diarrhœa and frequent micturition, after which *a very high fever* sets in with a relatively slow pulse, followed by early unconsciousness, laboured (sometimes stertoreous) breathing, lividity of the face, warmth of the skin and relaxation of the muscles. In fatal cases, with dyspnœa and delirium the coma deepens, pulse becomes more rapid and feeble, finally ending in death within a few hours—36 hours to the utmost.

85. Describe some of the atypical temperature-curves of Typhoid Fever.

See Ans. to Q. 45.

86. Give the prodromal symptoms suggestive of Typhoid Fever.

A general feeling of illness accompanied by restlessness and discomfort, headache, anorexia, constipation or diarrhœa and epistaxis. The onset is often suggestive, particularly when *epistaxis* and the *step-like ascending fever* are present. The presence of *dicrotic pulse* is also a valuable indication.

87. Describe the second week of Typhoid Fever.

The symptoms ameliorate or aggravate according to the severity of the attack in this period. In MILD CASES, the temperature subsides to the normal in the end of this week with the accompanying symptoms. In MODERATE CASES, the virus spends its force in this period, which leads the case on to recovery, which usually happens a week later. In SEVERE CASES, all the symptoms become aggravated in this period and new complications set in.

88. What are the most common complications of the heart in Typhoid Fever?

The granular parenchymatous degeneration of the myocardium and the true Myocarditis. The heart becomes soft and flabby.

89. What is the condition of spleen in Typhoid Fever?

The spleen enlarges during the early stage and increases rapidly to 2 to 3 times of its normal size, attaining the maximum during the height of the fever, and retaining its abnormality till the convalescence begins, gradually diminishing with the fever.

90. Describe the so-called "Rose-spots" of Typhoid Fever.

The erythematous eruptions (2 to 4 m. m. in diameter and slightly convex) of a rose-red colour (fading on pressure) coming on during the 2nd week, above the surface of the skin (usually on the abdomen and lower portion of the chest or upon the back) in successive crops, are known as the Rose-spots. Each crop lasts for about 4 days and may persist till the end of the disease, usually disappearing within a couple of weeks. It is one of the most characteristic symptoms of Typhoid Fever and has much diagnostic value. Their abundance does necessarily signify the more severity of the disease.

91. Of what value are urinary examinations in the diagnosis of Typhoid Fever?

They have little or no practical diagnostic value.

92. Give the abdominal symptoms of Typhoid Fever.

Loss of appetite, diarrhœa, constipation, nausea, vomiting, flatulence, pain, tenderness, tympanites, intestinal hæmorrhage and perforation, peritonitis and ascites.

93. How would you diagnose a hæmorrhage of the bowels in Typhoid Fever and what information might the condition of the blood furnish you (a) as to extent of lesion; (b) amount of ulceration?

Its onset is usually characterized by a sudden fall in temperature (upto 10° F.), a drop of 10 to 20 m. m. in the systolic blood-pressure, and quickening of the pulse and the general features attending all internal hæmorrhage. Its usual time of occurrence is in the earlier part of the 3rd week, when occurring earlier i. e., in the later part of the second week it is a *dangerous* omen, signifying the rapidity and virulence of the attack.

Information from the blood—

(a) as to the extent of lesion, it is nearer to the anus if the colour approaches the normal, remote when presents a tarry or pitch-like appearance.

(b) as to the amount of ulceration, if the discharge is little, the ulceration is small, if diffused, the size is large.

94. What symptoms suggest Intestinal Perforation?

A sudden severe pain in the hypogastric region and to the right of the middle and local tenderness in the same. Rapid and extreme distension and rigidity of the abdomen. The pulse is very rapid. Tremor of the tongue. Silencing of the peristaltic movements over the site of the perforation. Hæmorrhage which may precede or accompany the perforation. Leucocytosis. See also Ans. to Q. 46 & 93.

95. Mention some respiratory symptoms of Typhoid Fever.

Epistaxis, Laryngitis, Bronchitis, Broncho or Lobar Pneumonia, Hypostatic congestion and Œdema of the lungs etc.

96. Describe some of the nervous symptoms of Typhoid Fever.

Headache, backache, vertigo, apathy, coma vigil, stupor, insomnia, delirium, psychoses, tremor, subsultus tendinum, etc.

97. Upon what features does the prognosis of Typhoid Fever depend?

The important elements in the prognosis of Typhoid Fevers are—pulse and temperature, quantity of urine, presence or absence of toxic features, and the period of illness from the time when absolute rest was first enforced.

98. Mention the characteristic symptoms of Scarlet Fever.

Sudden onset with rapid rise of the temperature, vomiting, sore-throat, disproportionately rapid rise in the pulse-rate, appearance of the characteristic rashes, white strawberry tongue and well-marked leucocytosis.

99. Describe the complications met with in Scarlet Fever.

Arthritis, Endorcarditis, Purulent Pericarditis, Toxic Myocarditis, Empyema, Pleurisy, Acute Bronchitis, Broncho-Pneumonia, Otitis Media, Nephritis, Adenitis, Measles, and sudden convulsions followed by Hemiplegia.

100. Describe the symptoms of Measles.

Fever (see Ans. to Q. 58), furred tongue, pulse rate increasing with fever, Koplik's Spots, characteristic rashes with catarrhal symptoms increasing in violence with the advent of the rashes.

101. Give the principal diagnostic features of Small-pox.

(i) History—as to the condition of vaccination in the patient.

(ii) Environment—as to epidemic condition or presence or absence of Small-pox in the locality.

(iii) Characteristic symptoms.—Sudden onset with more or less severe chill, moderate fever, severe headache and backache ; initial rashes may appear on the 2nd day disappearing within 24 to 48 hours ; characteristic eruptions as papules on the 3rd or 4th day, in one crop, first upon the forehead, near the hairline and wrists, involving the whole body within 24 hours. The odor of the Small-Pox patients are very distinctive from the early stage.

102. Differentiate the eruption of Small Pox from that of Varicella (Chicken Pox).

The eruption of Small-pox comes out first as a papule turning into vesicles after 24 hours, whereas the eruption of Varicella is vesicular, almost from the beginning. The eruptions of Small-pox are circular in shape and indurated, while those of Varicella are ovoid in shape and look more superficial. The eruptions of the former are surrounded by distinct areola, which is wanting in Varicella. The eruption of Small-pox presents a shotty feel to the examining hand, while that of Chiken-pox is soft to the touch.

103. Give the diagnostic symptoms of Erysipelas.

Rapid onset. Rapid rise of fever preceded by a severe chill. Induration of the local lesion, surrounded by an irregular line of demarcation—the edges being raised and hard.

104. Mention the varieties of Tuberculosis.

Acute Miliary Tuberculosis. Tuberculosis of the lymphatic system. Acute Pulmonary Tuberculosis. Chronic Fibro-caseous Tuberculosis. Fibroid Tuberculosis. Also Tuberculoses of the brain and chord, alimentary canal, liver, mammary gland, circulatory system and genito-urinary system.

105. Describe the types of Malarial Fevers to time of occurrence of the paroxysm.

Paroxysm occurring regularly at intervals of 48 hours i.e., on every third day is known as *Tertian*, and that which occurs on every fourth day has been named *Quartan*. The paroxysm which occurs daily is known as *Quotidian*.

106. Give the stages of the Malarial attack.

(1) *Cold Stage*—marked by more or less severe chills with violent shiverings and shakings ; (2) *Hot Stage*—is marked by occasional flushes of heat and the disappearance of the chill. (3) *Sweating Stage*—when the temperature subsides, sweat at first appears on the head and face, which soon becomes general and usually very profuse.

107. Give the diagnostic symptoms of Cerebro-spinal-Meningitis.

(1) General features—sudden onset, fever, severe headache, retraction of the neck, rigidity of the muscles particularly of the neck and back, tremor and delirium the spinal symptoms are very marked.

(2) *Special features*—(a) *Kernig's Sign*—if the thigh is flexed at right angles to the abdomen, the complete extension of the leg at the knee in a straight line with the thigh is imposible, which under normal conditions is possible ; *Brudzinski's Sign*—if the head is flexed on the chest, involuntary flexion of the legs at the hip and knee-joints follows. Also flexing one leg on the trunk, produces the same movement in the other.

(3) Clinical tests—(a) *Lumbar Puncture*—if the puncture is dry, the indication is negative ; if a fluid comes out and is distinctly turbid in appearance the sign

is positive. (b) *Leucocyte Count*—pronounced leucocytosis.

108. Give some symptoms suggesting Yellow Fever.

Abrupt onset. Fever with chill—temperature 101°—104°F., sometimes higher, continuing for 3 or 4 days falls to (or below) normal by crisis ; followed by a period of remission of 2 or 3 days, reactionary fever appears, which follows an irregular course for 3 or 4 days, usually disappearing by lysis. Pulse at first full and strong but slow relatively to the temperature ; *during the reactionany fever pulse retards while the temperature rises.* Flushing face. Highly albuminous scanty urine. Tenderness of the epigastrium. Jaundice. Black vomit. Epistaxis. Hæmorrharge from the bowels. Metrorrhagia.

Unfavourable symptons—high temperature (105° 106°F.) ; persistent vomiting ; black vomit ; suppression of urine and great epigastric distress.

RIGORS.

109. What do you understand by the term Rigor ?

A sensation of coldness that causes tremor or shivering.

110. Give the symptoms usually associated with Chill.

General distress ; headache ; nausea and vomiting; various pains ; shivering or tremor ; coldness of the surface of the body.

111. Give the Physiological causes of Rigor.

(1) Exposure to cold and (2) sensory irritation through the skin and ears.

112. Give the Pathological causes of Rigor.

Suppuration aud septic infections.

113. What is the greatest diagnostic value of Rigors as a symptom ?

They indicate suppuration in the course of an illness in which septic infection is a possibility.

114. Occurring in the course of a continued fever Rigors usually suggest what?

Usually suggest a suppurative complication, generally of abscess or phlebitis.

115. What do you understand by the so-called Nervous Chills?

Cold and creepy sensations in which the objective phenomena of a chill are absent.

SUB-NORMAL TEMPERATURE

116. What constitutes a Sub-normal Temperature?

The exhaustion or withdrawal of heat from the body causes a sub-normal temperature.

117. Mention some pathological states associated with a Sub-normal Temperature.

Exhausting hæmorrhages, shock, collapse, toxæmia, Pernicious Anæmia and circulatory weakness.

118. Name some constitutional diseases associated with a Sub-normal Temperature.

Diabètes, Cancer, Cholera Asiatica, Cholera Morbus, and Tuberculosis.

119. What nervous conditions have a Sub-normal Temperature?

Melancholia, Apoplexy, Brain tumor, Tubercular Meningitis, etc.

120. A morning Sub-normal Temperature with an evening rise without other symptoms makes one suspicious of what?

An incipient tubercular disease of the lungs.

SWEAT

121. What do you understand by the term Hyperidrosis?

A functional disorder of the sudoriferous glands characterized by *excessive secretion* of sweats.

122. What do you understand by the term Anhidrosis?

An altered condition of the sweat in which *deficiency* is marked.

123. What do you understand by the term Bromidrosis?

An offensive sweat.

124. What do you understand by the term Chromidrosis?

Coloured sweating usually black or sepia in colour.

125. What do you understand by the term Hæmatohydrosis?

A bloody sweat.

126. Give some diagnostic features of Anhidrosis.

(1) Deficiency in the regulation of the bodily temperature whenever heated from any cause.

(2) Partial detention of the excrementitious substances in the system.

(3) Abnormal excretion from the other organs.

127. Mention some conditions suggested by Hyperidrosis.

(1) *A sign of exhaustion*—when occurring at the end of convalescence from acute and long-lasting illness.

(2) *A sign of collapse*—when occurring in cases leading rapidly towards a fatal issue.

(3) *A critical phenomenon*—in Intermittent Fever and Croupous Pneumonia.

(4) *A prominent feature*—in acute inflammatory Rheumatism.

128. What condition of sweat is usually found in Diabetes?

Anhidrosis.

CHAPTER III.

THE PULSE.

1. How do you examine the Pulse—(a) by Hand; (b) by Instrument?

(a) Conducted by palpating usually one of the radial arteries of the patient with three fingers, in a way, so that the index finger is placed towards the circulatory centre, subject to precautions as enumerated in answer to Q. 4 of this chapter.

(b) Conducted by *Sphygmograph* and *Polygraph*.

2. Give the methods for recording information learned from the Pulse.

(a) When by *hand*—the pulse-rate, its rhythm, the size, force and character of the waves, the resistance of the artery to pressure between the pulse-beats and difference in the two radial pulses in their beats are recorded in plain or printed sheets.

(b) When by *instrument*—recorded in a sphygmogram.

3. When examining the Pulse to what points should you pay attention.

(1) The frequency, (2) regularity, (3) force or strength and (4) tension of the pulse. (5) The thickness and size of the arterial walls. (6) The condition of the arterial walls. (7) The character of onset and subsidence of the individual beats.

4. What precautions are necessary in order to avoid errors in taking of the Pulse?

Avoidance of the time of physical or mental excitement of the patient. The counting should be for full one minute to find its average frequency.

5. What is the Normal Pulse Frequency?

The normal pulse frequency of an adult is *72 beats* per minute.

6. What Physiological factors vary the Pulse?

Age. Sex. Posture. Exercise. Excitement. Temperature. Diet. Time of day.

7. What is the effect of Age?

At birth—140, at one year—120, at two years—108, at ten years—90, in the old age 80 or thereabout, beats per minute.

8. What is the effect of Sex?

With the advent of puberty the female pulse becomes slightly greater in frequency which continues till the old age.

9. What is the effect of (a) Posture: (b) Exercise?

(a) The sitting posture increases the pulse rate by about 10 beats per minute than while lying; standing, by about 10 beats more than sitting.

10. What is the effect of Temperature on Pulse?

Intense heat may increase the pulse frequency to a great extent, it may even double the pulse-rate. With the cold it is the reverse.

11. Name the Pathological causes for increase in the Pulse Rate.

Fevers. Asthenia. Pain. Reflex irritation. Pulmonary diseases. Alcoholic excesses. Excessive indulgence in Tobacco. Convulsions. Irritable heart Tachycardia. Organic heart diseases.

12. What is the general rule for increase in the Pulse Rate for every degree of rise in the temperature?

As a rule, each degree increases the pulse-rate by 8 to 10 beats per minute. Notable exceptions may be found in Typhoid Fever, Meningitis, Scarlatina, Diphtheria and Peritonitis. In the first two, it is disproportionately slow, while in the last three, disproportionately rapid.

13. What effect has Pain on the Pulse Rate?

Increased frequency.

14. What is Tachycardia?

A cardiac disturbance in which the movement of the heart quickens abnormally owing to the disorder of the nervous regulatory apparatus and is characterized by a much higher frequency in the pulse rate, hence quick pulse.

15. What conditions produce persistent Tachycardia?

Anæmia, Dyspepsia, Neurosis, Mitral Stenosis, Mediastenal Tumor, Paralysis of Vagus in Peripheral Neuritis, febrile conditions, effects of certain drugs (Belladonna, Thyroid extract, etc.), abuse of tea, coffee or tobacco, Exophthalmic Goitre, and diseases of the Medulla Oblongata.

16. What conditions produce Paroxysmal Tachycardia?

Dilatation of the heart, nervous instability, infective processes (such as Rheumatism, Gout, Scarlatina and Syphilis), Mitral Stenosis, Myocardial degeneration, Aneurysm, Arterio-sclerosis, and cardio-renal disease. It may also be spontaneous or may be excited by digestive disturbances, muscular or mental strain, excitement or the like.

17. Mention some general conditions associated with Tachycardia.

Some anxiety and præcordial distress; slightly accelerated respiration; a sense of weakness; fainting attack, etc.

18. What is Bradycardia?

A form of cardiac disturbance in which the action of the heart is slow and infrequent and is characterized by a fall in pulse frequency much below the normal, and hence, a slow pulse.

19. Name some conditions associated with Bradycardia?

Dyspnœa, Palpitation, sense of constriction in

the chest, nausea, vomiting, severe abdominal pain, pain simulating Angina Pectoris, etc.

20. Name some of the brain diseases associated with Bradycardia.

Meningitis, Hpdrocephalus, Tumor and Abscess of the brain, Paralytic Dementia, etc.

21. What disease of the heart is especially liable to be associated with a slow Pulse ?

Stokes-Adams Disease.

22. What is the usual condition of the Pulse in Uræmia ?

The pulse is slow.

23. What is the prognostic value of a slow Pulse in Diptheria ?

Unfavourable—fore-runner of the Paralysis of the heart.

24. Name some of the poisons causing slow Pulse.

Digitalis, Opium, Carbonic Acid Gas, Lead.

25. Describe the Pulse usually associated with Jaundice.

The pulse is slow, often as low as 40 beats per minute.

26. What is meant by the term "Linked Beats" ?

Beats due to secondary ventricular contractions immediately after the normal ones.

27. What may be considered as safe limits of Pulse Frequency during an attack of Typhoid Fever ?

60 to 120 beats per minute.

28. Describe the Pulse of Miliary Tuberculosis.

In the early stage, weak and disproportionately rapid in comparison with the temperature. Slow and irregular when old.

29. What is Arrhythmia.

Irregularity in the rhythm of the pulse, characterized by pulsations of unequal duration or breaches in their continuity by occasionally dropping a beat, is known as arrhythmia.

30. Name some of the causes of Arrhythmia.

Lesions of the brain affecting the accelerans or pneumogastric nerves, affections of the heart, various Toxæmiæ, reflex irritation from the abdominal viscera and functional nervous disturbances.

31. What is an Intermittent Pulse?

When the pulse is characterized by breaches in the continuity of its pulsations by omitting a beat now and then, or at regular intervals, is said to be an intermittent pulse. It displays irregularities also in force—the pulsation immediately following the intermission is stronger than the others.

32. What is Pulsus Alternans?

An irregular pulse, in which every alternate beat is weaker and smaller than that which precedes it.

If continuous, it indicates the gravity of the situation; if present only for a few beats at a time, it is a signal of cardiac failure.

33. Describe the Pulsus Bigeminus.

This is an irregular pulse characterized by alternate quick and slow intervals between pulsations. A longer pause follows every two beats.

34. Describe the Pulsus Trigeminus.

This is an irregular pulse exhibiting longer intervals at the end of every third beat.

35. Describe the Pulsus Bigeminus et Alternans.

This is an irregular pulse in which two pulsation of unequal force are noted to occur quick together and are followed by an abnormal pause.

36. Describe the Pulsus Allorhythmia.

This is an irregular pulse which intermits or is irregular at every third or fourth beat.

37. Name some of the toxic causes of Arrhythmia.

Excessive indulgence in tea, coffee, tobacco and

alcohol; effects of drugs (Muscarine, Digitalis, Belladonna and Aconite) and certain infectious diseases in which Toxæmia is marked.

38. Give some of the reflex causes of Arrhythmia.

Indigestion, Flatulence, Renal colic, Biliary-calculi.

39. What valvular lesion is usually associated with an Arrhythmia?

Mitral Regurgitation.

40. What subjective symptoms may suggest an Arrhythmia?

Nervous disturbances—as effort syndrome, neuro-circulatory asthenia; respiratory irregularities; disagreeable sensation or discomfort in the præcordium; intense anxiety.

41. What does an Arrhythmia occurring during convalescence suggest?

Perverted nutrition of the heart muscle.

42. What are the features of Pulse in Miliary Tuberculosis?

The pulse-frequency increases beyond the average pulse temperature ratio, and the beat character is notable for its weakness and low tension in the early stage. After a few days it presents characteristic slowness and irregularity.

43. What is the Pulsus Paradoxus?

An irregular pulse characterized by weakness of the beats during inspiration, while strong during expiration or vice versa is called the pulsus paradoxus.

44. Give some of the conditions which may cause irregularity of the Pulse.

Meningitis, Neurasthenia, Hysteria, Shock Arterio-Sclerosis, Myocarditis, Mitral Regurgitation, etc.

45. Name some of the causes of irregular pulse.

Vide Ans. to Q. 38 of this chapter.

46. Describe the method of examining the Pulse for determining its tension.

The radial arteries is to be compressed with the examining fingers. To palpate the same, the vessel should be emptied at a point above the wrist, after which its wall must be rolled under the examining fingers to determine its tension, which may be soft or hard according to the condition of the patient. If soft the tension is low, if hard, it is high.

47. Name the general causes of increased vascular tension.

Increased volume of the blood. Frequent and powerful action of the heart and arteriole, and capillary contraction.

48. Give examples of increased arterial tension due to increased quantity of blood.

After partaking a very heavy meal the tension increases. In Nephritis, when the urine is scanty the tension is high. In plethora, the tension of the pulse is high.

49. What are the general causes of Arterio-capillary Resistance?

Old age. Heredity. Chill. Action of poisons in the blood. Over-eating. Pregnancy. Over-straining. Alcoholism. Deficiency of blood in the system. Abnormal collection of air in the arteries. etc.

50. Name some conditions producing high tension from increased Arterio-capilliary Resistance.

Old age. Heredity. Renal diseases. Gout. Diabetes. Lead-poisoning. Pregnancy. Anæmia. Emphysema.

51. What personal habits lead to High Arterial Tension?

Excessive indulgence in highly nitrogenous food, as meat. Drinking of small quantities of water. Too little or no exercise. Alcoholic drinks.

52. Name some of the evil results of High Arterial Tension.

Rupture of the blood-vessels. Cramps. Hypertrophy of the heart. Valvular diseases and Dilatation of the heart. Arterio-Sclerosis.

53. Name some of the causes of Low Arterial Tension.

Heredity. Obesity. Exposure to heat. Anxiety and worry. Debility. Food (improper quality and low quantity). Pyrexia. Dilatation of the capillaries and arterioles. Weakness of the cardiac action. Diminution in the quantity of blood.

54. Name some of the changes discoverable in the arterial walls by examining the radial arteries.

Thickness and undue hardness. May be tortuous. Rolls under the finger like a hard cord. Rough local patches of hardness. Gives the impression of a rigid, rough-walled tube.

55. With what conditions is Arterio-Sclerosis usually associated?

Interstitial Nephritis. Syphilis. Atheroma.

56. Describe the Pulse of Aortic Stenosis.

A hard, slow and infrequent pulse of moderate volume and fairly good tension.

57. Describe the Pulse of Aortic Insufficiency.

The pulse is more rapid in its rise and fall and the pulse-wave strikes the examining fingers forcibly with a bounding and throbbing impulse which immediately recedes or collapses.

58. What is the Water-hammer Pulse?

An irregular pulse which is characterized by bounding and throbbing pulsations, the rises of which are as sudden as the falls. To the examining finger the artery feels as if its contents had been suddenly projected against it, being immediately followed by a sudden falling away.

59. What is the Dicrotic Pulse?

An irregular pulse which imparts the sensation of a double beat at each pulsation. See also Ans. to Q. 80 of this chapter.

60. In which of the acute diseases is the Dicrotic Pulse apt to occur as a prominent feature?

Typhoid Fever.

61. What is the effect of heat on vascular tension?

Heat brings about vascular relaxation and hence the dilatation of the capillaries and arterioles, which causes the vascular tension to be diminished.

62. What is the effect on vascular pressure from the withdrawing quickly of large quantities of fluid?

The arterial tension is suddenly lowered. Often leads to fatal collapses.

63. How do you recognise changes in the vessels?

The pulse deviates from its normal course. Tension, size and structure of the arteries alter. Visceral disturbance of the particular vessel affected. By failing of the nutrition. By more or less general functional incapacity. By renal disturbance.

64. Name some of the causes of Arterio-Sclerosis.

Old age. Heredity. High arterial tension and blood pressure. Excessive physical exertion. Overstrain. Over-eating. Alcoholism. Lead-poisoning. Gout. Renal disease. Syphilis. Certain acute infections, viz., Influenza, Typhoid Fever, Malaria, Yellow Fever, Diphtheria, and Pneumonia.

65. What symptom should lead us to suspect Arterio-Sclerosis, when it is associated with an Interstitial Nephritis?

A persistent renal inadequacy with a deficient elimination of the urinary solids, specially of urea.

66. What is the characteristic of Arterio-Sclerosis dependent upon Syphilis i.e., what vessels are usually attacked?

The cerebral blood-vessels.

THE PULSE

67. What cause might result in a unilateral disturbance of the Pulse?

A congenital anomaly—due entirely to anatomical differences.

68. Name some causes for delay of radial Pulse.

Pleurisy, Pneumothorax, Embolism, Thrombosis, Tumors of the neck and axilla and aneurysm of the sub-clavian, axillary or brachial arteries.

69. Describe the Sphygmograph.

It is an instrument for ascertaining and recording graphically the character and differential features of the pulse. It gives an accurate record of the variations in arterial tension.

70. Describe the Polygraph.

It is an instrument by which simultaneous tracings of the radial pulse, of the pressure-changes in the jugular vein and their time are noted. It reveals the delay between auricular and ventricular events.

71. Describe the method of preparing smoked films and fixing them.

The smoked film is prepared by fixing a slip of paper in one of the tinholders of the instrument (a clinical polygraph), which is held over a piece of burning camphor, till it is evenly smoked.

72. Describe the method of application of the Sphygmograph.

The button of the instrument is placed over the radial artery just above the styloid process and strapped firmly therein, the patient lying or sitting with the arm supported.

73. What information can a pulse-tracing give one?

It gives an accurate record of the variations in arterial tension.

74. Give the component parts of a pulse-tracing.

(1). The chief ascending wave, (2). Percussion or summit wave, (3). A notch preceding the tidal wave,

(4). The tidal wave, (5). The Aortic or predicrotic notch, (6). The dicrotic wave, (7). The base line.

75. Describe the Chief Ascending Wave, giving its use and describing some of its alterations.

The chief asscending wave is the upstroke of the tracing-needle of the sphygmograph produced by the contraction of the left ventricle, denoting the force or pressure with which it is emptied. It is the tallest line in the tracing and normally a vertical one with small, rounded deflection at its either end.

It slants more or less if the ventricle is weak and abnormally when there is aneurysm. When there is high arterial tension its height is lower than normal, but in low arterial tension higher. The summit is flattened, if the discharge of blood into the arteries is retarded. Its amplitude is scant when the blood forced into the arteries with each systole is small in quantity, but unduly marked if the blood forced is large in quantity.

76. What determines the height of the up-stroke.

The height depends upon the suddenness with which the left ventricle becomes emptied.

77. Apsymmetry of Tracings may be due to what conditions?

Aneurysm. Unilateral vaso-motor changes. Lack of vascular symmetry. Deeper situation of one of the radial arteries. Lack of experience in the use of the sphygmograph.

78. Describe the Summit Wave and give some of its variations with their significance.

The small rounded deviation, in the form of an acute angle at the summit of the upstroke in the tracing when the downward movement of the needle begins, is known as the summit or percussion wave. When there is prolonged effort of the left ventricle to overcome an obstruction the summit is lower than the secondary or the tidal wave and when the discharge of blood into the arteries is retarded the summit becomes flattened.

79. Describe the Tidal Wave and give some of its variations with their significance.

When the tracing-needle after reaching the base-line or in the midst of its descent again forces upwards, causing slight elevations in the line of descent, these elevations are known as the tidal or secondary waves. Its position is normally below the summit wave. When it is higher it indicates a prolonged effort of the left ventricle to overcome an obstruction. It is small or absent when the heart is weak or in cases of Mitral or Aortic Regurgitations.

80. Describe the Aortic Notch and its variations.

A depression in the line of descent of the needle is known as the aortic notch. It is associated with a dicrotic wave. It occupies a high position in the line of descent when there is a post systolic tension and a low one in the presence of a systolic tension. When it touches the base-line it is characterized as full dicrotic and hyper-dicrotic when falls below the base-line.

81. Outline the sphygmographic evidence of High Arterial Tension.

The line of ascent is slanting. The summit is broad. The tidal wave is higher than the summit wave. The aortic notch with the dicrotic wave is less prominent and remains in a higher position than in a normal tension.

82. Outline the sphygmographic evidence of Low Arterial Tension.

The line of ascent is high and almost vertical. The summit wave is pointed. The dicrotic wave prominent with the aortic notch displaying full or hyper-dicrotism.

83. Outine the sphygmographic evidence of Aortic Stenosis.

The line of ascent is slanting; its height is less than the average. The summit is broad. There is dicrotism in the curve.

84. Outline the sphygmographic evidence of Aortic Regurgitation.

The line of ascent is long and vertical. The summit is pointed. The line of descent is rapid.

85. Outline the sphygmographic evidence of combined Stenosis and Regurgitation.

When not in an advanced stage the sphygmograph presents a tracing which bears neither the influence of Stenosis nor that of Regurgitation. When the regurgitation is in an advanced stage the tracings are of a somewhat collapsible character.

86. Outline the sphygmographic evidence of Mitral Regurgitation.

The line of ascent is small. Dicrotic waves. The curve is wavy and disturbed.

87. Outline the sphygmographic evidence of Mitral Stenosis.

The line of ascent is small. Signs of increased aterial tension. Every possible curve. Linked beats on the downstroke, may be irregular.

88. What is the great predisposing cause of Arterio-Sclerosis?

Heredity.

89. What is the influence of nervous activity on the tension and resulting Sclerosis?

The nervous activity has a direct influence over the tension but on the resulting Sclerosis it is a reflex one.

90. Name some of the symptoms resulting from Arterio-Sclerosis.

(a) In the EARLY stage—failure of the physical or mental health ; moderate loss of flesh ; a peculiar pallor suggestive of Anæmia and high arterial tension.

(b) In the ADVANCE stage—A high blood pressure ; hypertrophy of the left ventricle ; thickening of the arteries ; dyspnœa, syncope, Angina Pectoris ; cerebra hæmorrhage ; cramping of the muscles of the extremities interstitial Nephritis, etc.

91. Give a disease dependent directly on sclerosed vessels of the heart.

Angina Pectoris.

PHLEBITIS.

92. Outline the causes of Phlebitis.

Traumatism. Rheumatism. Gout and other infections.

93. Give some of the varieties of Phlebitis.

Simple, Traumatic, Rheumatic, Gouty, Infective and Suppurative Phlebitis.

94. Give the symptoms of Phlebitis.

Gradually increasing pain followed by swelling and induration of the affected vein with redness of the skin over the same. Moderate fever rising upto 102°F. Embolism.

95. Give the symptoms of Suppurtive Phlebitis.

The constitutional symptoms are severe. The fever may rise upto 106°F. Septic embolism.

VENOUS PULSATIONS.

96. Give the symptoms of Venous Pulsations.

Undulation or flicker in the affected veins. Tricuspid or Aortic or Mitral Insufficiency. Engorgement of the right side of the heart. More readily visible than palpable.

97. Give an instance of Physiological Venous Pulsations.

An undulation or flicker in the jugular veins at the root of the neck, in pronounced Anæmia is an instance of Physiological or presystolic venous pulsation.

99. Mention the Pathological Venous Pulsations.

In Tricuspid Regurgitation in the jugular veins,

in Aortic Insufficiency or undue pateney of the arterioles and capillaries in the arms, occur the pathological or systolic venous pulsations, which may also be detected in the inflamed and œdematous parts and beneath the finger-nails.

100. How do you detect a Venous Pulsation?

It is detected when the patient is in lying position with his neck slightly horizontal.

101. On which side is it most pronounced?

It is generally most pronounced in the right ride.

102. What is the indication of Systolic Venous Pulsation in jugular veins?

The presence of Tricuspid Insufficiency.

CHAPTER IV.

RESPIRATION.

1. What is the normal frequency of respiration?

Varies from 16 to 20 per minute in an adult.

2. In observing the respiration, of what factors do we take note?

Frequency and quality. The method of performance.

3. Give the Physiological variations.

More rapid in children and infants. The method of performance differs markedly in two sexes. The frequency is slightly increased after eating; it is greatly increased by exercise and greatly diminished during sleep. Rarefied atmosphere increases the frequency. The cold air increases both the number and the depth of the respiration, while the reverse is the case in hot weather.

4. What effect has exercise on respiration?

See answer to the previous question. The depth is reduced.

5. What effect has rarefied air on respiration?

The frequency is increased. The breathing is deep.

6. What effect has eating on respiration?

The frequency is slightly increased.

7. What effect has cold air on respiration?

See answer Q. 3 above.

8. What effect has sleep on respiration?

The frequency is greatly diminished and the operation is less forcible than while awake.

9. **What factors are necessary for the proper performance of respiration?**

   Inhalation of an adequate quantity of air of normal composition. Proper air passages. Good pulmonary surface. Free pulmonary circulation. Normal blood. Proper function of the lungs.

10. **What nervous causes are there for interference in the respiration?**

    Affections of certain cranial nerves. Disorders of the upper portion of the spinal cord. Central nerve-lesions. Affections of the pneumogastric and recurrent larengeal nerves. Reflex influences of the nerves derived from stomach and skin.

11. **How may Paralysis of the Diaphragm be recognised?**

    It may be recognised by the inactivity of the diaphragm during respiration; the respiration becomes entirely costal and its function disturbed; the epigastrium recedes instead of being inflated during inspiration.

12. **Affections of what cranial nerves will give rise to interference in respiration?**

    Olfactory or the 1st. cranial, Trigeminus or the 5th cranial, Facial or the 7th cranil, Glosso-pharyngeal or the 9th cranial, Pneumogastric or the 10th cranial and the Spinal Accessory or the 11th cranial nerves.

13. **What disorders of the blood may interfere with respiration?**

    Chlorosis. Leukæmia. Secondary Anæmia. Pernicious Anæmia. Hodgkin's Disease. Hemophilia. etc.

14. **What diseases of heart may interfere with respiration?**

    Angina Pectoris, Endorcarditis, Pericarditis, Myocarditis, Hypertrophy and Dilatation of the Heart, Valvular lesions, etc.

15. **Name the pulmonic causes of interference in the respiration.**

    Destruction of the lung tissues. Disturbance of

of the pulmonary circulation. Disordered innervation. Obstruction of the air-passage and diminution of the breathing surface.

16. Give some of the pleural causes for interference with respiration.

The pain in the Pleura. Pressure for the diminution of air-space in the lungs.

17. Give some of the obstructions of the air-passages resulting in interference with the respiration.

Obstruction of the nose by adenoids, Rhinitis, etc. Obstruction in the back of the throat by diseases of the fauces and pharynx. Obstruction in the larynx due to Laryngitis, Laryngismus Stridulus, etc. Obstruction in the trachea due to Tracheocele, etc. Obstruction in the bronchi due to Bronchitis, etc., and foreign bodies in the air-passages.

18. What is deficient respiration? Give some of its Causes.

The respiratory activity whose movements and character are defective is known as deficient respiration. It is either slow, or restricted or shallow and feeble or ineffectual.

CAUSES----Slow breathing is caused by sleep, certain nervous affections (as Hysteria, Apoplexy, etc.), Toxæmia and some reflex disturbances. Restrained breathing is caused by pain or mechanical obstruction in the chest and some pathological conditions (as Pleurodynia, Pleurisy or Angina Pectoris). Shallow and feeble breathing is caused by Hysteria, trance or shock and impending dissolution due to pulmonary œdema. The ineffectual breathing is due to the distension of the pleural cavities and air-vesicles of the lungs.

19. Give the varieties of Dyspnœa.

Inspiratory or obstructive; ordinary, excessive or short breathing; expiratory; paroxysmal; Orthopnœa.

20. Describe the Cheyne-Stokes respiration.

It is a peculiar respiratory disorder in which the

rhythm is disturbed and follows a cyclic course. From slow and shallow breathing, there is a rhythmical increase, step by step with each set, upto a certain degree of rapidity then decreasing gradually, as the increase to a temporary cessation of several seconds followed again by the recurrence of the phenomenon, each cycle consisting from 12 to 30 respirations.

21. Describe the Hiccough.

It is a contraction of the diaphragm, due to clonic spasm, causing inspiration, followed by a sudden closure of the glottis, manifesting itself by a peculiar clucking sound. When obstinate, it may be a matter of considerable alarm.

22. Describe the hysterical respiration.

It is a rapid breathing of a peculiar type, which is a common phenomenon of all sorts of hysterical paroxysm.

23. Describe the sighing, yawning respiration.

SIGHING is a peculiar long, deep and audible respiration.

YAWNING is a changed condition of the natural movements of respiration, in which the inspiration is deeper than the normal, accompained by a spasmôdic contraction of the muscles which depress the lower jaw making the mouth wide open. It ends with a loud respiration.

24. What do you understand by Inspiratory Dyspnœa?

It is a morbid condition of the respiration, in which the inspiratory movements are obstructed due to the weakness of the chest-walls ard the inspiratory muscles.

25. What do you understand by Expiratory Dyspnœa?

It is a labored state of breathing, when the expiratory movements of the respiration are interfered with, due to the impairment of the elastic expiratory force of the chest and lungs and also to an obstruction by any movable growth which acts as a ball-valve in the respiratory passage.

26. Mention some diseases and conditions accompanied by Hiccough.

DISEASES.—Peritonitis. Typhoid Fever. Hysteria.

CONDITIONS.—Gastric disorders. Excessive use of tobacco. Gluttony. Eating of highly-seasoned foods.

27. Mention some diseases and conditions accompanied by slow breathing.

DISEASES.—Hysteria, Apoplexy, Uræmia, etc.

CONDITIONS.—Sleep, trance, shock, coma, irritation of the inspiratory fibres of the superior laryngeal nerve during swallowing. Irritation of the trigeminal fibres. Opium-poisoning. Acute Alcoholism. Etc.

28. Mention some diseases and conditions accompanied by restrained breathing.

DISEASES.—Phthisis (early stage), Pleurodynia, Pleurisy, Pneumonia, Pulmonary infarction, Angina Pectoris.

CONDITIONS.—Pain and the mechanical condition which restricts the chest movement in its entirety or over a limited area.

29. Mention some diseases and conditions accompanied by shallow breathing.

DISEASES.—Hysteria, Epilepsy, Œdema of the lungs.

CONDITIONS.—Hysterical conditions. Impending dissolution due to pulmonary œdema.

30. Mention some diseases and conditions accompanied by ineffectual breathing.

DISEASES.—Hydrothorax, Empyema, Pleurisy, Asthma, Emphysema, Paralysis and Rigidity of the respiratory muscles.

CONDITIONS.—Distension of the pleural cavities with fluid. Distension of the air-vesicles with loss of elasticity of the lungs.

31. Mention some diseases and conditions accompanied by Inspiratory Dyspnœa.

DISEASES.—Paralysis of the diaphragm. Rachitis.

CONDITIONS.—Paralysis of the laryngeal abductors. Weakness of the chest-walls and the inspiratory muscles.

32. Mention some diseases and conditions accompanied by ordinary Dyspnœa.

DISEASES.—Fevers. Anæmias. Toxæmias. Pleurisy. Dropsy. Pneumonia. Bronchitis. Diseases of the heart. Tuberculosis.

CONDITIONS.—Violent exertion. Weakness of the respiratory organs. Pleuritic and abdominal effusions.

33. Mention some diseases and conditions accompanied by expiratory Dyspnœa.

DISEASES.—Emphysema. Asthma.

CONDITIONS.—Loss of elasticity of the chest and lungs. Obstructions due to movable growths in the respiratory tract. Rigidity of the chest-walls.

34. Mention some diiseases accompanied by Orthopnœa.

Asthma. Acute Croupous Pneumonia. Aneurysms. Advanced Heart Disease. Intra-thoracic Tumor.

35. Mention some diseases and conditions accompanied by Cheyne-Stokes Respiration.

DISEASES.—Cerebral Hæmorrhage. Intra-cranial Tumor. Abscess of the brain. Meningitis. Peritonitis (diffuse). Endocarditis. Chronic Nephritis. Renal Toxæmia. Typhoid Fever. Heart diseases and ruptured compensation. Morphia-poisoning. Etc.

CONDITIONS.—Brain, heart and kidney disorders. Gastric and hepatic troubles. Acute infectious diseases. Sleep.

36. What is the clinical significance of Cheyne-Stokes Respiration?

It is a sign of most unfavourable character.

CHAPTER V.

THE DIGESTIVE TRACT.

LIPS—MOUTH—GUMS—TEETH—TONGUE—
LINGUAL TONSIL—SALIVA—OFFENSIVE BREATH
FAUCES—PHARYNX—TONSILS—ŒSOPHAGUS—
STOMACH—INTESTINES & RECTUM.

THE LIPS.

1. **Name the Anatomical Structures entering into the composition of the Mouth.**

    Mucous membrane. Connective tissue. Muscles. Glands and Teeth.

2. **Name the Pathological Lesions of the Mouth.**

    Congestions. Inflammations. Eruptions. Ulcerations. Tumors. Caries and necrosis of the maxillary bones.

3. **To what points or conditions should you pay attention in examining the Lips?**

    Color. Movements. Shape and size. The presence or absence of eruptions, fissures, etc.

4. **What various alterations in the Colour of the Lips occur as the results of disease?**

    Pallor. Blueness. Cyanosed hue. Yellow hue.

5. **What is the clinical significance of the "Pallor" of the Lips?**

    Effect of Anæmia.

6. **What is the clinical significance of "Blueness" of the Lips?**

    Effect of general chilling of the body.

7. **What is the clinical significance of "Yellow Color" of the Lips?**

   Effect of Jaundice.

8. **What is the significance of the Tremor of the Lips?**

   One of the early signs of General Paralysis of the Insane.

9. **What disease is suggested by Restlessness or Twitching of the Lips?**

   Chorea.

10. **What is suggested by Paralysis of the Lips on both sides?**

    Glosso-labio-laryngeal Paralysis (Bulbar Paralysis).

11. **What is suggested by Unilateral Paralysis of the Lips?**

    Disease or injury of the facial nerve on the corresponding side.

12. **What is the significance of Abnormal Thickness of the Lips?**

    Myxœdema (Thyroid cachexia).

13. **What is suggested by Congenital Thickness of the Lips?**

    Idiocy and cretinism,

14. **What conditions are suggested by Swelling of the Lips?**

    Cheilitis. Cheilites glandulares. Epilepsy.

15. **What is suggested by Abnormal or Acquired Thinness of the Lips?**

    Abnormal thinness suggests Glosso-labial Palsy or unilateral Facial Paralysis.

    Acquired thinness is a racial peculiarity.

16. **What are Hydroa and what is their clinical significance?**

    Fever-blisters around the mouth and the nose. Their clinical significance is not bad.

17. What is the suggestion of Linear Cicratices and Fissures on the Lips of Infants?

They are suggestives of hereditary Syphilis.

18. What is the appearance presented by Chancre of the Lips?

It is usually round or oval with an indurated base. It presents a mucous patch of a greenish-white surface and is surrounded by a pinkish red areola.

THE MOUTH.

19. To what points should you pay attention when examining the Mouth?

(1) Condition of the mucous membrane. (2) The presence or absence of swelling and (3) the character of the secretions.

20. What is suggested by undue Pallor of the Mouth?

Anæmia.

21. What acute infectious diseases are attended by undue Redness of the Mouth?

Scarlatina.

22. What condition of the Mouth is suggested by the appearance of a dark or bluish-red, hard spot, rapidly increasing in size and deepening in colour, with general induration and formation of beblets, fœtor and breaking down of tissue?

They are suggestives of an inflammation of the mouth known as Gangrenous Stomatitis or Noma.

23. What condition of the Mouth is suggested by the appearance of raised white patches looking like the Milk-curds?

The characteristic lesion of Thrush or mycotic Stomatitis.

24. How would you differentiate Thrush from deposit of Milk-curds upon the Mucous Membrane of the Mouth?

The Thrush adheres so strongly with the mucous membrane that to remove it, it must be scraped off.

The milk-curds can be removed easily.

25. What is the Mouth Lesion characteristic of Scarlatina?

The mouth lesion of Scarlatina presents an intense or undue redness of the mucous membrane of the mouth.

26. Describe the Mouth Lesion of Measles.

In the EARLY STAGE—*Koplik's spots* (see Q. 39), usually on the mucous membrane of the cheek, rarely of the mouth.

DURING and AFTER the attack—mucous membrane of mouth patchy red ; and may be associated with stomatitis of any one of the varieties.

27. Describe the Mouth Lesions of Variola.

Appear as hyperæmia of the mucous membrane of the mouth which is afterwards infested with eruptions of numerous rounded elevations of pinhead size, soon becoming elevated or papular ; they follow the course pursued by those of the skin, forming into vesicles, which break down early and form small ulcers causing much soreness of the mouth.

28. Describe some of the features of Syphilitic Ulcerations of the Mouth.

May be met with as ERYTHEMA, FISSURES, PAPULES or PUSTULES or TUBERCLES forming later into MUCOUS PATCHES and ULCERATIONS, in the secondary and the tertiary stages of the acquired Syphilis, differing in the latter by their greater tendency to dryness, deeper infiltration and obstinacy to treatment. The mucous patch, in the tertiary stage, may degenerate into conditions known as LEUCO-KERATOSIS. In this stage GUMMATA or Gummatous tumors may appear, which rapidly tends to ugly and destructive ulcerations and sometimes PERFORATION.

In the congenital Syphilis in infants, it is found as FISSURES commonly known as RHAGADES and also there may be marked ulcerations in the muco-cutaneous surfaces. They occur within three months from the birth, which is a conclusive evidence of their congenital origin.

29. What alterations in the shape of the Mouth result from Post-Nasal Adenoids?

Arching of the hard palate; superior dental arch altered and narrowed; the roof of the mouth considerably raised; and the lips are thick.

30. What is the clinical significance of the Pallor of the Gums?

The existence of Anæmia.

31. What is the clinical significance of the Blueness of the Gums?

Heart diseases with ruptured compensation.

32. What is the clinical significance of a Blue Line along the edge of the Gums?

Lead-poisoning.

33. What is the clinical significance of Bluish-Red Discolorisation of the Gums, which are swollen and bleed readily on touch?

It is significant of Seurvy or Scorbutus.

34. What are some of the Mouth symptoms of Scurvy?

A red line of congestion around the neck of a tooth, which spreads afterwards, and the affected portion becomes greatly swollen with bluish-red discolorisation of the same. The gums are soft, greatly swollen and bleed readily on touch. Hæmorrhage from the gums and the mucous membrane of the mouth, specially on the hard palate Pain in the gums.

35. What is the clinical significance of Swelling and Sponginess of the Gums with Salivation?

It is indicative of Mercurial-poisoning.

36. What are Sordes?

Foul secretions on the teeth and gums deposited as thin yellowish or thick brown crusts, in low forms of fevers are known as SORDES.

37. What is the composition of the Thick-Brown Crusts appearing on the Gums in cases of Typhoid Fever and allied conditions?

They are composed of particles of food, epithelial debris and various micro-organisms.

38. What do they indicate?

A profound asthenia.

39. Describe the Koplik's Spots.

Eruptions of white or bluish-white specks surrounded by bright red, irregular areolæ on the mucous membrane of the cheek, in the early stage of Measles are known as the Koplik's Spots. They are of short duration and occur less frequently upon the mucous membrane of the lips and rarely on the entire mucous membrane of the mouth.

40. What infectious disease is suggested by a patchy Redness of the Mouth?

It is suggestive of Meales.

41. What local diseases are suggested by undue Redness of the Mucous Membrane of the Mouth?

All the varieties of Stomatitis and Scarlatina.

42. What condition is suggested by Yellowish Discolorisation of the Mouth?

It is suggestive of Jaundice.

43. What is suggested by a Cyanotic Hue of the Mucous Membrane of the Mouth?

Heart diseases with ruptured compensation.

THE MOUTH

44. What is Stomatitis?

The inflammation of the interior of the mouth, followed by increased salivation and swelling of the tongue is known as the Stomatitis. It may be limited to the gums and lips or may extend over the whole interior surface of the mouth including the tongue.

45. What is suggested by the undue Redness of the Mouth without Ulceration, and with Soreness, Heat and Swelling?

Suggestive of Catarrhal Stomatitis.

46. What form of Stomatitis is characterized by Small Yellowish-white Spots breaking down to form shallow Ulcers with raised edges?

Aphthous Stomatitis.

47. At what period of life is an Aphthous Stomatitis most frequently observed?

In children during their first dentition.

48. What form of Stomatitis is suggested by the beginning of the lesions in the folds of the mucous membrane between the gums and the cheeks, associated with Swelling and Sponginess of the Gums, which bleed easily, and break down, and form Ulcers, with horrible Fœtor of the Breath?

An ulcerative Stomatitis.

49. Describe the simple Ulcerations of the Mouth.

(a) SIMPLE ULCERATIONS of the Dyspepsias sometimes known as the CANKER-SORES.

(b) PERLICHE......beginning as a small fissure, it forms into an intractable ulcer, at the angle of the mouth, being infected by constant licking due to irritation. Usually runs a course of 2 to 4 weeks.

(c) MAL PERFORANT BUCCÆ or the perforating ulcer of the mouth. They are preceded by a progressive absorption of the alveoli, with falling of the teeth and followed by perforations of the palatine arch.

(d) BEDNAR'S APHTHÆ.........small, superficial ulcers, surrounded by redness of the adjacent mucous membrane and accompanied by some pain. It is found on either side of the median line of the hard and soft palate. It is a common children's disease and is not serious.

50. Describe a False Membrane as it makes its appearance in the Mouth.

A fibrinous exudation on the mucous membrane of the mouth, as an extension of the diphtheritic process of the fauces. It is at first grayish or dirty white, which becomes brownish with the progress of the disease, being surrounded by an area of intense congestion.

It is also known as Buccal Diphtheria.

51. Name the Tumors found in the Mouth.

Gummata. Ranula. Salivary Calculi. Epithelioma. Etc.

52. Describe the Ranula.

A painless cystic tumor beneath the tongue or in the floor of the mouth caused by an accumulation of saliva and other causes, presenting bluish, pellucid appearance.

53. Describe Catarrhal Stomatitis.

A mild form of inflammation of the mouth, without any ulceration, presenting a very red and raw surface with soreness in the mouth.

54. Describe the Mercurial Stomatitis.

The inflammation of the mouth, with sponginess of the gums, profuse flow of the saliva, metallic taste in the mouth and ulcerations. It is caused by the internal use of Mercury.

55. Describe the Aphthous Stomatitis.

The inflammation of the mouth characterized by the presence of Aphthæ or numerous small, yellowish-white spots, breaking down into shallow ulcers with raised margins, upon the mucous membrane of the cheeks, lips and tongue and may extend upto the pharynx, involving the same. They usually appear in successive crops and are dependent upon constitutional causes.

56. Describe the Mycotic Stomatitis.

Small and round patch or patches in the mucous membrane of the mouth and pharynx, of milk-white or greyish-white appearance, though at first adherent, can be readily scraped off later, presenting small bleeding ulcerations. They coalesce together involving a greater area.

57. Describe Ulcerative Stomatitis.

The inflammation of the mouth which begins, as indicated in Q. 48 of this chapter and formation of ulcers with horrible fœtor of the mouth and breath. The ulcers are covered with a yellowish membrane and have irregular, swollen blusih-red edges. The entire gums may be involved and in extreme cases the floor of the mouth. The ulcers though at first superficial extend deeply, loosening the teeth and exposing the alveolus. It strongly resembles the Mercurial Stomatitis.

58. Describe Gangrenous Stomatitis.

It is also known as CANCRUM ORIS or NOMA. The inflammation starts as a small diphtherial patch of dark or bluish-red color and surrounded by general inflammation of the surface. It extends rapidly and becomes browny in appearance and indurated in nature, with the formation of one or more blebs in it, which soon ruptures resulting in ulceration and rapid destruction of the tissue, with perforation and extreme damage of the soft parts. The gangrenous process may extend upto the jaw, malar bone. tongue, etc., ending fatally within a very short time. The breath is horribly offensive and profound prostration from an early stage. The constitutional symptoms are very grave, but the fever is moderate and pain is absent, A typical typhoid state usually brings in the fatal end rapidly.

59. Describe Bednar's Aphthæ.

See Answer to Q. 49 of this chapter.

THE GUMS.

60. In observing the Gums of what conditions do you take note?

The color of the gums. The presence or absence of swelling, crusts, ulcerations, abscesses or tumors.

61. What do you understand by the term Gingivitis?

Inflammation of the Gums.

62. Describe the appearance of the Gums in Scurvy.

Greatly swollen with bluish-red discolorisation of the affected portion.

63. Describe the conditions of the Gums in Mercurial Poisoning.

The gums are swollen and become spongy in appearance. There may be ulcerations and Stomatitis attended with the same.

64. Describe the appearance in Lead-Poisoning.

There is a blue or bluish-black line at the margin of the gums close to the teeth. The gums are usually more or less ulcerated and irregular in outline.

65. What is the cause of the Sordes on the Gums?

The inactivity of the mouth, due to profound asthenia.

66. In what conditions do the Gums recede from the Teeth?

Stomatitis, Gingivitis, Pyorrhœa Alveolaris and Scurvy.

67. What is Pyorrhœa Alveolaris?

The inflammation of the alveolo-dental membrane, with inflammation of the gums adjoining the affected teeth, associated with a discharge of flow of pus from the alveoli, characterised by receding of the gums and exposure of the upper portion of the roots of the teeth, sometimes attended with considerable pain is known as the Pyorrhœa Alveolaris. It loosens the teeth in the long run and causes them to fall out.

68. What conditions produce Localised Swelling of the Gums?

Abscesses, Gum-boils and Tumors.

69. Give the usual causes of the Receding of the Gums from the Teeth.

Scurvy, Stomatitis, Gingivitis and Pyorrhœa Alveolaris.

70. Name the Tumors found in the Gums.

The various tumors of the gums are known as Epulides.

71. What is the appearance of Syphilitic Ulcerations of the Gums?

The surface is grayish-white and is surrounded by a pinkish-red areola.

THE TEETH.

72. Describe Dentition as it appears in the 1st set.

The first four or the *central incisors* appear at about the 7th month, the second four or the *lateral incisors* at about the 9th month, the third four or the *first molars* at about the 12th month and four *canines* and four *second molars* at about the 18th month complete the first set.

73. Describe the causes of Delayed Dentition.

Rachitis and ill-health from any cause.

74. Name the reflex disturbances occuring in children as a result of Dentition.

Convulsion. Diarrhœa.

75. Describe the appearance of the Gums during Dentition.

Unduly red.

76. Mention the Deformities met with in the Teeth

Jumbling or crowding. Unsystematic growth. Displacements. Furrowing. Irregularity in form—stunting and pitting. Rocky enamel. Syphilitic teeth.

77. What are the characteristics of Syphilitic Teeth?

They are peg-shaped; their bases are broader than their cutting edges and along the latter is found a single semi-lunar shaped notch.

78. What is the significance of Grinding of the Teeth in children?

A gastro-intestinal disorder.

79. What are the conditions favouring Caries of the Teeth?

Constitutional conditions as Rachitis, Syphilis, etc. Defective structure of enamel and dentine. Irregular growth favouring the deposit and decomposition of food. Want of cleanliness. Taking of such medicines as Iron, Mercury, etc.

THE TONGUE.

80. When examining the Tongue to what points should you pay attention?

Size. Shape. Colour. Degree of moisture. Movements. Coatings. Surface as to the presence or absence of fissures, ulcerations, eruptions and elevations.

81. In what conditions is the Tongue enlarged?

Glossitis, Hemi-glossitis, Macroglossia, Myxœdema, Chronic Heart disease, Anæmia, Liver affections, Mercurial poisoning, Cancer, Gummata and Cysts. In the last three, the enlargements are circumscribed.

82. What disease of the Tongue is suggested by enormous Swelling, with Pain, Heat and increased Redness?

Glossitis.

83. What disease of the Tongue is suggested by great Swelling of one-half of the Tongue with Pain, increased Redness and Heat?

Hemi-glossitis.

84. In what conditions may Macroglossia or Enlarged Tongue be observed?

In idiocy and other mental deficiencies.

85. What is the reason for the Enlarged Tongue in Myxœdema?

It is due to mucinoid infiltration of the sub-cutaneous tissue caused by the atrophy of the cellular elements of the thyroid gland, associated with Fibrosis.

86. What is the reason for Enlarged Tongue in Heart Diseases?

It is due to venous engorgement of the organ.

87. What is the appearance of the Tongue in the Anæmias?

The tongue is large and flabby.

88. What is the condition of the Tongue in Liver Diseases?

The tongue is slightly enlarged—takes the imprint of the teeth.

89. In what conditions does the Tongue present a Diminution in Size?

Peritonitis. Chronic Gastritis. Atrophy of its muscular substance.

90. Name the lesions or diseases which may produce Atrophy of the Muscles of the Tongue.

Injuries or diseases of the hypoglossal nerves or their nuclei. Glosso-labio-laryngeal or Bulbar Paralysis. Atrophy of disuse in old Hemiplegias.

91. What is the clinical significance of Pallor of the Tongue?

Anæmia.

92. What is the clinical significance of Blueness or Cyanosed Hue of the Tongue?

Heart disease with failing compensation.

93. What is the clinical significance of Purplish or Blackish Spots on the Tongue?

Addison's Disease.

94. What is the clinical significance of reddish, later becoming bluish to black subcutaneous Blotches on the Tongue.

They indicate hæmorrhage in the sub-cutaneous tissues.

95. What drugs may stain the Tongue black?

Biniodide of Mercury. Various Bismuth preparations and Iron.

96. What substance may stain the Tongue yellow?

Tobacco.

97. What substance may stain the Tongue orange-yellow?

Tea.

98. In what diseases or conditions may the Tongue present an abnormal redness?

In the early stages of most of the febrile and inflammatory diseases.

99. In what conditions may the Tongue be dark-red merging almost into black?

In Typhus, Typhoid Fever and Typhoid conditions generally.

100. What is the clinical significance of Raw, Red and Denuded Tongue?

Great depression of vital forces.

101. What are the Physiological agencies producing Dryness of the Tongue?

Mouth-breathing. Dehydration of the body,

THE TONGUE

102. What is the Prognostic significance of Dryness of the Tongue?

In acute diseases it is a certain indication for liquid diet, in chronic disorders an unfavourable issue.

103. In what Pathological conditions may the Tongue present an abnormal Dryness?

It is present in the course of fevers.

104. In what conditions is the Tongue protruded with abnormal readiness?

Hypochondriasis and Hysteria.

105. In what conditions is the Tongue protruded slowly?

In typhoid condition and in cases where mental condition is blunted, as, in the beginning of stupor.

106. What is the clinical significance of Tremor of the Tongue?

Deep intestinal perforation.

107. How would you recognise Unilateral Paralysis of the Tongue?

The tongue while at rest deviates from the paralyzed side, but when protruded it tends towards the paralyzed side.

108. How would you recognise Bilateral Paralysis of the Tongue?

The tongue lies motionless in the floor of the mouth.

109. Name some conditions in which Paralysis of the Tongue occurs.

Brain lesions, particularly in Apoplexy. Disease or injury of one or both hypoglossal nerves, Glosso-labio-laryngeal or Bulbar Paralysis, Disseminated Sclerosis, Post-diphtheritic paralysis.

110. Which of the acute infectious diseases is specially liable to have Paralysis of the Tongue as sequel?

Dipththeria.

111. In what diseases may Spasm of the Tongue occur?

Chorea. Hysteria. Epilepsy. Thomson's Disease. Disseminated Sclerosis. Irritation of the hypoglossal nerves.

112. Describe the different Coatings of the Tongue.

(a) COATING OF MINUTE WHITE SPOTS scattered over the surface of the tongue which is known as the STIPPLED TONGUE.

(b) LIGHT WHITE COATING, like deposit of frost, with minute white spots or dots as described above over the surface of the tongue known as STIPPLED PLUS COATED TONGUE. It signifies a constutional state which demands a liquid diet.

(c) WHITE COATING (thicker), even and continuous in tongue known as the COATED TONGUE. It is indioative of aggravation of the disease in which it is present.

(d) THICK WHITE FUR with projecting red fungiform papillæ in tongue known as the STRAWBERY TONGUE

(e) UNIFORM, THICK WHITE COATING, with tendency to become brown, or dirty yellowish in the long run in tongue known as the PLASTERED TONGUE. It signifies the severity of the disease and prostration. The coating becomes more thicker with the progress of the disease.

(f) COATING OF HORNY EPITHELIUM with a furred and rough surface of the tongue known as FURRED AND SHAGGY TONGUE. It is suggestive of failure of nutrition and decline of vital powers.

(g) COATING CF A DRY BROWN CRUST which is often broken and fissured, covering the papillæ in tongue known as the ENCRUSTED DRY AND BROWN

(h) MALPIGHIAN LAYER in tongue known as the DENUDED RED TONGUE. It is significant of exhaustion. TONGUE. It is significant of lowered vitality.

113. What is the significance of the Encrusted Dry and Brown Tongue?

Lowered vitality.

THE TONGUE

114. What is the significance of the Plastered Tongue?

Severity of the disease and prostration.

115. What conditions may produce Fissures of the Tongue?

Irritation from the broken or rough edge of a tooth.

Secondary Syphilis. Carcinomata. Tuberculosis.

116. Name some of the common forms of Ulceration of the Tongue?

Simple ulcers. Aphthous ulcers. Dyspeptic ulcers. Traumatic ulcers. Syphilitic ulcers. Carcinomatous ulcers. Tubercular ulcers.

117. Of what value is the presence or absence of Moisture in the Tongue?

The presence of moisture on the tongue indicates the favourable progress of the disease, while its absence is regarded as having an unfavorable significance.

118. Describe the "Stippled Tongue" and tell its significance.

See answer (a). to Q. 112 above.

119. Describe the "Stippled plus Coated Tongue" and tell its significance.

See answer (b). to Q. 112 above.

120. Describe the "Coated Tongue" and tell its significance.

See answer (c). to Q. 112 above.

121. Describe the "Strawberry Tongue" and tell its significance.

See answer (d). to Q. 112 above.

122. Describe the "Plastered Tongue" and tell its significance.

See answer (e). to Q. 112 above.

123. Describe the "Furred or Shaggy Tongue" and tell its significance.

See answer (f). to Q. 112 above.

124. Describe the "Encrusted Dry Tongue" and tell its significance.

See answer (g). to Q. 112 above.

125. Describe the "Denuded Dry Tongue" and tell its significance.

See answer (h). to Q. 112 above.

126. Describe the "Cyanosed Tongue" and tell its significance.

The cyanosed tongue has a bluish or purple color, the surface of the tongue being smooth, wet and slippery. It signifies heart diseases with ruptured compensation.

127. Describe the Fissured and Furrowed Tongue and tell its significance.

The fissures or furrows of the tongue may be single or multiple interlacing each other in every conceivable way.

It signifies disturbances in the cellular structure of the tongue.

128. Describe the Syphilitic Ulceration of the Tongue.

It signifies disturbances in the cellular structure Syphilis as large or small, single or multiple usually the latter with copper-colored surface surrounded by pinkish red areola and is painless unless there is secondary inflammation. In the *tertiary stage*, it is more deep and is prone to be followed by Sclerosis of the tongue.

129. Describe the Tubercular Ulceration of the Tongue.

The lesions are irregularly shaped, stellate or oval, usually the former, with sharp-cut or bevelled edges, without any inflammatory surroundings, deep and uneven bases of coarse pinkish granulations filled with purulent grayish or yellowish discharges. They are exceedingly painful and attended by salivation and always involve the sub-maxillary lymphatics. They are usually found on the dorsum near the tip of the tongue, and are always associated with Tuberulosis elsewhere.

130. Describe the Dyspeptic Ulcerations of the Tongue.

They are very painful small ulcers, which occurs on or near the tip of the tongue, and are surrounded by reddish inflammatory surfaces.

131. How do you test the Gustatory Sense?

To test the gustatory sense, the tongue is protruded and the substance is applied, in turn, to the back of the tongue—first on one side, then on the other. The tongue is not permitted to touch the lip or drawn back into the mouth during the experiment.

132. In what conditions do we find Perverted Taste?

The perverted taste or Paragencia may be found in Hysteria, Insanity, gastric disorders and by the presence of abnormal substances in the saliva.

THE LINGUAL TONSIL

133. Name all the possible disorders of the Lingual Tonsil.

Catarrhal inflammation. Abscess. Hypertrophy. Varicose veins.

134. Give symptoms of Abscess of Lingual Tonsil.

Severe pain with swelling of the affected parts, sufficient not only to obstruct the passage of food but also the normal respiration. It is attended with high fever. The inflammation may extend to the adjacent parts such as the larynx and the floor of the mouth.

135. Describe the Varicose Veins of the Lingual Tonsil.

The condition rarely produces any serious effect, but sometimes there may be pains, morbid sensation at the base of the tongue or in the throat, Torticollis, cough, hemming, dyspnœa, dysphagia, faucial tenesmus and haemorrhage for its diagnosis laryngoscopic examination should be made.

SALIVA.

136. What drugs produce Salivation?

Mercury and Pilocarpine.

137. Name all the conditions where the Salivary flow is increased.

The mouth and throat inflammations. Pregnancy. Certain nervous affections, particularly in Acute Mania. Hydrophobia. Certain drugs as Mercury and Pilocarpine.

138. Name all the conditions where the Salivary flow is decreased.

Diseases of the salivary glands. Fever. Diarrhœa. Diabetes. Certain drugs as Atropin.

139. Give some conditions where the Saliva is acid in reaction.

Inflammation and ulceration of the mouth, Fevers, Diabetes, Gout and Rheumatism.

140. Give the composition of Saliva.

It contains mainly the Albumin and Ptyalin.

OFFENSIVE BREATH.

141. Name the causes of Offensive Breath.

Pyorrhœa Alveolaris. Tonsillar diseases. Indigestions with catarrhal disturbances. All forms of stomatitis and ulcerations of the mouth. Decayed teeth. Affections of the brain. Pyrexia. Necrosis of the jaw. Chronic sinus disease. Diseases of the nose, larynx, bronchi and lungs. Diabetic Coma. Syphilitic ulceration of nares, pharynx, and larynx. Certain drugs. Anhilosis. Gangrenous Pharyngitis. Sloughing Cancer.

142. What respiratory diseases cause Offensive Breath?

Vincent's Angina, Bronchiectasis, Gangrene and Abscess of the Lungs, and putrid Bronchitis.

143. Name the drugs causing Offensive Breath.

Mercury. Phosphorus. Opium. Alcohol.

144. How do affections of the brain cause Offensive Breath?

The retained secretions being decomposed cause offensive breath.

145. How do affections of the stomach cause Offensive Breath?

The gaseous decompositions are absorbed by the blood ond exhalation by the lungs.

146. What is the peculiar Odor of the Breath in Diabetes?

A flavory odor—a peculiar, sweetish, apple-like odor.

147. What is the peculiar Odor of the Breath in Uræmic Coma?

A very foul breath—odor of Carbonate of Ammonia.

148. What is the most common cause of Offensive Breath?

Pyorrhœa Alveolaris.

FAUCES—PHARNX—TONSILS.

149. In what conditions do we observe Swelling of the Pharynx?

Acute Catarrhal, Phlegmonous, Erysipelatous and Gangrenus Pharyngitis. Retro-pharyngeal, Antero-pharyngeal and Peri-pharyngeal Abscesses.

150. In what conditions may we observe localised Swelling of the Pharynx?

Retro-pharyngeal, Latero-pharyngeal and Antero-pharyngeal Abscesses.

151. In what conditions may we observe the Swelling of the Tonsils?

Acute Catarrhal Pharyngitis. Phlegmonous Pharyngitis. Acute Suppurative Tonsillitis. Acute Follicular Tonsillitis. Post-nasal Adenoids. Latero-pharyngeal Abscess. Acute Herpetic Tonsillitis. Peri-tonsillar Abscess. Tonsillar Hypertrophy.

152. What are the objective appearances presented by Suppurative Tonsillitis?

Great tonsillar swelling; the affected gland presents *a peculiar redness* which is characteristic.

153. What are the objective conditions observed in Herpetic Tonsillitis?

Small vesicles are observed on the tonsils and pharyngeal walls.

154. What are the objective conditions observed in Follicular Tonsillitis?

The swelling of the tonsils and their follicles are inflamed and covered with dried and thickened mucus.

155. What are the objective appearances in Catarrhal Tonsillitis?

The tonsils are red and swollen, but the swelling is limited to mucous and sub-mucous tissues. The adjacent portions of the soft palate and pharynx are also inflamed.

156. What condition in the post-nasal space is often observed in connection with Enlarged Tonsils?

Acute inflammation.

157. In what conditions is the Pharynx abnormally roomy?

In congenital or acquired deformities and atrophy of the mucous and muscular structures of the pharynx.

158. What is the clinical significance of Œdema of the Uvula?

It is significant of some renal disease.

159. Differentiate Follicular Tonsillitis and Diphtheria.

In FOLLICULAR TONSILLITIS, the membrane is divided into *patches of yellowish-gray* colour and can be removed easily. It is limited to tonsils only.

In DIPHTHERIA the membrane is *ashy-gray of one single mass and not patchy*. It is adherent to the mucous membrane and cannot be removed easily, which when forcibly removed leaves a bleeding, eroded surface. It may be limited to the tonsils, but usually extends on the adjacent parts.

160. In what conditions may the Palate be paralysed?

Post-diphtheritic Paralysis. Bulbar Paralysis and Spinal Accessory Paralysis.

161. What parts are paralyzed in Bulbar Paralysis?

Tongue, lips, palates, pharynx, glottis and larynx.

162. How is the Paralysis of Palate manifest clinically?

The palate hangs lower than the normal and is not raised when the patient tries to pronounce a long "ah."

163. Of what conditions is Paralysis of the Pharynx symptomatic?

Nuclear Disease. Post-Diphtheritic Paralysis.

164. In what diseases may we observe the Spasm of the Pharynx?

Hysteria. Hydrophobia.

165. In what conditions may we observe increased production of mucus in the Pharynx?

In the early stages of all pharyngeal and tonsillar inflammations.

166. What lesions may give rise to Pharyngeal Hæmorrhage?

Abscesses. Ulcerations. Post-nasal Adenoids. The rupture of enlarged veins in the pharynx. Traumatism. Anæmias Bright's Disease and certain infectious diseases due to alterations in the composition of the blood.

167. In what conditions may pus be observed in the Pharynx?

In Retro-pharyngeal. Latero-pharyngeal. Antero-pharyngeal and Peri-pharyngeal Abscesses.

168. In what disease is False Membrane observed in Pharynx?

Diphtheria.

169. Describe the Follicular Ulcerations of the Pharynx.

The ulcers are small and superficial and located on the posterior pharyngeal wall. Sometimes they are preceded by vesicles, which ruptures into ulcers as above.

170. Give the method of examination of the Pharynx.

To examine the pharynx, the patients should be placed in a lighted position and to ensure that the parts to be examined will be exposed to view the tongue must be well-depressed. If the patient is unable to depress the tongue himself, a tongue-depressor may be employed for the purpose. If for any reason it is undesirable to use the depressor, the patient should be asked to show the tongue and take a deep breath or to pronounce the

Chap. V.] FAUCES—PHARYNX—TONSILS 71

sound "Ah", when the palate will be raised, the tongue depressed and the entire pharynx and tonsil will be seen.

171. What is there to observe about these parts?

The *colour* of the mucous membrane. Whether there is any *swelling*? The conditions of the uvula, palate, fauces, pharynx, and tonsils, as to their *shape*, movements. secretions, etc. Exudations. Ulcerations. The condition of the vessels of the Pharynx.

172. Describe some of the variations of Color of the Throat.

Increased redness. Patch redness. A cyanosed hue or lividity. Pallor. Yellowish hue.

173. What does a Cyanosed Hue of the Pharynx indicate?

It is indicative of a venous congestion.

174. What is the clinical significance of capillary pulsations in the Pharynx?

It is suggestive of Tricuspid Regurgitation.

175. Name the acute infectious diseases which make their appearance, known by some change in colour, in the mucous membrane of the Pharynx.

(a) By increased redness—Scarlatina. (b) By patchy redness—Measles. (c) By pallor—Tuberculosis.

176. What is the clinical significance of Pallor of the Pharynx?

Anæmia.

177. What does a yellowish hue of the pharynx indicate?

Jaundice.

178. Name some of the alterations in the Shape of Pharynx.

Diminution of the lumen of the tube. Dilatation of the lumen or diverticula.

179. Describe the appearance of a Retro-pharyngeal Abscess.

It appears as a swelling which is unilateral, red or purplish in colour, projecting out towards the buccal cavity as a tumor in the middle line, which can be seen or felt with the finger on the posterior walls of the pharynx.

180. Describe the Latero-pharyngeal Abscess.

The lesion presents a projecting and inflamed tonsil, with surrounding inflammation and swelling of the pharyngeal wall, extending specially in a backward direction. Externally there is a swelling of the neck corresponding to that in the throat. The natural depression beneath the angle of the jaw is replaced by a swelling which gives a boggy sensation to palpation. The underlying skin may be red and œdematous. It may be associated with chill, fever, pain and prostration. It interferes materially with deglutition and respiration.

181. Describe the Antero-pharyngeal Abscess.

It appears as a swelling of the pharyngeal mucous membrane in the layer of the connective tissue lying between the larynx and the pharynx.

182. Describe the Peri-pharyngeal Abscess.

It appears as a general swelling and the whole neck externally becomes greatly swollen. It is noted for the rapidity of its progress and deglutition and respiration become next to impossible.

183. Name some of the conditions producing Pain in the Pharynx.

Acute inflammations of the pharynx and the tonsils. Muscular rheumatism of the pharynx.

184. Outline some of the conditions producing Dryness in the Pharynx.

Acute inflammatory affections of the throat—in their initial stages. Majority of the cases of chronic catarrhs.

185. Name the variety of conditions which cause Enlargement of the Tonsils.

See Answer to Q. 151 of this chapter.

186. Differentiate true and false Tonsillar Hypertrophy.

The true tonsillar hypertrophy is differentiated from a false one in that it rarely interferes seriously with respiration.

187. Define Herpetic Tonsillitis.

It is an acute *inflammation* of the tonsils characterized by the presence of numerous small vesicles on the tonsils and pharyngeal walls. The inflammation is prone to involve the fauces and the entire pharyngeal walls.

188. Define Suppurative Tonsillitis.

An acute suppuration of the tonsillar tissues characterized by *chronic enlargement of the glands* and *great tonsillar swelling*, with *intense pain*. The deglutition is difficult and the affected gland presents a *peculiar redness* in appearance.

189. Define Catarrhal Tonsillitis.

It is an inflammation of the Tonsil, characterized by *severe soreness of the throat*, aggravated by the act of swallowing and is due to exposure to cold or wet. The tonsil is red and swollen, but the swelling is limited to the mucous and sub-mucous tissues.

190. Name the conditions which would increase the capacity of the Pharynx.

Pharyngocele. Dry or atrophic Pharyngitis.

191. What is the most frequently observed Deformity of the Palate?

The failure of union of the palate, usually at the median line.

192. Perforation of the Soft Palate may arise from what condition?

From ulcerations, specially of Syphilitic origin

193. Name the conditions causing Paralysis of the Palate.

(a) When the inflammatory infiltration is immoderate, and (b) various paralytic affections.

194. How is Paralysis of the Pharynx manifested clinically?

By the failure of deglutition. There is less difficulty in swallowing pulpy food than either fluids or solids.

195. The Spasm of the Pharynx is observed in what conditions?

In Hysteria and Hydrophobia.

196. Describe the Spasm of the Pharynx as observed in Hydrophobia.

After a few days of uncomfortable sensation about the throat, which results into attacks of choking and difficulty in swallowing liquids, the spasm sets in. It increases in severity and finally becomes general with widely distributed muscular rigidity. Opisthotonos, etc.

197. Describe the Hysterical Spasm of the Pharynx.

It constitutes the basis of the "Globus Hystericus"—the lump or choking sensation caused by the spasmodic contraction of the œsophagus and pharyngeal muscles.

198. Describe the appearance of Exudation of Mucus on the Pharynx.

The mucus appears in an increased quantity on the pharynx in the early stages of all its inflammatory affections. It forms into crusts later.

199. Describe the appearance of an Exudation of Pus on the Pharynx.

Pus appears on the pharyngeal mucous membrane only when discharged from an abscess connecting with the tube.

200. Describe the appearance of False Membranes on the Pharynx.

See Answer to Qs. 50 and 159. They appear on the pharynx as a reeult of the toxic action of the bacilli growing on the throat, which proliferate the nuclei of cells, bringing about the necrosis of the epithelium, changing the same into refractive hyaline masses. They may be caused by Klebs-Loeffer, Streptococcus, Staphylococcus, Pneumococcus or the Colon bacilli.

201. Name the causes giving rise to Pharyngeal Hæmorrhage.

Abscesses. Ulcerations. Traumatism. Postnasal Adenoids. Varicosities or the rupture of the enlarged veins in the pharynx. Conditions in which the composition of the blood is altered—as Anæmias, certain infectious dlseases, and the Bright's Disease.

202. Describe the Syphilitic Ulcerations of the Pharynx.

They occur in the secondary and tertiary stages.

In the SECONDARY STAGE, they appear as small, shallow excavations and are usualiy situated in the posterior walls of the pharynx frequently associated with mucous patches.

In the TERTIARY STAGE, they are more deep and serpiginous. Due to the erosion of Gummata (see Ans. to Q. 28) the entire soft palate and the pharyngeal wall may be involved, which on healing leave white *cicatrices*.

203. Describe the Tubercular Ulcerations of the Pharynx.

They are irregular in outline with ill-defined edges, and generally grayish in color. They are *exceedingly painful* and are always associated with *glandular involvement*. The posterior walls of the pharynx have an eroded and worm-eaten appearance.

204. Describe the Malignant Ulcerations of the Pharynx.

They are distinguished by their *marked infil-*

tration of the surrounding structures and *rapidity of their psogress*—spreading, in both surface and depth. The discharges from them are sanious and offensive. They are always secondary to the formation of tumor.

205. What is Dysphagia?

Dysphagia is difficult or painful swallowing which may be due to pain or obstruction, usually the former.

206. Describe and tell in what conditions Anæsthesia of the Pharynx may be found?

It may be the effect of some organic disease or may be due to lesions interfering with the function of the glosso-pharyngeal nerves or appear as one of the phenomena of Hysteria.

207. Describe and tell in what conditions Paræsthesia of the Pharynx may be found?

It is found in chlorotic or anæmic young women and in women during climacteric. It is usually of hysteric origin, but may constitute one of the initial symptoms of a malignant disease and also of many organic diseases.

208. Desrcibe and tell in what conditions Hyperæsthesia of the Pharynx may be found?

It may occur in Hysteria, mental affections and Hydrophobia and frequently as one of the initial symptoms of Gout, Phthisis and Pharyngeal Cancer. It may also be idiosyncrasy with some people.

209. Give the symptoms and appearance of the Gouty Pharyngitis.

SYMPTOMS.—Sudden onset with pain and fulness in the throat with a rigid and stiff feeling of the same. Aggravated during deglutition. When fully developed the pain is disproportionately severe. Fever slight or absent.

APPEARANCE.—The fauces and the pharynx are of a bright red colour. The inflammation is of a decidedly patchy character. The uvula may be œdematous.

210. Give symptoms and appearance of Rheumatic Pharyngitis.

SYMPTOMS.—The pain on swallowing is pronounced. Sensitiveness of the throat.

APPEARANCE.—Its objective appearance slight or absent.

211. Give symptoms and appearance of Herpetic Pharyngitis.

SYMPTOMS.—Much pain on deglutition. General prostration and moderate fever.

APPEARANCE.—Numerous vesicles on the pharyngeal walls. Their occurrence in successive crops. They rupture in the course of 24 to 48 hours giving rise to small, shallow ulcers, which usually coalesce and become covered with false membrane.

212. Give symptoms and appearance of Phlegmonous Pharyngitis.

SYMPTOMS.—Sudden onset with severe pain on deglutition, dyspnœa, soreness of the throat, swelling of the neck, rigors, high fever, headache, and profound prostration. The throat is filled with offensive mucus.

APPEARANCE.—The pharyngeal mucous membrane highly inflamed and injected and rapidly passes on to suppuration taking a slouhing character with consequent hæmorrhage. The tonsils also are highly inflamed.

213. Give symptoms and appearance of Gangrenous Pharyngitis.

SYMPTOMS.—Onset with high fever and severe pain in the throat. The prostration is profound from the beginning. The breath is horribly offensive. Fœtid Diarrhœa.

APPEARANCE.—Mucous membrane highly inflamed, the parts assuming a *dusky color*, which is soon followed by an eschar.

214. Give symptoms and appearance of Tubercular Pharyngitis.

SYMPTOMS.—In the early stage *the pain is severe,*

which may make deglutition impossible. Other symptoms dependent upon primary Tubercular lesion elsewhere are also present. In the chronic stage, it is less painful.

APPEARANCE.—In the early stage, eruptions of muddy-gray, slightly elevated miliary granules on the posterior walls of the phraynx, which break down within a few days and form ulcers. It is preceded by inflammatory infiltration of the parts. In the chronic stage, the granules are less prominent, and the ulcerations more so, than in the acute form. The ulcers are indolent.

215. Give symptoms and appearance of Syphilitic Pharyngitis.

See Answer to Q. 202 above.

216. Give symptoms and appearance of Catarrhal Pharyngitis.

SYMPTOMS.—In the acute stage, sudden onset with high fever. More or less pain in the throat, aggravated during attempts at swallowing. Sometimes general prostration and pain or aching all over the body. There may be pain shooting from the throat to the ears. In the chronic stage. burning, stuffy, pricking, tickling, and other sensations in the pharynx. Persistent accumulation of mucus in the same, forcing the patient to make frequent attempt at clearing the throat, by hemming and hawking. An irritating hawking cough is not unusual. Sometimes the hearing is involved. Pain is rare.

APPEARANCE.—In the acute stage, increased redness of the mucous membrane of the pharynx and adjacent parts, with slight puffiness and swelling. Externally the cervical glands are sometimes enlarged. In the chronic stage, the walls of the pharynx are studded with many small elevations. The mucous membrane is more or less congestd and is covered with mucus.

217. Give symptoms and appearance of Atrophic Pharyngeal Catarrh.

SYMPTOMS.—Local discomfort forcing the patient to clear the throat, at short intervals.

APPEARANCE.—The mucous membrane and the glandular structure present a dried appearance, the crust of inspissated mucus-collects in the pharyngeal walls is unusually roomy.

218. Give symptoms and appearance of Follicular Pharyngitis.

It is also known as Gangrenous Pharyngitis or Clergyman's Sore-throat.

SYMPTOMS.—The secretion at first increases, which after a short period lessens and alters in quantity. Dryness of the throat.

APPEARANCE.—The enlargement of distension of the muciparus glands of the pharynx. Later the glands inflame.

219. Describe and tell all you know of the appearance of Diphtheria.

It first manifests as a small grayish or dirty white spot, which within a few hours enlarges and developes into a false membrane (see Answers to Qs. 50, 159 & 200, above), covering the entire fauces, soft palate and pharynx, or it may be localised. It does not always remain limited to the throat, but may extend to the larynx, trachea or bronchi below, or to the nasal cavities, conjuctivæ or ears, above.

220. Describe the Post-Diphtheritic Paralysis.

It is frequently observed during convalescence, in the 2nd or 3rd week and has its origin in the toxic Neuritis. It may be of various types, and in the majority of cases eyes, throat and heart are involved producing Paralysis of Accommodation, Paralytic Dysphagia and Heart failure, respectively.

ŒSOPHAGUS.

221. Give the Medical Anatomy in brief of the Œsophagus.

The œsophagus or the gullet is a musculo-membraneous tube or canal from $\frac{3}{4}''$ to $1''$ in diameter and about $9''$ in length extending from the pharynx to the stomach, whose function is to carry food from the mouth to the stomach. It had its origin opposite the Circoid cartilage.

222. Describe the methods of examination of the Œsophagus.

Examination with the sound. Auscultation. Inspection. Palpation.

223. Describe the manner of passing the Œsophageal Tube or Sound.

After moistening the sound with milk or water, it should be passed, over the dorsum of the tongue to the pharynx. When in this position the patient should be asked to swallow, and as he attempts to do so, the tube should be pushed inward with a little force. The patient should be in a sitting posture.

224. What points are necessary to pay attention to in passing the Sound?

(a) The presence or absence of pain. (b) Detection of any obstruction. (c) Diverticula. (d) Movement of the instrument.

225. Name contra-indication to use of the Œsophageal Tube or Sound.

Recent vomiting of blood or Hæmatemesis.

226. How is organic obstruction recognised?

(a) By symptoms of persistent dysphagia and (b) by the detection of narrowing of the œsophageal calibre by the sound.

227. Give the symptoms of Œsophageal Cancer.

Increasing dysphagia—becomes severe. Rapid emaciation. Regurgitation of food mixed with mucus and blood, sometimes cautaneous fragments. Cervical lymph-glands are frequently enlarged.

228. Diagnose interferenec in passing due to Œsophageal Abscess.

The sound will contain pus in its body, after it withdrawal

229. Describe an obstruction caused by Aneurysm of the Aorta.

It causes obstruction by putting pressure on the œsophagus from outside.

230. Disease of what glands may cause Œsophageal Obstruction?

Mediastinal glands.

231. To what is Hæmorrhage from Œsophagus due?

The rupture of the Aortic Aneursym or varicose veins about the cardiac orifice.

232. What may be learnt by Auscultation of the Œsophagus?

The function and condition of the organ may be ascertained by the nature, time of recurrence and periodicity of the sound it gives out.

233. What may be learnt by Inspection of the Œsophagus?

The condition of the lumen in the neck.

234. What may be learnt by Palpation of the Œsophagus?

Information about subcutaneous Emphysema or of an enlargement behind the trachea.

235. Name the subjective symptoms referred to the Œsophagus.

Pain and dysphagia.

236. Give the causes and symptoms of Paralysis of the Œsophagus.

CAUSES.—Cerebral hæmorrhage. Brain Tumor. Bulbar Paralysis. General Paralysis of the Insane.

SYMPTOMS.—Difficulty in swallowing, but there is no eructation, flowing or throwing back of the things taken. The sound passes easily without any obstruction.

STOMACH.

237. What methods of inflating the Stomach may be used to aid its examination by Inspection and Palpation?

(a) By pumping of air by means of a specially-constructed instrument. (b) By administering 2 teaspoonfuls of Tartaric Acid dissolved in water, to be followed by the same quantity of Bicarbonate of Soda solution within a few seconds, the gas thus produced distends the stomach.

238. Describe the Method of Palpating the Stomach.

The examination is made systematically first with the fingers only, later when the abdominal wall is relaxed, with the whole hand, if necessary every portion of the abdomen. If the abdominal wall is rigid, the patient should be directed to breathe deeply, with the mouth wide open. When the abdominal wall is relaxed the stomach should be pushed by the left hand towards the right hand to get necessary information. The patient should remain in a recumbent position and the physician in the right side of the patient.

239. When Palpating the Stomach to what points should you pay attention?

(a) As to the *size* of the organ. (b) *Abnormal growth*, if there is any. (c) *Pulsation*, if there is any.

240. What is suggested by Increased Resistance, when Palpating the Stomach?

Hypertrophy of the muscular coat of the stomach.

241. What is the usual situation of the Palpable Tumor in Cancer of the Pylorus?

It is between the ensiform cartilage and the umbilicus to the right of the median line.

242. What are the conditions which may cause

Diminution of the area of Gastric Tympany?

Enlargements of the neighbouring organs and tissues.

243. What are the causes which may increase the Area of Gastric Tympany?

Cirrhosis and diseases of the liver, attended by diminished size of that organ. Retraction of the lungs. Flatulent distension and dilatation of the stomach.

244. What conditions contra-indicate the use of Stomach-tube?

Heart diseases, with failing compensation. Aortic Aneurysm. Advanced arterial degenerations. Advanced stages of any chronic disease. Febrile affections. Suspected ulcer. Haematemesis. Acute Gastritis.

245. Describe the obtaining of Gastric Contents by Expression.

A stomach tube, with which is attached a piece of glass-tube about 4" long, is made to pass through the mouth in the same way as an œsophageal sound. The end in which the glass tube is attached is placed in a bottle held by the patient. After these, the patient is advised to bear down, as if at stool, the physician also exerts firm pressure on the epigastrium, at the same time. The gastric contents come out promptly through the tube as a result of these manipulations.

246. Describe the Ewald's Test-Breakfast.

It consists of a roll and a half pint of plain tea or water. It becomes ready for test one hour after the meal.

247. Describe the test for Hydrochloric Acid in Gastric Contents.

A weak solution of congo-red turns blue, in the presence of Hydrochloric Acid in the gastric contents.

248. What is the significance of Increased Hydrochloric Acid in Gastric Contents?

It is significant of Hyper-chlorhydria.

249. Describe the method for determining the Total Acidity of the Gastric Contents.

10 c. c. of filtered gastric contents should be placed in a beaker, and with the same be added one drop of a one p.c. alcoholic solution of Phenol-phthalein. A decinormal solution of Sodium Hydrate is required to mix with it, drop by drop from a graduated burette, until the contents in the beaker turn out red permanently i.e., the quantity necessary for neutralisation of the Acid. By multiplying the quantity of the Sodium Hydrate with ten, the total acidity is determined. For example, if 7 c.c. of Sodium Hydrate is required for the purpose, the total acidity is 7 x 10 i.e., 70.

250. Describe the method for determining the Total Hydrochloric Acid of the Gastric Contents.

By multiplying the total acidity with ·00365 the percentage of the Acid is obtained and from the percentage the total is worked out.

251. In what diseases of the stomach is the free Hydrochloric Acid is diminished or absent?

Cancer in the stomach. Chronic Gastric Catarrh. Atrophy of the stomach. Achylia Gastrica.

252. What disease of the stomach is suggested by the presence of free Lactic Acid in Gastric Contents?

The Cancer of the Stomach.

253. What is the most reliable test for determining the Motor Power of the Stomach?

Leube's Test. The stomach is washed out after 6 or 7 hours of taking a meal. If no food-particles are detected in the washing, the motor power of the stomach may be regarded as normal.

254. What is suggested by Increased Gastric Motility?

Suggestive of certain motor neuroses.

255. In what conditions is the Hydrochloric Acid diminished?

Chronic catarrhal inflammation. Absence of gastric secretion. Contraction of the stomach.

256. Give quantitative test for free Hydrochloric Acid.

Vide Answer to Q. 249. Instead of Phenol-phthalein solution 2 or 3 drops of Topfer's solution is to be mixed with 10 c.c. of filtered gastric contents, which will produce a rose-red color of the whole thing. Then the decinormal solution of Sodium Hydrate, in the way as indicated previously (in Ans. to Q. 249) is to be mixed with the same until the rose-red reaction of the Topfer's solution disappears. Multiplying the quantity of Sodium Hydrate with ·00356, the result will indicate the actual percentage of free Hydrochloric Acid.

257. In what conditions is the Hydrochloric Acid increased?

Irritative Dyspepsia. Ulceration in the stomach. Neuroses of the stomach.

258. Give tests for free Lactic Acid.

(a) UFFELMANN'S TEST.—The mixture of a few drops of Carbolic Acid with a weak solution of Ferric Chloride will change the color of the gastric contents into canary yellow if Lactic Acid is present in the contents.

(b) ARNOLD'S TEST.—If with a few drops of gastric contents is added a mixture of 1 c.c. Gentian Violet Solution with one drop of Ferric Chloride, the whole thing will be changed into a yellowish or greenish solution if Lactic Acid is present in the contents.

(c) KELLING'S TEST.—If with a mixture of 2 c.c. gastric contents with 20 c.c. of water is added 1 or 2 drops of 1 p.c. aqueous solution of Perchloride of Iron, it will change into distinct green color perceived by holding the tube against a white background, if Lactic Acid is present in the contents.

(d) STRAUSS' TEST.—A funnel marked at 5 and 25 c.c., is filled with 5 c.c. filtered gastric contents and 20 c.c. of Ether. 20 c.c. of the solution is allowed to escape after it is well-shaken. The remaining 5 c.c. is again mixed with 20 c.c. of distilled water and 2 drops of Tinct. of Chloride of Iron (1 : 10). If the proportion of Lactic Acid in the gastric contents is more than 1 : 1000, a marked green solution will be observed in the funnel after it is well-shaken. If the proportion is lower the solution will be pale green.

259. What is the significance of free Lactic Acid?

It is significant of the Cancer of the Stomach.

260. Give a test for Propeptone.

By mixing some gastric contents, with an equal quantity of a saturated solution of common salt, the mixture will be *turbid*, if propeptone is present in the contents. In doubtful cases one or 2 drops of Acetic Acid should be added.

261. Give a test for Peptone.

If with mixture of gastric contents and the saturated solution of common salt in equal quantities, a few drops of a 1 p.c. solution of Cupric Sulphate is added, it will be turned purplish or violet red in the presence of peptone in the gastric contents.

262. How do you determine the absorptive power of the Stomach?

It is determined by administering the patient with 3 grains of Iodide of Potassium covered in a gelatine capsule. If the absorptive power is normal, strips of starched paper will give a blue reaction of Iodine, when they are moistened in the saliva taken after $6\frac{1}{2}$ to 10 minutes of the administration of the powder.

263. How do you determine the Motor Power of the Stomach?

See Answer to Q. 253 of this chapter.

264. In what conditions do we find increased Motor Power?

In cases of certain motor neuroses.

265. In what conditions do we find diminished Motor Power?

Gastric atony. Gastrectasia. Pyloric obstruction.

266. What information is afforded by the Microscopical Examination in Gastric Contents?

The information is limited to the detection of certain organisms as the Sarcinæ Ventriculi (responsible for fermentive processes) and Oppler-Boas Bacilli (indicative of Carcinoma or free Lactic Acid). Sometimes solid particles such as detached portions of gastric mucous membrane or tumor may be detected.

267. What is Hæmatemesis?

Vomiting of blood from the stomach—the blood is usually clotted and mixed with food.

268. To what is profuse Vomiting of Blood due?

Gastric ulcers.

269. Describe the Hæmatemesis of Cancer.

The bleeding is rarely free. It presents a "coffee-ground" color.

270. Describe the Hæmatemesis of Cirrhosis of the Liver.

It is due to the rupture of the gastric and œsophageal blood-vessels. The vomiting is severe and liable to recur.

271. Describe the Hæmatemesis of Renal Disease.

It is due to Sclerosis of the blood-vessels and increased arterial tension.

272. Name the constitutional diseases which may give rise to Hæmatemesis.

Scurvy. Small Pox. Yellow fever. Purpura. Acute Yellow Atrophy of the Liver. The essential Anæmias.

273. What are the characteristics of Cerebral Vomiting?

(a) It is easy and not attended with nausea or retching. (b) It is usually preceded by cerebral symptoms. (c) It is notably of projectile character. (d) Its frequency is greater in young subjects. (e) It is one of the cardinal symptoms of Meningitis, and one of the nitial symptoms of Apoplexy.

274. Describe the characteristics of Uræmic Vomiting.

It usually occurs in the morning and is associated with nausea, depression, high pluse tension, accentuated aortic second sound and cardiac hypertrophy.

275. What are the clinical sugggestions of Marked Thirst ?

It suggests loss of fluids by dehydration or evaporation. When it is associated with emaciation it is suggestive of the presence of sugar in the urine.

276. What is Anorexia ?

The loss of appetite.

277. What is Bulimia ?

Exeessive hunger.

278. Under what conditions does Bulimia occur ?

Convalescence from fevers and other acute disorders. Diabetes. Gastric irritation. After-effect of alcoholic beverages. Relaxation of Pylorus. Worms.

279. What is the clinical significance of Loss of Appetite ?

Signifies diminished gastric secretion.

280. In what conditions does Perverted Appetite occur ?

It occurs during pregnancy and Hysterical tacks in women and among the idiots and the insane.

281. What is Pica ?

Alterations of appetite.

282. Give an example of Perverted Appetite.

Under the morbid impulses, the patient eats most disgusting or indigestible article.

283. What Gastric Affections are characterized by Pain?

Acute Catarrhal and Toxic Gastritis. Gastralgia. Gastric ulcers. Cancer of the Stomach. Crises. Hyperchlorhydria. Atony of the Stomach. Gout of the Stomach. Chronic Gastric Catarrh.

284. Describe the Pain of Gastralgia.

The pain comes on in paroxysms and is notably cramping and gnawing. It occurs frequently when the stomach is empty, when food affords temporary relief.

285. Name some of the conditions, other than Gastric, which may produce Pain in the Epigastrium.

Localized Peritonitis. Affections of the Pancreas. Aneurysm of the Aorta. Gall-stones. Caries of the 6th or 7th Dorsal Vertebræ. Addisons's Disease. Acute Yellow atrophy of the Liver. Pericarditis. Strain or Rheumatism of the abdominal muscles and Neuralgias.

286. Describe the Pain of Gastric Ulcers.

Often a localised sensitiveness. The pain is aggravated after eating, but greatly relieved when the stomach has been emptied by vomiting.

287. Describe the Pain of Gastric Cancer.

Pain is constant and aggravates after eating, being milder than gastric ulcer, and not relieved to an appreciable extent after vomiting the contents of the stomach.

288. Describe the Gastric Crises and tell in what disease they occur.

They occur in Loco Motor Ataxia and constitute one of its early symptoms in some of its cases. The pains are characterized by thier severity and their resistance to treatment.

289. What is Pyrosis?

Water-brash which is commonly known as Heartburn. Burning pain or distress in the stomach, relieved on the ejection of a small quantity of clear, tasteless fluid which comes off without vomiting.

290. Name some of the symptoms referred to the Intestinal Tract, and dependent upon a Pathological Lesion involving that Tube.

Pains both dull and colicky, intestinal stenosis, early ulceration, meteorism and ascites, all dependent upon a tumor involving the intestine.

291. Name a symptom dependent upon Altered Functions of the Intestines as a Conducting Tube.

Constipation.

292. Describe the Anatomy, in brief, of the Stomach.

It is a dilated portion of the digestive tract situated between the œsophagus and small intestines and connected with them. $\frac{3}{4}$th of it is on the left of the median line and $\frac{1}{4}$th to the right.

293. Give the Dimensions of the Stomach.

Between Fundus and Pylorus 10″ to 12″; between Lesser and Greater Curvature 4″ to 12″; between interior and posterior walls $3\frac{1}{2}$″ and between Cardia and Pylorus 3″ to 6″.

294. Give the Landmarks for Diagnosis in diseases of that organ.

(a) EXTERNAL landmarks for physical examination are the ensiform cartilage and the costal cartilage.

(b) Characteristic symptoms for investigation are those related to the perverted function, those dependent upon pathological process and the constitutional symptoms mostly arising from malnutrition.

295. Name the general divisions of Disease of the Stomach.

(a) PRIMARY—due to perverted function and and secretory disturbance of the stomach. (b) SECONDARY—due to pathological processes of the lesions of other portions of the abdomen or the body and motor disorders.

296. Mention the diseases classed under Perverted Function.

Gastritis and Linitis Plastica.

297. Mention the diseases classed under the Secretory Disturbance.

Gastric ulcer. Hyperchlorhydria. Gastro-Succorrhœa. Achylia Gastrica Nervosa. Hypochlorhydria. Nervous Dyspepsias.

298. Mention the diseases classed under Pathological Processes.

Tuberculosis of the Stomach. Cancer of the Stomach. Dilatation of the Stomach or Gastrectasia. Hæmatemesis. Gastroptosis or Displacement of the Stomach.

299. Mention the diseases classed under Motor Disorders.

Isochymia. Regurgitation. Pneumatosis. Nervous Vomiting. Cardiospasm. Atony of the Stomach.

300. To what points should attention be paid when examining a case of Gastric Disorder?

(a) Systematic enquiry into the history of the case, and (b) careful physical examination.

301. Tell, what may be learnt from Inspection in diseases of the Stomach.

By inspection of the patient in general, malnutrition or emaciation suggests some serious disease, which is either Cancer, if the emaciation is rapid, or any organic disease, if it is progressive. By inspection of the epigastrium, usually, no information is gained.

302. How is Palpation of the Stomach performed and what value it is on examination?

See Ans. to Q. 238 of this chapter. It is the most useful means of physical examination of the stomach.

303. How is Percussion of the Stomach performed, and what value is it in examination?

The percussion is performed by striking lightly the portions of the stomach which lies in contact with the thoracic walls and the portion of the abdominal wall beneath which lies the anterior walls of the stomach, with the fingers for ascertaining the nature of the sound resonated by the stroke, which in *normal condition* elicit *a clear, low-pitched, tympanitic note, in the presence of solids or liquids a dull note* and in *flatulent distension* a *metallic note.*

The value of percussion in gastric disorders depends upon a consideration of facts bearing in the varying physical conditions of the normal stomach.

304. How is Auscultation of the Stomach performed, and what value is it in examination?

It is performed either by directly placing the ear over the organ or by the aid of a stethescope for examining the nature of the sound it gives out, from which information of the function and condition of the same are gained.

The value of auscultation in the examination of the diseases of stomach, though not so great as the other methods, it occasionally provides some important information.

305. What is the usual location of a palpable Tumor of Pylorus?

See Answer to Q. 241 of this Chapter.

306. Name the conditions giving rise to a decrease in the Gastric Area of Tympany.

See Answer to Q. 242 of this Chapter.

307. Gastric Tympanitic Area is increased in what conditions?

The contraction of the liver and the lungs and displacement of the thoracic viscera.

308. Describe the two Deglutition Sounds.

They are heard over the ensiform cartilage. The

Chap. V.] STOMACH 93

FIRST sound occurs at the time of swallowing, while the SECOND one is heard after an interval of 7 or 8 seconds. Their absence indicates the stenosis of the cardiac orifice.

309. Tell the methods for obtaining the Gastric Contents.

(a) By Expression or Aspiration through the stomach tube (vide Ans. to Q. 245 above). (b) By Einhorn's Stomach-bucket. (c) By Spallanzani and Edinger's Sponge methods.

310. Describe the Stomach Bucket.

It is a small silver vessel of the size of a gelatine capsule, having large holes on the top, bound in a long silken thread. It is used for obtaining gastric contents by swallowing it, by the patient and allowing it to remain in the stomach for 5 minutes, after which it is withdrawn. Specially useful for making a simple test for the presence of Hydrochloric Acid.

311. What constitutes a complete Gastric Analysis ?

The determination of the following points constitutes a complete gastric analysis, viz. Quantity of the contents. Chemical reaction. Total acidity. Presence and percentage of free Hydrochloric Acid, free Lactic Acid, Propeptone, Pepsin, Peptone, Rennet Ferment, Dextrine, Erythrodextrin. Achroadextrin and Maltose in the contents.

312. What is the normal quantity obtained from a Test Meal ?

Not more than 40 c.c. nor less than 20 c.c.

313. How is the Chemical Reaction obtained ?

It is obtained by the neutralisation of the Acid by the alkalis.

314. Describe the test for Total Acidity.

See Answer to Q. 249 of this Chapter.

315. What does Diminished Total Acidity mean ?

It indicates diminished gastric secretion.

316. What does Inlreased Total Acidity mean?

It indicates gastric hypersecretion.

317. Name all the Disorders of the Stomach.

See answers to Qs. 296 to 299 of this Chapter.

318. Give in brief the symptoms and signs of Gastric Catarrh.

Acute onset with moderate fever. Furred tongue. Foul and heavy breath with bitter or disagreeable taste in the mouth. Severe epigastric pain, shooting through to the back and deep diffuse tenderness. Nausea followed by vomiting. The pain is relieved when the stomach becomes empty.

319. Give in brief the symptoms and signs of Acute Toxic Gastritis.

SYMPTOMS.—Intense burning pain in the mouth, throat and stomach, salivation and dysphagia. The abdomen is tender, distended and painful on pressure. Constant vomiting and retching. Pain not relieved by emptying the stomach but is intensive. Intense thrist.

SIGNS.—The mucous membrane of the mouth and pharynx exhibits *corrosive effects*.

320. Give in brief Symptoms and Signs of Phlegmonous Gastritis.

SYMPTOMS.—Severe pain in the epigastrium, attended by a violent burning in the stomach, intense thirst, dry tongue, vomiting, and a septic fever which is usually high and irregular and associated with repeated rigors. The pulse is rapid and there is profound prostration.

SIGNS.—Occasionally a large tumor mass is felt in the stomach.

321. Give in brief the Symptoms and Signs of Chronic Gastric Catarrh.

SYMPTOMS.—Gradual onset. Abdominal discomfort soon after eating which may become aggravated and amount to actual pain. Flatulence—the eructed gas gives tasting of food or a foul flavour. The tongue is coated. Associated with these there are nervousness, headache, vertigo, disturbed sleep, general torpor, mental depression and drowsiness particularly after eating. In more advanced cases there may be nausea and vomiting—the ejected matter contains abundant quantity of mucus besides more or less digested food and little Hcl or Pepsin. There may be palpitation of the heart.

SIGNS.—The tip and margin of the tongue are very often red and there is pain on pressure over the stomach, usually diffuse and not severe.

322. Give in brief the Symptoms and Signs of Gastric Ulcer.

SYMPTOMS.—Continuous or intermittently progressive, severe *pain* which shoots through to the back and is aggravated after eating (within an hour or so) or by firm pressure. *Tenderness* over the site of ulcer. Vomiting after meals particularly of solid foods, which affords temporary relief from pain. *Constipation. Hæmatemesis. Hyperchlorhydria.* Slight fever. Anæmia.

SIGNS.—Points of tenderness and the presence of muscular rigidity of the affected area.

323. Give in brief Symptoms and Signs of Dilatation of the Stomach.

SYMPTOMS.—Diffuse burning pain in the epigastrium, relieved after a lavage. Pronounced *flatulence* and epigastric *distension.* Dyspnœa. Intense *thirst. Vomiting* at long intervals, of abnormal quantity of mucus and particles of food, of dark-grayish color with a sour odor; all symptoms are relieved after vomiting.

SIGNS.—Patient's appearance betrays a dangerous condition. The upper portion of the abdomen is prominent. Outlines of the stomach becomes enormously increased—perceived through palpation. The presence of a large quantity of fluid—perceived through succussion. All the signs disappear after a thorough lavage.

324. Give in brief the Symptoms and Signs of Cancer of the Stomach.

SYMPTOMS.—Digestive *disturbances*. *Loss of weight, strength and flesh*—Cachexia develops rapidly. Pain more or less continuous, not much relieved by vomiting which is not frequent but profuse. Nausea. Hæmatemesis—coffee-ground vomiting. Constipation. *Tumor* in the epigastric region. Fever.

SIGNS.—The appearance of tiny specks of blood and pus in the vomitus. Palpable Tumor in the gastric region. A localized sense of resistance. Rapid emaciation.

325. Give in brief the Symptoms and Signs of Gastroptosis.

SYMPTOMS.—Gastric disturbances in general.

SIGNS.—The stomach occupies a lower position than the normal and makes the lower abdomen unduly prominent while the epigastrium is depressed.

326. Give in brief the Symptoms and Signs of Hyperchlorhydria.

SYMPTOMS.—A sinking feeling before the meals. A sense of weight and burning in the episgastrium, often with *sour eructations*, one to three hours after meals, more pronounced after the chief meal—disappears soon after taking some food. Constipation. The episgastrium is often sensitive to pressure.

SIGNS.—High acidity of the vomited matters.

327. Name the Neuroses of the Stomach.

(a) The MOTOR neuroses—Hypermotility. Peristalitic unrest. Eructatio Nervosa. Nervous vomiting. Rumination. Regurgitation. Cardiospasm. Pyloric Spasm. Atony. Insufficiency or incontinence of the Pylorus. Insufficiency of the Cardia. Hyperkinesis Ventriculi. Akinesis Ventriculi. Nervous Dyspepsia. Pneumatosis.

(b) The SENSORY neuroses—Hyperæsthesia. Gastralgia. Bulimia. Akoria. Anorexia Nervosa.

Parorexia. Polyphagia. Sitophobia. Gastralgokines s Paræsthesias. Gastric Idiosyncrasis.

(c) The SECRETORY neuroses.—Hyperchlorhydria. Gastro succorrhœa—periodiac or continua chronica. Achylia Gastric Nervosa. Hypochlorhydria.

INTESTINES.

328. What methods are used in the Examination of the Intestines?

(a) Inspection. (b) Palpation. (c) Percussion. (d) Auscultation. (e) Inflation of the organ with gas. Test-lavage.

329. Tell what may be learnt from Inspection.

(a) From the SURFACE.—The evidence of intra-abdominal pressure by the formation of Striæ. About venous or epigastric arterial enlargements.

(b) From the CONTOUR—About the enlargement, both uniform or localized. About the retraction of the abdomen.

(c) From the increased PERISTALTIC ACTIVITY—Occlusion of the intestines, or Visceral Neurosis or about the Lead-Colic.

330. Give the causes for an uniform Enlargement of the Abdomen.

Accumulation of fat in the abdomen. Tympanites or Meteorism. Ascites.

331. Give the causes for a localized Enlargement of the Abdomen.

Tumors, or Herniæ, or localized accumulation of flatus.

332. Give causes for Retraction of the Abdomen.

Extreme emaciation, or colic of Lead-poisoning or Bacillar Meningitis or spastic contraction of single intestinal loops.

333. Tell what may be learnt by Palpation of the Abdomen.

About (a) the presence or absence of sensitive points or localized muscular rigidities, (b) the condition of special portions of the intestines, (c) œdema emphysema and corpulence of the abdominal walls, (d) splashing and friction vibrations, (e) herniæ, or (f) the presence or absence of tumors.

334. Describe Muscular Rigidity and tell what it indicates.

The general muscular rigidity is commonly dependent upon the nervousness of the patient and as such it has no clinical importance. A localized one is dependent on local tenderness and has the same clinical significance.

335. Describe the Test-lavage of the Colon.

It is a process for washing out the colon, by means of a large Langdon tube 80 c.m. in length, introduced through the rectum and causing water to flow while it passes; with care, it may be pushed through as far as the ileo-cæcal valve. Normally the water comes out clear, but in Colitis mucus is abundant. It is used for the diagnosis of Colitis.

336. Give the constitutional causes of Constipation.

Sluggishness of function. Sedentary habits. Irregularity in going to stool. Improper diets. Dehydration. Diseases of the heart, stomach, liver, etc. Indigestion. Fevers. Excessive use of Alcohol, Tobacco, Coffee, etc. Frequent use of purgatives.

337. Give the local causes of Constipation.

Weakness of the abdominal muscles. Atony of the large bowel. Atony of the colon. Intestinal obstruction. Painful affections of the abdominal walls. Mechanical obstacles. Local condition of the anus. Pelvic pain. Fæcal impaction.

338. Name the Pathological conditions giving rise to Bowel Obstruction.

(a) Conditions originating in the intestine itself—Intussusception. Volvulus or Twist and Knots. Strictures. Obstruction of the lumen by Gall-stones or Enterolith or hardened fæces or round worms. Paralytic Ileus.

(b) Conditions external to the intestine—Strangulation by bands or adhesions. Strangulated Hernia. Compression and traction by tumors of the adjacent organs.

339. Give Symptoms of Intestinal Obstruction.

Sudden *colicky pain* which later becomes continuous and very intense. *Vomiting* constant and most distressing, at first gastric, then bilious (greenish bile-stained matter) and finally stercoraceous containing brownish-black fluid having a fæcal odor. Complete and absolute constipation. Constitutional symptoms severe from the very outset. Distension of the abdomen. Paroxysmal peristaltic movement. Tenesmus often marked.

340. Describe the symptoms of Fæcal Impaction.

Long-continued constipation. General hardness of the lower bowel, due to accumulation of fæcal masses. Fæcal obstruction. Intense Colitis. Peritonitis.

341. What are the causes of Diarrhœa?

(a) When it is a PRIMARY CONDITION—Improper food. Cold drinks. Gastric indigestion. Chemical irritants. Putrefactive decomposition in the large intestine. Sudden atmospheric changes. Defective Hygiene. Changes in the constitution of the intestinal secretion. Constipation. Irritation of parasites. Ruptured abscsses. Certain nervous influence such as worry, fear, pleasurable emotions, etc. Rectal and anal irritation.

(b) When it is SECONDARY or SYMPTOMATIC—Certain infectious diseases. Extension of the inflammatory processes from adjacent parts. Portal congestion. Cachectic conditions. Acute intestinal catarrh.

342. Give a list of diseases in which Diarrhœa may be Symptomatic.

(a) INFECTIOUS DISEASES.—Dysentery, Cholera Infantum, Cholera Morbus, Cholera Asiatica, Typhoid Fever, Toxæmia, Pyæmia, Septicæmia, Tuberculosis and Pneumonia.

(b) INFLAMMATORY DISEASES OF THE ADJACENT

PARTS.—Peritonitis, Colitis, Intussuception, Hernia, Tuberculosis, and Cancerous ulceration.

(c) PORTAL CONGESTIONS.—Cirrhosis of the Liver. Valvular affections of the heart and lungs.

(d) CACHECTIC CONDITIONS.—Carcinoma, Anæmia, Addison's Disease and Chronic Nephritis.

(e) ACUTE INTESTINAL CATARRH.

(f) ACUTE MEMBRANEOUS ENTERITIS.

343. Give the causes of Intestinal Hæmorrhage.

Traumatism by foreign bodies. Intestinal ulcerations. Gouty Kidney. Changes in the composition of the blood.

344. How may the Colour of the Blood give an idea as to the the location of the Intestinal Hæmorrhage?

(a) When the blood discharged is pure and merely coats the fæces, it comes from the rectum.

(b) When the color approaches the natural—the lesion is nearer to the anus. The blood mixes with the fæces less intimately.

(c) When the stool presents a tarry pitch-like appearance, the blood is intermingled with it and the lesion is more remote from the anus.

345. Give the causes of Abdominal Pain.

(a) Intestinal causes.—Colic or Enteralgia. Intestinal indigestion. Acute Enteritis. Chronic Lead Poisoning. Duodenal ulcer. Malignant diseases of the intestines. Hernia. Appendicitis. Cholera morbus and Asiatica. Dysentery. Enteroptosis. Fæcal Impaction. Intestinal obstuction. Intestinal Perforation.

(b) Non-intestinal causes.—Spinal cord diseases. Neuralgia and Rheumatism of the abdominal walls. Gall-Stone Colic. Renal Colic. Cystitis. Aneurysm of the abdominal Aorta. Pelvic disorders in the female. Peritonitis.

346. Describe the Pain of Intestinal Indigestion.

Colicky in character. Subsides when the bowels are cleared of the offending matter.

347. Describe the Pain of Acute Enteritis.

Pains of varied nature, the most common form is colicky. It recurs in paroxysms and between them sensation of distress, discomfort or actual soreness. It precedes an evacuation and is relieved when bowels are cleared.

348. Describe the Pain of Lead Colic.

The pain is severe and colicky in nature, and is usually of sudden onset and being centred about the umbilicus spreads over the whole of abdomen. It may be paroxysmal or constant and often preceded by gastric or intestinal symptoms. The pain is relieved by pressure.

The history, the presence of *blue lines on the gums* and the blood-changes are important factors, in differential diagnosis.

349. Describe the Pain of the Duodenal Ulcer.

It is the most constant and distinctive feature of the ulcer and varies greatly in character—from a burning or boring sensation it may assume a more characteristic form, in which it comes on in paroxysms, radiating downwards or to the back and to the sides. The characteristic period of its aggravation is about *2 to 4 hours after every meal* and often at night. It is also aggravated by lying on the right side. During pain the victim is usually bent forward, and finds relief from pressure over the epigastric region. It is also *relieved temporarily by taking some food*, hence it is known as the "hunger-pain". The location of the pain is somewhat below the gall-bladder on the right para-sternal line (in the right hypochondrium).

350. Describe the Pain of Hernia.

The abdominal pain of Hernia is mild and fugitive. It is not associated with tenderness, but excited or aggravated by sudden muscular exertion.

351. Describe the Pain of Appendicitis.

It has a more fixed position than the other abdominal pains. Its onset is sudden with violence, manifesting itself first in the epigastrium, spreading down through the abdomen, soon becomes localized to the right iliac fossa—*the point of maximum intensity being at McBurney's point* (a point midway on the line drawn between the right anterior superior iliac spine and the umbilicus). Sometimes it may be localised from the beginning. It is spasmodic and colicky in nature, and is usually very intense, but it may also be a dull ache—a connective tissue pain, which ceases after a time and is replaced by a feeling of soreness in the appendix region.

352. Describe the Pain of Cholera Morbus.

The pain is griping and colicky in nature and in most cases, it is very intense. It precedes an evacuation and is relieved after it, but some soreness or discomfort, more or less constant, is always left.

353. Describe the Pain of Dysentery.

From a mere abdominal discomfort it may amount to actual agony. It is relieved temporarily with the passage of the stool. With the progress of the disease, it is constant and paroxysmal, and becomes griping in nature. It is associated with great straining and tenesmus.

354. Give the Non-intestinal causes of Abdominal Pain.

See Answer (b) to Q. 345 this chapter.

355. What character of the Diet produces Constipation?

Insufficiency. Dryness. Deficiency of vegetable matters. Coarse diet. Highly nutritious foods.

356. What symptoms may result from Constipation?

(a) The CARDINAL SYMPTOMS.—Infrequent or insufficient evacuation of stools. Hardened fæces.

(b) ASSOCIATED SYMPTOMS.—Sometimes practically absent. Usually, ineffectual urging, local discomfort, anorexia, a furred or coated tongue, foul taste in the mouth in the morning, foul breath, depression and loss of energy. Sometimes, sensation of fulness and distension of the abdomen or flatulence—relieved following a good evacuation. IN NERVOUS OR NEURASTHENIC SUBJECTS —debility, lassitude, headache, vertigo, sleeplessness, abnormal drowsiness at all times, mental irritation, Hypochondriasis, Melancholia, indigestion, palpitation of the heart, cardiac irregularity and fever. IN GIRLS— muddy skin, Acne, Chlorosis and there is a flabby state of the system, in general.

(c) UNUSUAL SYMPTOMS—Colic or abdominal pain. Pain down the back or front of the left thigh. Œdema of the feet. Intestinal inflammations. Weakening of the intestinal walls. Emphysema. Cardiac strain. Hernia. Hæmorrhoids or varicocele. Ulceration of the Colon. Formation of large tumors. Formation of Enteroliths. vic congestion in women, Intestinal Toxæmia, and the generation of a colonic wave. Intestinal infections. Diarrhœa.

357. What is Diarrhœa?

By Diarrhœa is meant, persistent purging or evacuation of fæces, which are watery and sometimes acrid. The stools are consisted of fluid fæces, mucus, serum, undigested food and even of blood and pus.

See also Answer to Q. 341 of this Chapter.

358. Name the symptoms usually associated with Diarrhœa.

Pain, flatulence and sometimes tenesmus.

359. Name some causes of Abdominal Pain.

See Answer to Q. 345 of this Chapter.

360. Describe the Pain of the Intestinal Colic.

The pain is griping in nature and recurs in paroxysms, disappearing when the troubles are relieved. The seat of its maximum intensity is about the navel. It is usually relieved by bending double or by making firm pressure with the hands.

361. Name the Situation of the Pain in Gall-Stone Colic.

The seat of its maximum intensity is in the region of the Gall-bladder; it may radiate to the back and shoulder.

362. Name the Situation of the Pain in Renal Colic.

The pain originates in the region of one of the kidneys and extends downwards along the course of the ureter into the bladder, to the pubes. In some cases the corresponding testicle and thighs also are involved.

363. Diagnose the Colic of Lead-poisoning.

See the last portion of the Answer to Q. 348 of this Chapter.

364. Describe the appearance of a Normal Stool.

A normal adult stool takes the shape of cylindrical masses of firm density, presenting a light dark-brown colour.

365. What is meant by a Formed Stool?

A normal adult stool.

366. What is the effect of long Retention of Fæces on the Color?

Becomes darker.

367. What is the effect of a Milk Diet on the Color of Stools?

Light-color.

368. What Drugs cause Black Stools?

Iron. Bismuth and charcoal.

369. What is the clinical significance of Clay-colored Stools?

Significants of absence of biles in the alimentary tract.

370. What is the significance of Mucus in the Stools?

Significant of a catarrhal condition of the intesnal mucous membrane.

371. What is the significance of Pus in the Stools?

It is significant of ulceration; when in large quantity, usually of the rupture of an abscess in the intestinal tract.

372. What is the significance of Fatty Stools?

A pancreatic disorder.

373. Give some nervous causes of Abdominal Pain.

A bilateral Neuralgia of the trunk, Loco motor Ataxia, Caries of the Vertebræ and Neuralgia of the abdominal walls.

374. Describe the pain of Rheumatism of the Abdominal Walls.

Superficial pains consisting of a steady soreness, aggravated during motion or attempts to move.

375. Mention all the causes of Meteorism or Tympanites.

Abnormal formation of gas in the intestinal tract. Retention of gas within the intestinal tract. Abnormal introduction of gas within the intestinal tract.

376. Give symptoms and diagnosis of Acute Catarrhal Enteritis.

SYMPTOMS.—*Diarrhœa* in the incipiency. *Abdominal pain* around the umbilicus, usually of a colicky nature. Flatulence. Intense thirst. Tongue is dry and furred. Disproportionately rapid pulse. Scanty urine. Nausea and vomiting in severe cases.

DIAGNOSIS.—The disease starts with gastric disturbances following a definite cause. When the large intestine is involved, the stools are pultaceous like thin gruel-grayish in color, with flakes of mucus, here and there or in large quantity—when the lower portion of the large intestine is involved, there is usually marked tenesmus. When the small intestine is involved, the stools contain undigested food and are more yellowish-green or grayish-yellow in color and flaky with less mucus. If the case is complicated with high fever it is to be viewed with much concern, keeping in view the individual peculiarities of the patient. There is no abdominal tenderness in Acute Catarrhal Enteritis, nor is there visible peristalsis. It is differentiated from

Typhoid Fever by its early Diarrhœa and from Appendicitis by its absence of pain in the McBurney's point.

377. Give symptoms and diagnosis of Phlegmonous Enteritis.

It involves all the coats of the bowel and is especially liable to attack the duodenum and leads to suppuration of the submucous layer and abscess formation. It is complicated with Peritonitis.

As an independent affection, it is very rare and cannot be diagnosed during life, except when it is associated with Hernia or Intussusception, which is its common cause.

378. Give symptoms and diagnosis of Diphtheritic Enteritis.

SYMPTOMS.—It may run its course without any symptom. In some cases, there are Diarrhœa, pain, tenesmus and passing of blood-stained mucus. In the toxic cases the intestinal symptoms are very marked.

DIAGNOSIS.—The stool contains shreds of membranes.

379. Give symptoms and diagnosis of Ulcerative Enteritis.

SYMPTOMS.—The ulcerative Enteritis having a most diversified etiology and different sites of origin, gives rise to a variety of intestinal conditions, which have *ulcerations* as their common characteristic, the general symptoms depending upon their etiological factors. In many cases, there is not only, the absence of symptoms entirely, any discomfort also is absent, even the existence of the trouble cannot be suspected; but the special clinical features of the ulceration are identical in all cases.

DIAGNOSIS.—The diagnosis is based upon the exclusion of the lesion disturbing the intestinal functions together with the finding of factors which may be the causes of the ulceration. The character of the discharges is of much importance, pus, sloughs and blood, if profuse, furnish valuable information. Tympanites, fever and wasting though not common are diagnostic.

380. Give symptoms and diagnosis of Membraneous Enteritis.

SYMPTOMS.—*Paroxysmal abdominal pains* with digestive and nervous disturbances. There are free intervals in which the abdominal symptoms are absent and nervous disturbances predominate. General nutrition is usually disturbed.

DIAGNOSIS.—Pseudo-membraneous formations varying in length from a few inches to several feet in the discharges from bowels. They are transparent, gelatinous and show fæcal staining. The discharges are preceded by colicky pains.

381. Tell under what circumstances Pus is found in the Secretions from the Bowel.

If the pus is pure, it is due to rupture of a pericæcal abscess or Cancer of the bowels or some local disease in rectum; in women, it may be due to an abscess in the broad ligament. Otherwise, it is frequently found when there is ulceration in the large intestine, the secretion being more, than when the bowel only is involved,

382. Give symptoms and diagnosis of Chronic Entero-Colitis.

SYMPTOMS.—Diarrhœa, flatulence and general *malnutrition*. Nervous symptoms are always prominent. There is little pain or fever. Mucus with stools.

DIAGNOSIS.—depends upon discovery of cause and presence or absence of ulceration. Examination of the stools—as to the amount of mucus, presence of blood or pus, the occurrence of parasites and above all the state of digestion, is essential.

383. Give symptoms and diagnosis of Cholera Morbus & Asiatica.

SYMPTOMS.—

(a) CHOLERA MORBUS—Nausea, abdominal pain, most violent and profuse *vomiting*. Purging—stools at first pultaceous, finally watery fluid. Cramps in the legs and other parts of the body. Suppression of urine,

Weak pluse, cold and clammy skin, profuse sweat and prostration.

(b) CHOLERA ASIATICA—Preliminary *Diarrhœa*, with headache, vertigo, depression of spirits and nausea. *Violent purging*—rice-water stools, usually attended with griping pains and flatulence, soon associates with *muscular cramps* and *severe vomiting*. Evacuations extremely copious and frequent. Suppression of urine. The pulse is rapid and weak, afterwards small and flickering. Thirst pronounced. Profound prostration. Typhoid state. Coma. Collapse.

DIAGNOSIS.—Both the diseases in their early stages simulate each other. The last named one is differentiated with the former by the knowledge of the presence or absence of the disease in the locality, and bacterial examination of the stools, which in case of the latter always contains Comma Bacilli. The former is less severe than the latter.

384. Give symptoms and diagnosis of Appendicitis.

SYMPTOMS.—Pain of sudden onset (as for its character see Answer to Q. 351), local *tenderness*—greatest at McBurney's point, *rigidity* of the right rectus and *Leucocytosis* are the cardinal symptoms. Associated with them are fever, accelaration of the pulse, furred tongue, nausea, vomiting, constipation frequent micturition, albuminuria, etc.

DIAGNOSIS.—The *pain, tenderness* and *rigidity* as described above, with *leucoyte count* and rectal examination (in the advanced stage) which reveals a *diffuse tumor* i.e., a tender mass to the right of the rectum help one to diagnose the disease. The patient lies on his back, with his right leg semiflexed. An increased leucocytosis is always an unfavourable sign. Diffusion of the pain, tympanites and marked aggravation of the general symptoms indicate its complication with Peritonitis.

385. Tell where is Cancer most frequently found in the Intestine. Give symptoms and diagnosis of Cancer of the Intestines.

The Cancer is most frequently found in the

lower portions of the intestinal tract, i.e., in the large intestines, particularly in the various flexures of the colon and the rectum.

SYMPTOMS.—Pain (continuous or paroxysmal), Constipation. Vomiting. Cachexia and general emaciation.

DIAGNOSIS.—The above symptoms aided with the examination of the bowels (after thorough evacuation) and discovery of the tumor, make the diagnosis absolutely certain. In doubtful cases X-ray gives conclusive evidence.

386. Give the causes for Dilatation of the Colon and Duodenum and describe their occurrence as far as possible.

(a) Dilatation of the COLON may be due to flatus, solid substances, organic obstruction and unknown causes.

(b) Dilatation of the DUODENUM may be due to dropping or displacement of the viscera, pressure by the root of the mesentery and tumors.

387. Name the Intestinal Neuroses.

Enterospasm. Peristaltic restlessness. Paresis or the Atony of the Intestines. Nervous flatulence. Enteralgia. Nervous Diarrhœa. Intestinal Neurasthenia.

388. Give the symptoms and diagnosis of Dysentery.

SYMPTOMS.—*Abdominal pain* (see Answer to Q. 353). *Evacuation*—beginning like ordinary Diarrhœa, the stools soon lose their fæcal character, finally consist of mucus or mucus and blood and become odorless and small in quantity ; when ulceration develops, clumps of gray and fœtid small sloughs appear in the stools and are very offensive. *Tenesmus recti*. *Straining*. Slight *Leucocytosis*.

DIAGNOSIS.—Its diagnosis is based upon the above symptoms. The abdomen is very sensitive even to the slightest pressure, which is sometimes associated with muscular rigidity. The differentiation of the types are made by bacterial examination.

389. Name an intestinal symptom dependent upon constitutional disturbance, the origin of the disease being in the intestines.

Diarrhœa dependent upon Typhoid Fever.

390. What is Constipation?

Retention and hardening of the fæces due to defective functions of the gastric organs, functional inactivity of the intestinal musculature or deficiency of the biliary or other secretions. See also Answers to Qs. 355 and 356 of this chapter.

391. In what way does frequent use of Purgatives produces Constipation?

The excessive excitation of the intestine by the frequent use of purgatives, paralyzes its normal function, making the same powerless to expel the fæces, in consequence of which they are retained in the bowels producing constipation.

392. What is Splanchnoptosis? Give its symptoms and diagnosis.

The displacements of the abdominal vessels from their normal position are known as the Splanchnoptosis.

SYMPTOMS—The visceral displacements in the majority of cases produce no symptoms. In some cases, the symptoms are mainly nervous, while in the others the dyspeptic symptoms are prominent.

DIAGNOSIS is based upon the whole clinical picture. X-ray gives positive evidence. In the case of gastroptosis the lower abdomen becomes unduly prominent, while the epigastrium is depressed.

RECTUM.

393. Attention to what particulars is necessary when examining a case of Rectal Disease?

The history of the case. The presence or absence of a Tubercular or Syphilitic infection. Condition of the bowels. Character of the discharges. Character of the pain, if there is any. Its association with any other disease. Conditions associated with defæcation. Power of the Sphincter ani. Effects of local examination by inspection and palpation. Findings of the digital and instrumental examination.

394. What points are included in the Examination?

The history of the case. Special interrogation for further enquiry as detailed above. Examination of the discharges. Local examination by inspection and palpation. Digital and instrumental examination in complicated cases.

395. Describe the preparation of the patient for Rectal Examination.

The examination should be conducted always in the daylight and in a place where sun-light will not cast any shadow over the place of examination, and he should be placed standing or in the knee-chest position.

396. Describe the method of Digital Examination of the Rectum.

The digital examination i.e., the examination of the interior of the rectum with the finger, is conducted in the following way :—

First the *anus* is thoroughly cleansed with Carbolated Green Soap or Synal, after which it is rinsed with a Bichloride solution. The *finger* is thoroughly lubricated with an antiseptic lubricant. Before introducing the finger, the *rectum* is anæsthetised by the injection of $\frac{1}{2}$ a dram of a 2 p.c. solution of Cocaine into it. The examination is conducted after the anæsthesis i.e., five minutes after the injection of the Cocaine solution. For examination of the upper third of the rectum, the middle finger is used, with the patient standing and directed to strain down. The depth of the hypertrophy of the sphincter is determined by taking it between the index finger in the anus and the thumb on the cutaneous surface outside. To note the condition of the mucous membrane, the examining finger should be well-introduced.

397. Of what are you to take note when examining the Rectum by the Finger?

The conditions of the sphincter and mucous membrane. The calibre of the rectum. The presence of new growths or abscesses, if there are any. The condition of the prostate gland. The presence of internal fistulæ, if there are any.

398. Describe the Instrumental Examination of the Rectum.

It is conducted by a cylindrical shaped Speculum, provided with a handle (set at such an angle as to permit of clearing the buttock during examination) and containing and obturator to facilitate introduction. Different sizes, both in calibre and length may be required to suit different condition.

To use the Speculum, it should be first made thoroughly antiseptic and after making it well-lubricated, it should be introduced into the rectum to its fullest extent i.e., above the pile-bearing inch. The obturator is then withdrawn and the exposed rectal surface thoroughly cleansed with cotton applicator. Then by a slow rotary motion while gradually withdrawing the instrument, all the conditions which prolapse into or present themselves at the end are noted.

399. Name the causes of the Rectal Pain.

Hæmorrhoids. Lesions in and below the pile-bearing inch, generally during or after defæcation. Strictures caused by ulceration above the pile-bearing inch in the rectum.

400. Give the Anatomy of the Pile-bearing Inch.

The sensory nerves derived from the sacral and lumbar plexuses are freely distributed in this region.

401. What are the causes of Bleeding from the Rectum?

Hæmorrhoids or fissure or malignant growths or ulceration.

402. Give symptoms of Cancer of the Rectum.

Along with the symptoms of other intestinal

Cancer detailed in Answer to Q. 385 above, pressure symptoms such as unilateral or bilateral Sciatica may be present. The stools in the early stages—"pipe-stem" or "sheep's-dung" stools—later mucus, blood, pus and sloughs with stools are frequent and are very offensive.

403. Give symptoms of Fissure of the Rectum.

Discharge of pure blood during and shortly after stools.

404. Give symptoms of Abscess of the Rectum.

Purulent discharges.

405. Give symptoms of Stricture of the Rectum.

Interference with defæcation. Ballooning of the rectum.

406. What is indicated by Ballooning of the Rectum?

It indicates the increasse in calibre of the cavity of the rectum, characterized by the non-elasticity of its wall.

407. Pruritus Ani may arise from what conditions?

Hæmorrhoids. Abscess of the rectum. Fissures. Ulcers. Fæcal impaction. Irritation by parasites (worms).

CHAPTER VI.

DIGESTIVE TRACT.

(continued)

LIVER—GALL-BLADDER—BILE DUCTS.

LIVER.

1. **Name the diseases characterized by Circumscribed Enlargement of the Liver.**

    Cancer or other tumors of the liver. Abscess of the liver. Hydatid Cysts.

2. **Name the Painful Enlargements of the Liver.**

    (a) DIFFUSE—Hyperæmia. Inflammation. Hypertrophic Cirrhosis. Catarrh or the obstruction of the gall duct.

    (b) CIRCUMSCRIBED—Tumors, especially those of malignant character. Abscess of the Liver.

3. **Name the Painless Enlargements of the Liver.**

    (a) DIFFUSE—Fatty & Amyloid degeneration of the liver.

    (b) CIRCUMSCRIBED—Hydatid cysts.

4. **What information may be obtained by Auscultation of the Liver?**

    Of the inflammation of the peritoneum of the liver by friction fremitus. Of the Cirrhosis of the Liver by a well-marked murmur. Of the compression or Aneurysm of the abdominal aorta by arterial murmurs.

5. **What is the usual character of Pain in Diseases of the Liver?**

    A dull, heavy, sensation in the right hypochondrium.

6. **Name the physical methods for examining the liver, and tell what information may be obtained by Inspection.**

   METHODS.—Inspection. Palpation. Percussion. Auscultation.

   INFORMATION by Inspection—*Undue prominence*, when diffuse, suggests hepatic enlargements; when localised, tumors. *Localized œdema—abscess. Pulsation—* Tricuspid Regurgitation or aneurysmal dilatation of the abdominal aorta. Venous *enlargements*—of the superficial veins.

7. **Differentiate Enlargement of the Liver and Downward Displacement.**

   Undue prominence and rising and falling of the lower margin of the liver suggest enlargement.

8. **Differentiate the prominence from Right-sided Pleural Effusion, and that of the Enlarged Liver.**

   In PLEURAL EFFUSION the spaces between the ribs bulge more or less prominently.

   In the LIVER ENLARGEMENT—undue prominence of the hepatic region.

9. **What information may be obtained by Palpation in Diseases of the Liver?**

   The recognition of the downward displacement and enlargement of the liver. The character of the liver surfaces. The consistence of the liver. Mobility during respiration. The presence or absence of friction fremitus or hydatid cysts.

10. **What is suggested by a Fremitus over the Liver?**

    Peritonitis.

11. **In what conditions is the method of examination, known as "Dipping" for the Liver, dangerous?**

    In Abscess, Hydatid Cysts and distended gall-bladder.

12. Describe the method of examination known as "Dipping" for the Liver.

It is conducted by holding the finger-tips perpendicularly over the abdominal walls and pushing it suddenly at a place where the location of the liver is expected. The fluids or gas, as the case may be, is thus pushed aside and the fingers come in contact with the hepatic surface. By repeating the experiment over different points, the margin of the liver can be located. This method is adopted (in palpation) when the enlargement is associated with Ascites or Tympanites.

13. What diseases are suggested by Round, Smooth Swellings over the Liver, fluctuating on Palpation?

Abcess of the liver and Hydatid cysts.

14. What conditions of Liver are suggested by Increased Hardness?

Hyperæmia. Cirrhosis. Amyloid disease.

15. What is the significance of Localized Œdema over the Right Hypochondrium?

Acute Suppurative Hepatitis (Abscess).

16. Name the Normal Percussion Outlines of Liver.

(a) The area of absolute dullness i.e., the area under which the liver comes in direct contact with the abdominal wall and over which absolute dullness or flatness is obtained by light percussion.

(b) The area of relative dullness i.e., the area in which the liver is separated from the overlying surface by the lung-tissue. It lies above the area of absolute dullness and its upper boundary runs parallel to and about 1¼″ above the upper line of absolute dullness. Deep percussion elicits the relative dullness.

17. What is suggested by the discovery of Diminished Liver Dullness?

Diminution in the size of the organ, or its separation from the abdominal walls, or the Pulmonary Emphysema, or the upward displacement of the liver.

18. What conditions may give rise to an apparent increase in Liver Dullness?

Right-sided Pleurisy with effusion. An abscess between the liver and the diaphragm. Inflammation of the lower lobe of the right lung. Distension of the stomach and colon by solid matters. Malignant growths of the adjacent structures downwards. Distension of the gall-bladder. In the first three, the increase is upwards, while in last three, it is downward.

19. What is the effect of Pulmonary Emphysema on the Liver Dullness?

It diminishes the area of superficial dullness and may even lessen the absolute area.

20. Differentiate Liver Displacements from alterations in the size of the organ.

In a DISPLACEMENT the position of the liver is either lowered or raised—both the ends lose their normal position.

In an ALTERATION, either one of the edges of the liver retains its normal position or both exceed their normal limits.

21. What are the causes of Displacement of the Liver?

Rachitic chest. Tight lacing. Subphrenic abscess. Tumors. Wandering liver. Pressure of tumors and effusion from below. Croupous Pneumonia. Pneumothorax. Pleuritic effusion.

22. Name the diseases characterized by general Enlargement of the Liver.

Hyperæmia. Inflammation. Hypertrophic Cirrhosis. Tumors. Catarrh or obstruction of the gall-duct. Abscess of the liver.

GALL BLADDER & BILE DUCT.

23. Give symptoms and course of Acute Infectious Cholecystitis.

SYMPTOMS.—Severe paroxysmal *pain* and *sensitiveness* in the region of Gall bladder. *Rigidity* of the over-lying muscles. *Distension of the gall-bladder* and if palpable, it appears as a pear-shaped lump. These are the cardinal symptoms of the disease.

COURSE.—An average case of Acute Infectious Cholecystitis depicts the above symptoms associated with extreme local tenderness, fever with sudden onset, etc. Serious cases may be confounded with Appendicitis or Acute Intenstinal obstruction, where history of the case, with the above-mentioned symptoms helps its diagnosis.

24. Give symptoms and course of Cancer of the Bile-passages.

The bile-passages include gall-bladder and bile duct; the Cancer in the former is not very uncommon, while in the latter it is rare.

(a) CANCER OF THE GALL BLADDER—

SYMPTOMS.—Its cardinal symptoms are, severe and paroxysmal *pain,* too much *tenderness* on pressure, *loss of weight, anorexia* and *Jaundice* (in the advanced stage). Associated with them, is distension of the gall-bladder and often gastro-intestinal disturbances.

COURSE.—It appears, either preceded by or accompanied with Gall-stone or indigestion, first as a sense of dicomfort or fulness in the right hypochondrium. It is then followed by gastro-intestinal disturbances and local pain. The real aspect of the disorder comes out with the distension of the gall-bladder and the symptoms noted above. Enlargement of the liver and ascites may appear due to secondary pathological changes. Extension of the growth to pylorus may lead to gastric disturbances, while to the colon, gradually increasing intestinal obstruction. In its diagnosis, along with symptoms noted in the preceding paragraph, the age of the patient (advanced middle life) is an important factor.

(b) CANCER OF THE BILE DUCTS—

SYMPTOMS.—A rapidly developing, intense and persistent Jaundice with little or no pain. Distension of the gall-bladder.

25. Give symptoms and course of Cholelithiasis (Gall Stone).

SYMPTOMS.—Dull & aching *pain*. Paroxysmal and excruciating *biliary colic*. *Indigestion* with flatulence. Stones or calculi in the stool. These are the cardinal symptoms of the disease. Associated with them are nausea and vomiting in the early stage, fever preceded by chill with sudden rise and remission, and Jaundice.

COURSE.—The main clinical pictures of Gallstones are those of indigestion and flatulence with the symptoms stated above and secondary visceral lesions. Symptoms disappear with the passing of the stone in the bowel. Though they are liable to relapse at short intervals, they may remain latent for many years. Family history and the history of previous illness plays important parts in diagnosis, which is based upon the presence of symptoms pointing to the gall bladder and its syndrome.

26. Give symptoms and diagnosis of Obstruction of Common Ducts.

The diagnostic symptoms of complete obstruction are—the Jaundice is deep, marked and persistent. The stools are of an ashy color and the urine contains bile.

27. Give symptoms and diagnosis of the Obstruction of the Cystic Ducts.

The diagnostic symptoms are—colic, dilatation or Dropsy of the gall-bladder, acute or suppurative Chole-cystitis, and calcification of the gall-bladder.

CHAPTER VII.
DIGESTIVE TRACT.
(continued)
SPLEEN.

1. **Describe the Situation of the Spleen.**

    It is situated immediately below the diaphragm in the left hypochondrium. Its upper portion is covered by the left lung which overlaps it, while its lower extremity extends to the 11th rib. Its anterior limit is upto the mid-axillary line, while the posterior extends to within an inch and a half of the median line.

2. **What physical methods have we for examining the Spleen?**

    (a) Inspection. (b) Palpation. (c) Percussion.

3. **Describe the normal limits of Splenic Percussion Dullness.**

    The area of splenic dullness is rounded in front and below. Above it is straight. Normally the area should measure $\frac{3}{4}''$ by $2''$.

4. **What are the causes of Displacement of the Spleen?**

    (a) DOWNWARD displacement.—Rachitis, left Pleural Effusion, Pulmonary Emphysema.

    (b) UPWARD displacement.—Ascites. Tumors of the abdominal and pelvic viscera. Flatulent distension of the stomach and intestines.

5. **Name the conditions producing Splenic Enlargements.**

    Many of the infectious diseases, particularly Typhoid Fever and Malaria. Some of the chronic infectious diseases as Tuberculosis and Syphilis. Anæmias. Amyloid degeneration of the liver. Cirrhosis of the liver. Rachitis. Tumors and Hydatid cysts. Abcess. Embolism.

CHAPTER VIII.

DIGESTIVE TRACT.
(continued)

PANCREAS.

1. Give the Anatomy of the Pancreas.

The Pancreas is a large conglomerate gland situated transversely across the posterior portion of the epigastric and hypochondriac regions behind the stomach. It is oblong, tapering in shape and about 6" to 8" long. Its right extremity is decidedly thicker and is called the *head*, fitted in the arch made by the curve of the duodenum, while the left one which is thinner and is in relation with the lower extremity of the inner border of the spleen, is known as the *tail*. The head has also important relations with the portal vein, the superior mesenteric artery, the common bile duct, the inferior Vena Cava and the Aorta. It secretes a limpid, colorless juice which is discharged into the duodenum through the duct known as the pancreatic duct, or the duct of Wirsung, joining the common bile duct in the Ampulla of Vater and pours with the bile into the digestive system and helps in the digestion of *oils* and *fats*.

2. Name some symptoms resulting from Pancreatic Diseases.

Pain—subjective discomfort or actual pain—deep-seated. Diarrhœa with clay-colored fatty stools, Urine, with increase of urea and diminution of sugar. Increased salivary flow. Emaciation.

3. Name some symptoms resulting from Deficient Pancreatic Secretion.

Fatty stools. Diminution of sugar in the urine. Increased salivary flow.

4. What is the association of Glycosuria with Pancreatic Diseases?

Effect of the disorder of the Islands of Langerhans.

5. Give symptoms and diagnosis of Pancreatitis.

Sudden and violent *left-sided* epigastric *pain*, associated with early vomiting and collapse, and a circumscribed epigastric distension with *rigidity* and tenderness are the cardinal symptoms. With leucocytosis they help to come to a correct diagnosis.

6. Give symptoms and diagnosis of Hæmorrhage into the Pancreas.

Sudden and severe left-sided epigastric pain with nausea, vomiting, collapse and anxiety. Tenderness sometimes absent.

Diagnosis—practically impossible.

7. Give symptoms and diagnosis of Chronic Interstitial Pancreatitis.

Its initial symptom is *indigestion* with loss of appetite, nausea, flatulence, heaviness and distension in the epigastrium. When the disease is due to the morbid condition of the bowels, gastric symptoms are predominant; when due to Cholelithiasis, hepatic symptoms with Jaundice; when to malignant diseases, etc., or Syphilis, it is secondary and to diabetic causes Glycosuria helps its diagnosis. Pain develops in the later stage as dull and boring in character and occurs after food. Emaciation and debility when the case is advanced.

8. Give symptoms and diagnosis of the Panreatic Calculi.

Many cases run a symptomless course. As a rule, the paroxysmal pain with symptoms of pancreatic disorder are the characteristic features. The discovery of stones in the characteristic stools removes all doubt. It closely simulates Gall-stone, with all the reflex and constitutional symptoms accompanying it.

9. Give symptoms and diagnosis of Pancreatic Cysts.

The history of the digestive disturbances followed by the apperance of an epigastric *tumor* (semicircular bulging and often visible externally), the major portion of which lies to the left of the median line and which appears, after examination, to lie behind the stomach and the colon and as a rule lies between them, is indicative of Pancreatic Cysts. The history of traumatism or of probable Acute Pancreatitis adds to its probability. The distension of the abdomen is progressive. Pain usually colicky.

10. Give symptoms and diagnosis of Cancer of the Pancreas.

The symptoms appear early and are most marked. *Rapid emaciation*, the presence of the *tumor* (sometimes increased resistance only) in the upper abdomen to the right of the middle line, intense and persistent *Jaundice*, with dilatation of the Gall Bladder and features of pancreatic disturbances (whose onset is gradual and progressive) are definite indications of the Cancer of the Pancreas.

CHAPTER IX.

THE RESPIRATORY ORGANS.

NOSE—PHYSICAL DIAGNOSIS—CHEST.

THE NOSE.

1. Describe the method of examining the Nose.

The nose is examined externally by INSPECTION and internally by RHINOSCOPE.

By INSPECTION externally *lip* and *bridge* of the nose, as also the *nostrils*, are examined.

By RHINOSCOPE both the *anterior* as also the *posterior* of the nose are examined. The examination of the *anterior* is conducted by a head-mirror, which helps the examiner to view, (i.) the opening of the cavity, which if obstructed, the nature and situation of the same, (ii.) the condition of the *mucous membrane* as to, color, discharges and ulceration, (iii.) the condition of the *turbinated bodies,* as to size, color and ulceration, (iv.) the condition of the *septum,* as to, shape, position, color and ulcerations, and (v.) the morbid growth (if there is any)—the essential points required for the purpose. The examination from the *posterior* is conducted by a smallest size throat-mirror to obtain a true picture of the post-nasal space.

2. Name some of the evil effects of Nasal Obstruction.

Mouth-breathing. Flatness or deformity of the chest. Adenoid facies. Recurring attacks of Tonsillitis. Pharyngitis. Bronchitis. Gastric disturbances—due to bolting of unsufficiently masticated food. Increased susceptibility to the acute exanthemata. Etc.

3. What is the characteristic appearance of the Face in Nasal Obstruction?

ADENOID FACIES—semi-idiotic face, pinched nostrils, lack of expression, open and dry mouth.

4. What diseases of the Nose have profuse Serous Discharges?

Acute Catarrhal Rhinitis, Hay Fever and nasal Hydrorrhœa.

5. Name the conditions which may produce Ulceration of the Nose.

Catarrh. Catarrhal Herpes. Eczema. Trauma. Neuro-Paralysis. Scurvy. Diabetes. Varicose Veins.

6. Describe a method by which you can differentiate Turbinated Enlargement due to Engorgement, and that due to increased Tissue-formation.

By applying a 4% solution of *Cocaine*, the enlargement due to engorgement is promptly reduced in size, but it produces little or no effect when the same is due to increased tissue-formation.

7. In what condition do we find a Purulent Nasal Discharge?

Abcess or ulceration.

8. Which of the Acute Infectious Diseases is characterized by profuse Nasal Discharge?

Infantile Syphilis.

9. What is Epistaxis?

Bleeding from the nose is known by the term Expistaxis or nose-bleed.

10. What is suggested by a unilateral Purulent Nasal Discharge in adults?

It is suggestive of abscess due to diseases of the accessory sinuses in adults.

11. What is suggested by a unilateral Purulent Nasal Discharge in children?

Suggestive of ulceration in any of the sinuses of the affected side.

12. Mention some of the conditions capable of producing Nasal Obstruction.

Adenoids. Hypertrophic Rhinitis. Deviations and spurs of the nasal septum. Polypi. Benign and malignant neoplasm. Swelling of the nasal mucous membrane. Enlargement of the turbinated bodies. Foreign bodies. Parasites.

13. Name and describe Ulcerations found in the Nose.

(i.) CATARRHAL—superficial, sometimes painful and readily heals. (ii.) HERPETIC—at the margin of the nostrils. (iii.) ECZEMATOUS—with cracks and fissures about the alæ nasi, occurs in association with Eczema of the face and skin about the nostril; itching. (iv.) TRAUMATIC—due to picking at the nose or presence of foreign bodies; readily heals. (v.) NEURO-PARALYTIC—painless and sluggish, without any discharge. (vi.) SCORBUTIC—the edges hard and thick and the surface susceptible to bleeding and attended with fœtor. (vii.) DIABETIC—at the nasal orifice. (viii.) VARICOSE—superficial, bluish in color, exceedingly sluggish and susceptible to bleeding. (ix.) SYPHILITIC—may occur at all stages. (x.) TUBERCULAR—mainly on the septum, whitish-gray surface, bleeding readily. (xi.) LUPOID—simulating tubercular ulcers. (xii.) LEPROUS—very destructive, watery and very offensive discharge. (xiii.) POST-FEBRILE—very irritable. (xiv.) ULCERATION OF THE MALIGNANT DISEASE—secondary to the formation of a tumor.

14. Give symptoms of Hay Fever.

Profuse coryza, which is watery at first, becoming purulent later. Constant sneezing. Chest symptoms may complicate the case, developing into Bronchitis, Paroxysms of Asthma.

15. Give symptoms of Acute Catarrhal Rhinitis.

Begins with a scanty mucous discharge, being more profuse with the progress of the disease, which excoriates the skin over which it flows.

16. Give symptoms of Antrum Highmore Disease.

A *purulent discharge* in which the patient feels an unpleasant odor, but unperceptible to others as such. It may become offensive exceptionally. It is yellowish in color, sometimes brownish-yellow or green and viscous. Nasal obstruction. In acute inflamation, there is intense pain in the cheek, with redness and œdema of the overlying parts. The pain may also be in the forehead.

ASSOCIATED SYMPTOMS.—Headache, neuralgia, indigestion, mental lassitude, and a feeling of general illness.

17. Give symptoms of Ethmoidal and Frontal Sinus Involvements.

(i.) OF THE ETHMOIDAL SINUS—Empyema, which may be closed or open; (a) *Closed Empyema*.—severe aching over the bridge of the nose and nasal obstruction; trigeminal neuralgia; iridocylitis; iritis and nerve involvement; (b) *Open Empyema*—in addition to pain over the bridge of the nose, there is purulent discharge from the nose.

(ii.) OF THE FRONTAL SINUS—may be acute or chronic. (a) *Acute involvement*—supra-orbital pain, which may be intense if the sinus is closed; tenderness on pressure over the lower part of the forehead; œdema and swelling of the upper eyelid and fever; headache; migraine; vertigo; somnolence; vomiting; etc.; (b) *Chronic involvement*—frontal headache, the discharge of pus; the formation of polypi and granulation tissue within the nasal cavity.

18. Give symptoms of Sphenoidal Sinus Disease.

The characteristic symptoms are severe pain in association with ocular symptoms and post-nasal purulent discharge which is usually not great. The ocular symptoms are—retro-bulbar neuritis, ocular pain and tenderness, rapid blurring of vision and slight exophthalmos.

19. Differentiate true and false Hypertrophy of the Turbinated Bodies.

The false hypertrophy is due to vascular turgescence. The application of a 4% *Cocaine solution* readily reduces its size; while in a true hypertrophy, which is due to connective tissue formation, *Cocaine* exerts little or no influence.

20. Name the causes of Perforation of the Septum.

Syphilis. Irritation of a dusty atmosphere. Chemical fumes. Traumatism. Malignant disease and ulcerations attended upon specific infectious fevers.

21. What is Anosmia?

A partial or complete loss of the sense of smell is known by the term *anosmia*.

22. What is Hyperosmia?

An abnormal increase in the sense of smell is termed as *hyperosmia*.

23. What is Parosmia?

Alteration in the sense of smell, usually unpleasant, is known as *parosmia*.

24. Give the relationship of Nasal Disease to the Menstruation.

The NASAL DISORDERS bear important relationship with MENSTRUATION—(i.) Nasal swelling may take the place of the menses; (ii.) the nasal mucous membrane becomes more susceptible to reflex-producing impressions during menstruation; (iii.) in women with healthy nares, congestion of the nasal cavernous tissue may take place during menstruation; (iv.) epistaxis may occur as a vicarious menstruation ; and (v.) nasal discharges may be offensive during the menses.

25. Name the causes of Nasal Obstruction.

(i.) Swelling of the nasal mucous membrane. (ii.) Enlargement of the turbinated bodies. (iii.) Deflection of the septum. (iv.) Synechiæ. (v.) Polypi and other tumors. (vi.) Foreign bodies. (vii.) Parasites. (viii.) Post-nasal Adenoids.

26. Name the causes of Pain in the Nasal Disease.

(i.) Sinus disease. (ii.) Glanders. (iii.) Foreign bodies in the nasal passages. (iv.) Primary Syphilis. (v.) Hypertrophic Rhinitis. (vi.) Malignant disease.

27. What constitutional diseases may have Nasal Symptoms ?

Diphtheria, Measles and Glanders.

28. What is the relationship of certain Neuroses to Disease within the Nose ?

They are the reflex action of the nasal disease.

29. Give symptoms of Abscess of the Septum.

It is associated with pain, extensive swelling of adjacent structures and sometimes suppurative fever. The pus localized at first, tends to spread beneath, between the perichondrium and the septal cartilage, extending even to the tip of the nose, and if not evacuated promptly, destruction of cartilage and deformity of the nose may ensue.

PHYSICAL DIAGNOSIS.

30. Define the meaning of the term Physical Diagnosis.

By the term PHYSICAL DIAGNOSIS is denoted the distinguishing of a disease from the corporal signs obtained by direct examination of the affected part or parts, by the recognised process as recommended by the teachers of the medical principles. In most instances, the examination of the organs having possible relationship with the symptoms, is necessary, to find their connection with the same.

The value of physical diagnosis in distinguishing a disease is not all-sufficient; the history of the case and the subjective symptoms also must be taken into account to come to a correct conclusion.

31. What is the difference between the "Sign" and "Symptom" of Disease?

See Ans. to Q. 6. of Chapter I.

32. What do you understand by "Objective Symptoms"?

The objective symptoms are those symptoms observed by the physician.

33. What do you understand by "Subjective Symptoms"?

Symptoms elicited by enquiry and observed or felt by the patients are known as subjective symptoms.

34. Name the methods in use in Physical Diagnosis.

Inspection. Palpation. Percussion. Auscultation. Mensuration.

What is Inspection and how it is performed?

By INSPECTION is denoted the examination of the body of the patient or a part of it by observation, in strong-light coming from the side. By this method the general condition of the patient and the local abnormalities are detected. The body or the part, should be bare.

36. What is Palpation, and how it is performed?

By PALPATION is denoted the exploration with the hand any part of the body, by depressing the same with fingers, to detect any morbid condition therein, by feeling the same with the examining fingers. The examiner takes the position, opposite to the parts, he is examining. The parts must be bare. To note the degree of resistance is important. Increased resistance is indicative of consolidation or fluid effusion.

37. What is Percussion, and how it is performed?

By PERCUSSION is denoted the method employed with a view to ascertaining the morbid condition of an internal organ (especially the chest or abdomen), by tapping the same to produce sounds by the resonance of the stroke. The character of the sounds elicited are either *dull* or *flat, resonant, tympanitic,* or *amphoric,* which varies according to the situation at which percussion is made, being normal in certain parts assigned for its frequency, abnormal when occurring in different ones —indicating organic changes there. The pitch, intensity and duration of the percussion sounds are indicative of their individual characteristics. The percussion can be performed directly upon the parts to be examined, when it is called *immediate* or over a finger placed for the purpose or upon an instrument, as the pleximeter, placed on the part, when it is called *mediate*. (The fingers are commonly used in preference to the instrument.) The force of the stroke should be moderately light and the uniformity of the same should be strictly observed.

38. What is Auscultation and how it is performed?

By AUSCULATION is denoted the method of discovering about the functions and conditions of the respiratory, circulatory, digestive or the other organs, by the sounds they themselves give out or that are elicited by percussion. It is called *immediate*, when the ear is directly applied to the part, or *mediate*, when a stethescope is used.

39. What is Mensuration, and how it is performed?

The method of ascertaining the quantitative dimension of any organ or part of the body by measuring the same is known as MENSURATION.

40. Tell in a general way what information may be had from Inspection.

See Ans. to Q. 35 above.

41. Tell in a general way what information may be had from Palpation.

See Ans. to Q. 36 above.

42. Tell in a general way what information may be had from Percussion.

See Ans. to Q. 37 above.

43. Tell in a general way what information may be had from Auscultation.

See Ans. to Q. 38 above.

44. Tell in a general way what information may be had from Mensuration.

See Ans. to Q. 39 above.

CHEST.

45. Give the lines forming the Division of the Normal Chest.

The lines forming the division of the normal chest are :—

(i.) IN FRONT.—
    (a) The median.
    (b) Sternal—running down the either border of the sternum.

(c) Mammillary—running through the nipples.
(d) Para-sternal—midway between the median and the mammillary.

(ii.) LATERALLY—
(a) The anterior.
(b) Middle.
(c) Posterior axillary.

(iii.) POSTERIORLY—
(a) The Scapular—in the inner border of the scapula.
(b) Vertebral.

(iv.) HORIZONTAL landmarks are furnished by the ribs.

46. Name the Regions of the Chest giving the Boundaries.

(i.) ANTERIOR—
(a) IN THE MIDDLE—SUPRASTERNAL, STERNAL and XIPHISTERNAL;
(b) ON EITHER SIDE—the SUPRA-CLAVICULAR, CLAVICULAR, and INFRA-CLAVICULAR (the last extending towards the third rib) followed by the MAMMARY REGION and INFRA-MAMMARY below the SIXTH rib.

(ii.) LATERAL—
(a) UPWARD—the AXILLARY region extending downwards to the sixth rib.
(b) DOWNWARD—the INFRA-AXILLARY below the sixth rib.

(iii.) POSTERIOR—the *Supra-scapular, Scapular, Infrascapular* and *Interscapular* regions.

47. Tell what Organs lie in each respective Regions.

(i.) In the ANTERIOR REGION—Heart and the Lungs.

(ii.) In the LATERAL REGION—Lungs, Spleen, Liver, Stomach and Kidneys.

(iii.) In the POSTERIOR REGION—Lungs, Spleen, Liver and Kidneys.

48. Describe the Normal Chest as learned by Inspection.

Normally the chest as viewed in inspection, is eliptical in shape, the transverse diameter being greater than the anterior posterior and its two sides are almost perfectly symmetrieal; in it the sternum is slightly more prominent than the rest of the thoracic walls, projecting forward from above downwards, and there is no depression in the supra or infra-clavicular spaces.

49. What is meant by the term Vocal Fremitus?

The VOCAL FREMITUS is the vibration imparted by the voice uttered in one unvaried tone, to the walls of the chest, through the columns of air in the bronchial tubes.

50. In palpating the Chest describe the changes in the Vocal Fremitus.

The vocal fremitus is changed both in health and as also the result of disease.

IN HEALTH it is more pronounced in the males and in those with thin chest-walls. It is modified, by the pitch of the voice, being more noticeable in a deep-voiced one. It is more marked over the right apex.

IN DISEASE, it may be (i.) INCREASED or (ii.) DECREASED or (iii.) ABSENT.

It is *increased* when the substance of the lungs consolidate as in Pneumonia and Phthisis.

It is *decreased* by air or fluid interposed between the lung and the chest-walls or by partial occlusion of a bronchus, as in Pleurisy (with slight effusion), Pneumothorax, and pulmonary Emphysema.

It is *absent* when a bronchus is entirely obstructed, as in Pleurisy (with marked effusion), Pneumothorax, Pyothorax and Hæmothorax.

51. On which side of the Chest normally is the Vocal Fremitus far intense?

It is more marked over the right apex.

52. What qualities of Sound do we use in Palpation?

Monotonous sound uttered in one unvaried tone.

53. Describe the terms Intensity, Pitch, and Duration of Percussion Sounds.

PITCH.—It is one of the three factors composing the sound which determines its degree of elevation or depression. It depends upon the number of vibrations made by the air inhaled and bears important relationship with *dulless, resonance* and *tympany*, the three varieties of the percussion-sounds. It is *high* when the sound is dull and *low* when tympanitic or resonant.

INTENSITY.—It determines the force of the sound and varies, with the amplitude of vibrations. It is greater when the pitch is low i.e., when the percussion-sounds are tympanitic or resonant.

DURATION.—It determines the range or extent of the sound. It is *long*, when the sounds are tympanitic or resonant, *short* when dull or flat.

54. How is Percussion of the Chest performed? Give Position of the Patient.

The PERCUSSION OF THE CHEST may be performed either by applying the blow directly to the chest, or to a finger or a pleximeter placed over the part to be examined. The last method gives better results than the former and to do the same, the second nger of the left hand is to be placed on the part o be examined, and the blow is to be struck, with a motion strictly from the wrist, by the 2nd or the 1st and the 2nd fingers of the right hand, perpendicularly on the finger placed over the part. The force of the blow as a general rule, should be moderately light, and care should be taken to strike with uniform force.

THE POSITION OF THE PATIENT, may be either sitting or lying on his back, but thoroughly relaxed and at the same time well-supported.

55. Describe the term Whispering Bronchophony.

The resonance of the whispered voice within the bronchi as heard by the stethesope, is termed whispering Bronchophony. The increased resonance of the same is a most delicate sign of consolidation than is breathing.

56. Describe the term Egophony.

EGOPHONY is a modification of Bronchophony (vocal resonance) characterized by sharp and tremulous sounds heard in auscultation, in cases of moderate pleuritic effusion. The best location of these sounds is at or below the angle of scapula. It may also occur in some cases of Pneumonia when the bronchial tubes are obstructed by plugs of fibrin.

57. Describe the term Amphoric Respiration.

The respiratory murmur producing a hollow empty sound like that of blowing into an empty bottle, which is caused by the reverberation of sound in a cavity of the lung is known as amphoric or cavernous breathing. It is always pathological and occurs in cases of Phthisis with formation of cavities and Pneumothorax.

58. Describe the term Pectoriloquy.

The very marked and articulate increase in the vocal resonance, due mainly to excavation of the lung substance, is termed as Pectoriloquy. The sounds, in auscultation, becomes so distinct that it seems as if they were emanated from the portion of the chest, immediately beneath the stethescope.

59. Tell in what cnditions we find Increased Vocal Resonance.

It is found in all conditions in which there is pulmonary consolidation, excepting when there is associated obstruction of the bronchial tube tributary to the affected area. It is also found, when cavities form during the course of Phthisis.

60. Tell in what condition we have Increased Bronchial Whisper.

Pneumonia.

61. What condition is represented by Cavernous Whisper & diminished and suppressed Vocal Resonance ?

The condition represented by CAVERNOUS WHISPER is tubercular in character with formation of cavities in the lungs.

The condition represented by DIMINISHED and SUPPRESSED VOCAL RESONANCE indicates either accumulation of secretion within a bronchial tube or pressure on it by a tumor from without, with consequent obstruction of the passage, either partial or complete. It is also due to thickening of the pleura or to pleuritic effusion and dense pleuritic adhesions.

62. What is the significance of suppressed Vocal Fremitus ?

It is significant of the complete destruction of a bronchus and as such it is indicative of either pleural effusion or Pneumothorax or Pyothorax or Hæmothorax.

63. What is the significance of Bronchial or Rhonchial Fremitus & Friction Fremitus ?

The significance of BRONCHIAL or RHONCHIAL FREMITUS is accumulation of mucus or other fluid in the bronchial tubes, which occurs in Asthma, Bronchitis and in Œdema of the lungs.

The significance of FRICTION FREMITUS is *infflammation of the pleural surfaces*, and is present in dry Pleurisy *i. e.*, in Pleurisy before the stage of effusion, being detected at the base of the axillary region.

64. What conditions of Voice are used in examining the Chest?

When examining the chest the patient should use either his whispered voice or his conversational voice uttered in a monotone, as counting "one" "two," "three" or repeatedly the words "ninety-nine".

65. By what Sound Qualities do you recognize Bronchial or Tubular Breathing?

In bronchial breathing there is always a distinct break between the sounds of inspiration and expiration and the two sounds closely resemble each other.

66. By what Sound Qualities do you recognise Broncho-Vesicular Breathing?

The sound emanated in the broncho-vesicular breathing are characterized by harshness of the inspiring act, which is shorter in duration than the expiration, which is of a blowing type.

67. What is the significance of Absent Vocal Fremitus?

The significance of absent vocal fremitus is entire obstruction of a bronchus which may occur in marked pleural effusion, Pneumothorax, Pyothorax or Hæmothorax.

68. Name the three of the twelve Respiratory Signs.

(i.) Brachypnœa or slow breathing, (ii.) Dyspnœa or the difficult breathing and (iii.) Orthopnœa.

69. Name the Vocal Signs.

Bronchophony, Egophony and Pectoriloquy.

70. Name the most imporatnt Loud Vocal Signs.

Pectoriloquy.

71. Describe the term Bronchophony.

The resonance of the voice, in the normal health, within the bronchi, as heard by the stethescope, is termed Bronchophony. It is buzzing when the voice is conversational, while feeble and blowing in whispered voice. When the vocal resonance is increased pathologically in other portions of the chest it is also called Bronchophony due to its similarity with the voice-sounds of the bronchi and trachea, which is heard in pulmonary consolidations.

72. Describe and tell in what conditions we may have Vesiculo-Cavernous Breathing.

It is best developed in Pneumothorax, but may also be observed In Pulmonary Tuberculosis with large cavities.

73. Describe and tell in what conditions we may have Shortened Inspiration.

We may have shortened inspiration in Emphysema and Asthma, which is due to lack of elasticity in the pulmonary structures in the case of the former and inability to expire in the case of the latter. Expiration in such cases is prolonged. The change is evident throughout the chest.

74. Describe and tell in what conditions we may have Prolonged Expiration.

The prolongation of the expiration may be observed in Emphysema and Asthma, and also in cases of commencing pulmonary consolidation, of which it is an initial sign. The term is usually used to denote, not the prolongation of the act, but the prolongation of the sound only, except in cases of Emphysema and Asthma, in which the act is prolonged, being often much longer than inspiration.

75. Describe and tell in what conditions we may have Interrupted Respiration.

Interrupted respiratory sounds termed as COG-WHEEL RESPIRATION may be detected either all over the chest or locally in the region of the lungs. We may have the former in some general or nervous conditions such as nervousness, fatigue or chill, while the latter in tubercular conditions due to occlusion of the bronchioles by tubercular deposits, which causes the air to reach the pulmonary vesicles at irregular intervals, transforming the inspiratory sound being interrupted by breaks, audible as a series of puffs or jerks and the expiratory murmur a prolonged one. In tubercular cases, it is usually associated with small, moist rales, especially after coughing or taking a full breath.

76. Describe and tell in what condition we may have Metamorphosing Breathing.

Sudden displacement of a plug of mucus in an occluded bronchus by the act of inspiration may transfrom vesicular breathing to bronchial or bronchovesicular breathing.

77. Tell in what conditions you find Bronchophony.

Bronchophony may be found in all conditions in which there is pulmonary consolidation.

78. Tell in what conditions you find Whispering Bronchophony.

See Answer to Q. 55 of this Chapter.

79. Tell in what conditions you find Egophony.

See Ans. to Q. 56 of this Chapter.

80. Tell in what conditions you find Increased Vocal Resonance.

See Ans. to Q. 59 of this Chapter.

CHEST

81. Tell in what conditions you find Cavernous Whisper.

See Ans. to Q. 61 of this Chapter.

82. Tell in what conditions you find Amphoric Vocal Echo.

See Ans. to Q. 57 of this Chapter.

83. Tell in what conditions you find Pectoriloquy.

See Ans. to Q. 58 of this Chapter.

84. Tell in what conditions you find Diminished and Suppressed Vocal Fremitus.

See Ans. to Qs. 50 & 62 of this Chapter.

85. Tell in what conditions you find Metallic Tinkling.

The metallic tinkling is observed in Hydro- and Pyo-Pneumothorax. It may also occur due to formation of large pulmonary cavities. The sounds observed may be compared to a dropping into a liquid confined in a cavity.

86. Give two divisions of Rales.

(i.) Rhonchi or dry rales, and (ii.) Mucous or moist rales.

87. Mention two varities of Dry Rales.

(i.) SONOROUS—occurring in larger tubes; and
(ii.) SIBILANT or WHISTLING or COOING produced in the bronchioles.

88. What physical condition does a Dry Rale represent?

Bronchitis and Asthma.

89. What physical conditions does a Moist Rale represent?

Bronchitis. Pulmonary Œdema. Pulmonary Hæmorrhage. Croupous Pneumonia. Localized Atelectasis. Pulmonary Tuberculosis. Etc.

90. Describe a Sub-crepitant Rale.

It is a fine moist rale which originates in the smaller bronchioles. It is audible during both inspiration and expiration. Its presence suggests Acute Bronchitis in the stage of secretion or Pulmonary Œdema or Pulmonary Hæmorrhage, or Croupous Pneumonia in the early stage or in the stage of resolution or when localized at either apex—Tuberculosis.

When occurring at the base of the lungs, without any other physical signs and when few in number it is suggestive of slight œdema or hypostatic congestion or disuse of the lungs in part.

91. Describe a Crepitant Rale.

It is a fine sound, owing its origin to an exudate in the air-vesicles being caused by the separation of the alveolar walls. It can be compared to the peculiar sound produced by rolling a lock of dry hair between the fingers closed to the ear. It is heard during inspiration and is not influenced by coughing. It may be observed in the first stage of Croupous Pneumonia, in Plumonary Œdema, in Hæmorrhagic Infarction in localized Atelectasis, in hypostatic congestion of the lungs, etc.

92. Describe the mechanism of a Crepitant Rale.

See the Ans. to the previous Question.

93. Describe and tell in what conditions are found Increased Respiratory Sound.

It is a pathological modification of the respiratory murmur, being due to an attempt by a healthy lung to compensate for the loss of function of other portions of the pulmonary structures. It is observed in Pneumonia and Pleurisy with effusion.

94. Describe and tell in what conditions are found Diminished Respiratory Sound.

DIMINISHED RESPIRATORY MURMUR may be found under the following conditions :—

(i) *Defective movements of the thorax* due to general ill-health or bad breathing habits. (ii.) *Obstruction of the air-passages* by a plug of mucus or outside pressure. (iii.) *Pulmonary Emphysema.* (iv.) *Pain in the thoracic walls.*

95. Describe and tell in what conditions are found Suppressed Respiratory Sound.

The presence of fluid or air in the pleural cavities may cause entire disappearance of the respiratory murmur over that portion of the chest invaded by the abnormal accumulation. It may also be due to complete *obstruction of the air-passages* caused by a plug of mucus or outside pressure, as in intrathoracic tumor.

96. Describe and tell in what pathological conditions are found Bronchial Respiratory Sound.

The bronchial respiratory sound is characteristically of tubular quality, and in normal condition it is heard over the lower portion of the neck and the upper portion of the manubrium sterni in the front and over the lower two cervical vertebræ in the back. It is both inspiratory and expiratory and between them there is a distinct interval of silence, and the pitch of the latter is somewhat higher than the former.

Pathologically it may be found over the pulmonary consolidations and as such it occurs in Croupous Pneumonia and Pulmonary Tuberculosis, of which it is a prominent symptom. It may also be observed in Pulmonary Syphilis, Hæmorrahagic Infarcts and Pleuritic Effusions.

97. Describe and tell in what pathological conditions are found Broncho-vesicular Sounds.

The broncho-vesicular respiratory sounds are heard normally over the lower portion of the manubrium sterni and the costal cartilages at their sternal junction at this level in the front and over the upper three or four dorsal vertebræ, and to a short distance to each side of the same in the back.

Pathologically, that is, when they are heard in other portion of the chest, they indicate a moderate degree of pulmonary consolidation and as such they occur in early Tuberculosis and the first and last stages of Croupous Pneumonia.

98. Describe and tell in what conditions are found Cavernous Respiratory Sounds.

The cavernous or amphoric respiratory sounds are observed in cases of Pulmonary Tuberculosis with formation of cavities and in Pneumothorax.

See also Ans. to Qs. 63 & 81 of this Chapter.

99. Describe and tell in what conditions is found Prolonged Respiratory Sounds.

See Ans. to Q. 74 of this Chapter.

100. Describe and tell in what conditions is found Interrupted Respiratory Sounds.

See Ans. to Q.75 of this Chapter.

101. Give the Percussion, Respiratory and Vocal Signs of slight Consolidation.

THE PERCUSSION NOTE : —The relative or marked dullness. It is first discovered in the lower portion of the chest.

THE RESPIRATORY SIGN :— Broncho - vesicular breathing.

VOCAL SIGN:—Bronchophony or the marked increase of vocal resonance.

102. Give signs of Beginning Consolidation.

The signs of beginning consolidation are :—
(i.) Slight or simple impairment of the normal resonance. Slight dullness on percussion. The percussion sound is higher in pitch and shortened in duration and intensity.
(ii.) The change of respiration type to broncho-vesicular breathing. Cog-wheel respiration. Small moist rales, especially after coughing or taking a full breath.
(iii.) Slight increase in the vocal resonance.

103. Give signs of Complete Consolidation.

The signs of complete consolidations are :—
(i.) Absolute dullness on percussion.
(ii.) Bronchial breathing.
(iii.) Marked increase in the vocal resonance.

104. Describe a Pleural Friction Sound.

It is also known as the FRICTION FREMITUS. It is produced by the rubbing of the two opposing pleural surfaces (roughened by firbrinous exudate) one on the other. It is usually best elicited in the lower most portion of the axillary region and is of a grating or cracking nature. Its diagnostic significance is undoubted, as *it indicates Pleurisy, before the stage of effusion.*

105. Give various Shapes of the Chest.

(i) ALAR or PTERYGOID CHEST—flattening of the anterior surface of the chest, depressions in the supra- and infra-clavicular fossæ, stooping shoulders, unusual projection of the scapular angles, and the angle at which the ribs join the sternum is unnaturally acute. It is also called the PARALYTIC THORAX. It is observed in phthisical subjects.

(ii). FLAT CHEST—the sternum is depressed below the level of the costal cartilages and the angle at which the true ribs join the sternum is almost at right angles. It indicates deficient respiration.

(iii). RACHITIC CHEST.-

(iv). BILATERAL DIMINUTION IN THE SIZE OF THE CHEST— the ribs are more obliquely placed, and the diaphragm higher.

(v). BILATERAL ENLARGEMENT— indicates enlargement of the thoracic contents.

CHAPTER X.

RESPIRATORY ORGANS.

(Continued)

LARYNX.

1. Describe the method in use for the Examination of the Larynx.

The apparatus required for examination of the larynx include *a reflecting head mirror*, several *laryngeal mirrors* (small circular mirrors ranging in size from ½ inch to an inch-and-a-quarter in diameter affixed to shank-handle at an angle of 130° to 135°), a *laryngial probe* and some *means for illumination*.

The patient is made to seat opposite the operator with the illumination in one side in level with the ear. The patient is directed to incline somewhat backward in a sitting position and protrude his tongue; then with the head mirror, the fauces are made well-illuminated. Before examining the larynx, the physician takes note of the lesions of mouth, soft palate, tonsils and pharynx, if there are any. Then after holding the tongue firmly with a small napkin, as large a laryngeal mirror as can be skillfully used, is introduced in the larynx, with its reflecting surface downwards, through the mouth. without touching any of the parts until it enters the fauces, when its posterior surface should rest against the soft palate and uvula, pushing the latter backwards and somewhat upwards. Care is taken not to permit its edge to touch the posterior wall of the pharynx. (Before introducing the mirror it is well-warmed over a flame, the face of the mirror being next to the source of the heat.) If the laryngeal image does not come at once into view, over the surface of the mirror, the hand holding the mirror is raised or the handle of the mirror rotated slightly until the proper position is obtained. Accuracy of the result, depends only by attention to minute details as to the position of the patient and examiner, the light and the manipulation of instruments.

2. Describe the Laryngeal Image.

The image of the structures rendered visible by laryngoscopy is known as the LARYNGEAL IMAGE. The structures that may be visible are :—

The EPIGLOTTIS, superior and lateral GLOSSO-EPIGLOTTIC FOLDS, the VALLECULAE, the VOCAL CORDS, the CLINK OF THE GLOTTIS, the ANTERIOR WALL OF THE TRACHEA, the BIFURCATION OF THE TRACHEA, the VENTRICULAR BANDS, the VENTRICLE OF MORGAGNI, the ARYTENOID CARTILAGES, the INTERARYTENOID SPACE, the ARYTENO-EPIGLOTTIDIAN FOLDS, the CARTILAGES OF WRISBERG AND SANTORINI, and the PYRIFORM SINUSES.

3. In examining the Larynx what do you take note ?

(i.) Color of the mucous membrane. (ii.) The *form* and *contour* of the individual structures. (iii.) The *activity of the vocal cords* during speech and breathing.

4. Mention the Affections of the Mucous Membrane of the Larynx.

ANAEMIA—marked by the pallor. HYPERAEMIA— marked by inceased redness. HAEMORRHAGES and HAEMORRHAGIC EXTRAVASATIONS, ŒDEMA. CATARRHAL INFLAMMATIONS—acute cases by a pale, lustureless grayish colour. SYPHILIS—marked by grayish-red or whitish-yellow elevations surrounded by an inflammatory areola.

> Note :— The normal color of the mucous membrane of the larynx is pale pink or red.

5. Mention the Affections of the Cartilages of the Larynx.

(i.) PERICHONDRITIS—inflammations of the membrane investing the cartilages. May be *primary* or *secondary*. *Primary* due to exposure to cold ; *secondary* to Syphilis, Tubercular or malignant ulceration, acute infectious diseases, Gout and Traumatism. (ii.) NECROSIS or ABSCESS.

6. Mention the Affections of the Vocal Cords.

Same as the affections of the mucous membrane. See Ans. to Q. 4 of this Chapter.

7. Mention the Affections of the Nerves of the Larynx.

(i.) PARALYSIS—Total unilateral paralysis, total bilateral paralysis, unilateral abductor paralysis and total or double abductor paralysis. (ii.) SPASM.

8. Mention the Affections of the Muscles of the Larynx.

(i.) Rheumatism. (ii.) Under- or overaction due to affections of the nerves, which influences the movements of the muscles.

9. What does a localized Anæmia of the Larynx indicate ?

Is indicative of the possible advent of Laryngeal Tuberculosis.

10. Describe the causes of Swelling in the Mucous Membrane of the Larynx.

(i.) A simple or acute catarrhal Laryngitis (ii.) Chronic Laryngitis. (iii.) Syphilitic infection—in the initial stage. (iv.) A renal disease. (v.) Venous obstruction arising from pressure of an aneurysm or tumor in the cervical or upper thoracic regions. (vi.) Angioneurotic causes. (vii.) Local tumors. (viii.) Some acute infectious diseases. (ix.) Excessive indulgence in tobacco. (x.) Inhalation of irritating vapors or of a dust-laden atmosphere.

11. Describe the causes of the Structural Alteration of the Larynx.

(i.) Tumefaction of the soft parts, due to general or localized swelling of the mucous membrane, nodules and tumors. (ii.) Abrasions and ulcerations. (iii.) Abscess. (iv.) Œdema. (v.) Malformation. (vi.) Foeign bodies.

12. Mention the Ulcerations of the Larynx. Describe the Syphilitic Ulcerations of the Larynx.

The ULCERATIONS OF THE LARYNX may be classified as :—

(i.) *Syphilitic*, (ii.) *Tubercular*, (iii.) *Lupoid*, and (iv.) *ulceration of the malignant disease*. Though a rarely-observed condition there may be ulceration associated with Laryngeal Leprosy.

The *Syphilitic Ulcerations* of larynx may occur in the *secondary* and *tertiary stages* of Syphilis.

THE ULCERS IN THE SECONDARY STAGE :—The Mucous plaques, usually superficial and very often multiple. Sometimes they extend and coalesce foming a large ulcer with well-defined edges, presenting a grayish base.

THE ULCERS IN THE TERTIARY STAGE :—They appear in the form of Gumma, tending to rapid destruction and the formation of deep ulcerations, with intensive surrounding infiltration and closely adherent exudate. It leads to Necrosis of cartilages and is followed by peculiar cicatrices causing deformity of the larynx.

13. Describe the Tubercular Ulceration of the Larynx.

The TUBERCULAR ULCERATION OF THE LYRINX usually develop on the posterior wall of the larynx and on the false and true cords. The ulcers are very characteristic and are usually preceded by a pale, lustureless, opaque thickening of the mucous membrane. The ulcers, themselves are broad and shallow, with gray bases and ill-defined outlines and worm-eaten appearance and there is a general thickening of the mucosa about them. It spreads slowly and severe pain is present throughout. It is usually associated with well-marked Tubercular disease of the lungs, which makes its diagnosis rarely difficult. In doubtful cases search for tubercle bacilli (*Koch's Bacillus*) in the secretion from the base of an ulcer is conducted.

14. Describe the Lupoid Ulceration of the Larynx.

It resembles the tubercular variety more closely and has its worm-eaten appearance. It is preceded by a nodule which takes on an "apple-jelly" appearance on softening, after which it ulcerates. It progresses slowly and forms cicatrix. Distortion is often a prominent feature and there is also dyspnœa.

15. Differentiate Tubercular and Syphilitic Ulceraitons of the Larynx.

IN TUBERCULAR ULCERATION :	IN SYPHILITIC ULCERATION :
The posterior wall is attacked first.	The epiglottis is attacked first.
The course in slow.	The course is rapid.
The ulcers are broad, shallow and ill-defined with worm-eaten appearance.	The ulcers are deep, clear-out with well defined edges.
Marked thickening and infiltration.	Little thickening.
Secretions are profuse, with peculiar sweetish odor.	Secretion is scant, and closely adherent with fetid odor.
Hæmorrhage in common.	Hæmorrhage rare.
Pain in severe.	Absent or slight pain.
Respiration is embarrased and voice feeble.	Voice not affected unless the vocal cords are affected.

IN TUBERCULAR ULCERATION (*contd.*)	IN SYPHILITIC ULCERATION : (*contd.*)
No tendency to cicatrization.	Cicatrices on pharynx and else-where. There is great and varied deformities.
General condition is impaired.	Less affected.
Peculiar lustureless, opaque thickening of the mucous membrane before the attack.	There is localized unilateral swellings or gummatous growths.

16. Describe the Malignant Ulcerations of the Larynx.

In CARCINOMA, the ulceration is fissured or crater-like, the preceding tumor appears as a badly infiltrating mass, irregular in outline, disturbing the parts.

In EPITHELIOMA, the ulceration is superficial but rapid ; may spread so as to involve the whole larynx.

17. Describe the common forms of the Malignant Growths of the Larynx.

(i.) PAPILLOMATA—may be either single or multiple (in vocal cords) and are usually pedunculated. They never infiltrate.

(ii.) FIBROMATA—usually occurs singly and may be either sessile or pedunculated. They appear as, white, pink, cherry-red or bluish tumors with a smooth surface, and are usually situated on the anterior half or at about the middle of the vocal cords.

(iii.) CYSTOMATA—appears usually on the dorsal surface of the epiglottis, as a smooth, tense, globular, semi-transparent tumor, covered with light-red or grayish-white mucous surface. They are usually small, but may be large.

(iv.) SARCOMATA—appears as a soft, irregularly rounded, pinkish or more often grayish, semi-opaque tumor, distorting the soft parts.

(v.) CARCINOMATA—appears as a broadly infiltrating mass, irregular in outline, distorting the parts and sooner or later accompanied by ulceration above-described, in the previous question.

18. What is the normal Position and Motion of the Vocal Cords?

The normal position of the vocal cords is between adduction and abduction.

The normal motion of the vocal cords, on quiet breathing constitutes on their converging anteriorly and separating posteriorly. On PHONATION, they come into close or exact apposition in the middle line. ON DEEP BREATHING they separate widely at their posterior extremities.

19. What is the normal Location of Foreign Bodies in the Larynx?

The location is suggested by localized tumefactions.

20. Describe some of the Paralyses of the Voacl Cords, giving the characteristic portion of the Cords in each.

(i.) PARALYSIS of the *crico-arytenoidei lateralis, arytenoidei tranversus* and the *thyro-arytenoidei internus and externus,* or *adductor muscles of the cords.*—Under this condition the vocal cords remain in the position of inspiration during phonation. It may be *unilateral* due to local causes, such as cold, Small-Pox or Syphilis or *bilateral* due to Hysteria, Anæmia, Phthisis or catarrhal Laryngitis.

(ii.) PARALYSIS of the *arytenoidei transversi muscles*—during phonation the anterior extremities of the cords come together, but not the posterior, leaving a small triangular opening in that locality.

(iii.) PARALYSIS of the *thyro-arytenoidei interni muscles*—the vocal cords come together at both extremities, but remain separated at the middle, forming an oval-shaped chink. It is due to over-straining or improper use of the voice or to catarrhal Laryngitis in anæmic or neurotic subjects.

(iv.) PARALYSIS of the *arytenoidei transversi* and the *thyro-arytenoidei interni muscles*—a double elliptie glottic chink is formed during phonation.

(v.) PARALYSIS of the *abductor muscles*—one or both vocal cords remain in the median line during quite respiration.

(vi.) PARALYSIS of one or both *recurrent laryngeal nerves*—one or both vocal cords remain fixed in the cadeveric position during quiet respiration, phonation and deep respiration.

21. Pain in the Larynx is symptomatic of what conditions?

The pain in the larynx is symptomatic of :—

(i.) Laryngeal Tuberculosis. (ii.) Perichondritis. (iii.) Malignant diseases (tumors)—the pain freqnently shoots into the ear.

> Note :— Pains in these cases are sharp and severe.

(iv.) Acute Catarrhal Laryngitis (in a patient of rheumatic diathesis). The pain may be severe.

(v.) Laryngeal Syphilis.—The pain is slight, exceptionally it may be severe.

22. Differentiate between Aphonia, Anarthria and Aphasia.

APHONIA—simple loss of voice, the patient can utter words, but with a whispering or choked voice.

ANARTHRIA—phonation is perfect, but the power of articulation is lost owing to the paralysis of the tongue.

APHASIA—complete loss of the power of speech from disease of the speech centres in the brain, the movements of the tongue and larynx are preserved.

23. Name some causes of Aphonia.

APHONIA recurs in—

(i.) Paralysis and Andyloses of laryngeal cartilages. (ii) Acute and chronic catarrhs. (iii.) Œdema of the larynx. (iv.) Tumors. (v.) Perichondritis. (vi.) Ulcerations—tuberculous, syphilitic, etc. (vii.) Emotional disturbances. (viii.) Hysteria.

24. What are the characteristics of the Sputum from Laryngeal Disease?

The sputum is scanty in quantity and clear and starchy in quality.

25. Name the causes of Laryngeal Dyspnœa.

LARYNGEAL DYSPNOEA is always due to *obstruction* which may be caused by—

Spasm. Paralyses of the muscles of the larynx. Œdema. Inflammatory swelling of the mucous membrane. Pseudomembraneous formations. Malignant growths. Foreign bodies. Cicatrical contractions after syphilitic or lupoid ulcerations. Diseases of the surrounding organs which compress the aperture of the larynx by pressure.

> Note :— The characteristic of laryngeal dyspnœa is that a loud, stridulous sound is observed on inspiration; the expiration is silent but prolonged. The larynx falls and rises with the acts of respiration.

26. Give symptoms and clinical course of Acute Catarrhal Laryngitis.

SYMPTOMS :—Swelling of the larynx with the vocal cords with feelings of soreness, dryness and tickling about the larynx ; occasionally there may be severe burning pain. *Coryza with dry cough*, which becomes somewhat moist later with scanty but clear expectoration. *Hoarseness or complete loss of voice*. There may be accompained a slight fever. In severe cases it may come on with much intensity with distressing cough, dysphagia and dyspnœa.

CLINICAL COURSE :—The onset of the symptoms is rapid. The stages follow no regular course.

See also Ans. to Q. 28 of this Chapter.

27. Give the symptoms and clinical course of Chronic Catarrhal Laryngitis.

SYMPTOMS :—Horseness, which in severe cases is marked by aphonia. Constant hawking and desire to swallow. The expectoration is muco-purulent. There is usually very little pain.

CLINICAL COURSE :—It may be the sequel of Acute Catarrhal Laryngitis, but as a rule, is a sequence of the chronic inflmmatory changes of the higher air-passages, viz., nose and pharynx, growing simultaneously with the same. The onset of the symptoms is slow. There is increased secretion. It runs an indefinite course and is very often associated with Bonchitis or Tracheitis. It should be differentiated with Syphilis. Tuberculosis and Carcinoma.

28. Give the symptoms and clinical course of the Laryngitis Sicca.

SYMPTOMS :— There may be severe burning pain with a more or less complete Aphonia. Sub-glottic swelling may cause more or less dyspnœa which is relieved by clearing the throat—greenish-yellow masses or crusts being expelled. The *breath is fœtid during oral respiration* (DIAGNOSTIC.)

CLINICAL COURSE :—When the initial or dry stage of the Acute C. Laryngitis lasts longer for several days, it is known as the LARYNGITIS SICCA. During this stage dry crusts may form on the larynx and there is a violent paroxysm of coughing and following the same greenish-yellow masses or crusts are dislodged with more or less hæmorrhage. There may be intense sub-glottic swelling with abundant crusts (greenish-gray masses) adhering to the sub-glottic mucous membrane. The disease follows a chronic course and is incurable. It is practically always associated with Atrophic Rhinitis or Pharyngitis.

29. Give the symptoms and clinical course of Acute Phlegmonous Laryngitis.

SYMPTOMS :—Chill followed by fever. Dyspnœa. Aphonia. Stridulous breathing. The mucosa is bright red, tense and semi-opaque.

CLINICAL COURSE :—Its symptoms are of rapid onset. The disease reaches its acme in about 3 or 4 days and is apt to terminate fatally. The less severe cases end in resolution or in formation of abscess.

39. Give the symptoms and clinical course of Membranous Laryngitis.

SYMPTOMS :—A slight or moderate fever with *croupy* and *non-productive cough* and hoarseness. *Dyspnœa* at first paroxysmal, later aggravates and becomes continuous : the inspiration being more difficult than respiration. Stridulous respiration. *Expectoration of membranous formations.* False membrane is detected on the laryngeal mucosa which may spread below or above the larynx. Cyanosis, unconsciousness and asphyxia.

CLINICAL COURSE :—The onset is insidious. It may be primary or secondary to Laryngeal Diphtheria. The *primary* variety follows at first a course identical with those of the Catarrhal variety. But symptoms of laryngeal obstruction (dyspnœa) very soon complicates the case. Pronounced constitutional symptoms are absent. The prognosis is highly unfavourable, the child dies of suffocation, unless detected early and steps taken as soon as the breathing becomes labored. The *expectoration as described above settles the diagnosis.*

31. Give the symptoms and clinical course of Tubercular Meningitis.

SYMPTOMS :—Hoarseness. Pain. Dysphagia. Cough. Dyspnœa. Ulcerations. Aphonia. There is frequently pallor and hyperæmia involving one side of the laryngeal mucosa (one-sided redness.)

CLINICAL COURSE :—It is usually secondary to tubercular involvement elsewhere, in most cases, to Pulmonary Tuberculosis. It leads to infiltration and ulceration, first of the posterior part of the cords and the inter-arytenoid fold and spreads to epiglottis and ventricular bands. The relative severity of the symptoms depends upon the situation of the lesions. In the later stages the laryngeal mucosa becomes one mass of ulceration, which may extend in depth destroying the cartilages.

32. Give symptoms of Laryngismus Stridulus.

It may be PRIMARY or SECONDARY.

When PRIMARY it is commonly seen with Rickets and the SYMPTOMS are—

Intense dyspnœa without any cough or hoarseness and the child struggles for breath, the face gets congested or livid and then with a sudden relaxation of the spasm, the air is drawn into the lungs with a high-pitched crowing sound (hence the name *child crowing*); convulsion may occur during the attack. With the Cyanosis, the spasm relaxes and respiration begins.

When SECONDARY it complicates the Acute Catarrhal Laryngitis after a few days and the SYMPTOMS are—Barking, croupy cough, *stridulous respiration* with congestion or lividity of the face— at night. The oppression and distress for the time being are very serious, and there are signs of approaching Cynaosis. The attack passes off suddenly, leaving behind it slight laryngeal symptoms and in some cases a brazen croupy cough. It is prone to recur on several successive nights.

33. What is Chorditis Tuberosa?

It is a variety of Chronic Laryngitis, occurring in singers, characterized by hoarseness and inability to sing the high notes. Laryngoscopically there will be seen a nodule on one or both vocal cords. It is also called the SINGER'S NODE.

34. What is Dysphagia?

Difficulty or inability to swallow.

35. Give the symptoms of the Œdema of the Glottis.

SYMPTOMS of the Œdema of the Glottis or the Œdematous Laryngitis are—

The initial symptom is dyspnœa which usually comes on suddenly and rapidly increases in intensity becoming critical within a few hours, threatening suffocation. The respiration becomes stridulous and the voice becomes husky, which is ultimately lost. There are dysphagia, cough and cyanosis of the face. The paroxysms are separated by intervals of partial relief.

Laryngoscopically, the *epiglottis is enormously swollen* ; the mucosa is much injected.

CHAPTER XI.
RESPIRATORY ORGANS.
(Continued)

GENERAL DISEASES.

1. Give symptoms and physical signs of Croupous (or Lobar) Pneumonia (First Stage).

SYMPTOMS :—Sudden and rapid rise of temperature, *preceded by a short and severe chill*. Pain on the affcted side of the lungs. Fever—*high and continued*; may reach 103° to 106°F. Heavily coated tongue. Dyspnœa—almost constant. Maniacal symptons may occur at the very outset simulating Acute Mania or Mania-o-potu.

> Note :— In the alcoholic and in the aged the onset is insidious.
> In the asthenic or typhoidal cases tonic symptoms are prominent from the very outset.
> In children the disease may set in with convulsions and followed by delirium and retraction of the head and neck, which may be confused with Meningitis.

PHYSICAL SIGNS :—

(i.) By INSPECTION—Diminished movement of the affected side. The respiration increases in frequency.

(ii.) By PERCUSSION—Slight dullness ; a slight hyper-resonance (tympanitic quality) may be present, below vesicular breathing—a faint tubular breathing may be detected.

(iii.) By AUSCULTATION—*Fine pleural crepitations heard towards the end of inspiration*. The breathing is quiet and suppressed in the affected part; the breath-sounds may be feeble.

This stage is called the *stage of congestion* or *engorgement* and lasts usually from 2 to 3 days.

2. Give symptoms and physical signs of Croupous (or Lobar) Pneumonia (Second Stage).

SYMPTOMS :—Fever, subject to very small diurnal variation, remains high and constant, pain in the chest continues, but less marked. *Respiration increases in frequency*. Slight dyspnœa. Pulse though soft is full and bounding. *Leucocytosis*. *Hacking cough* associated with severe pain in the side. *Expectoration* at first mucoid, but it becomes thick, viscid and often blood-tinged or *rusty* and *very tenacious*. *Hydroa* or the *fever blisters*. Constipation more common than diarrhœa. *Dilation of the pupils*. Delirium—often present. *Urine-high coloured*, high specific gravity and increased acidity. Heart, spleen and liver also may be affected.

PHYSICAL SIGNS :—

(i.) By INSPECTION—The characteristic pneumonic countenance i. e., injected face, molar lividity, dilated pupils and fever-blisters in the face. Diminished movement of the affected side. The respiration increases in frequency.

(ii.) By PALPATION—The vocal fremitus increases greatly over the affected lung.

(iii.) By PERCUSSION—Decided dullness.

(iv.) By AUSCULATION——The dullness is well-defined.

(a) IN THE LUNGS——Tubular breathing, the vocal resonance is increased to the pitch of Broncophony or Egophony.

(b) IN THE HEART—The heart-sounds are usually loud and clear and murmurs in the mitral and pulmonary area are common during the intensity of the fever.

The second heart-sound in the pulmonary area is sometimes found to be accentuated indicat.ng the interference of the pulmonary circulation.

The second stage is called the *stage of red hepatization*, which may last from the 2nd to the 5th day. To get the physical signs the entire chest including the axilla and the apices must be examined.

3. Give symptoms and physical signs of Croupous (or Lobar) Pneumonia [(A) Third and (B) Fourth Stages].

THE THIRD STAGE—

SYMPTOMS :—The symptoms of the second stage continue. If they are aggravated, the patient falls into a typhoid state with rises of temperature, more rapid pulse, dry and brown tongue, viscid and prone-colored expectoration and aggravation of the heart symptoms, which may end fatally, frequently from collapse and heart failure. Sometimes prolonged exhaustion or œdema of the sound lung may bring about a fatal issue,

PHYSICAL SIGNS :—This stage is scarcely differentiated from the previous stage by physical exa. mination.

(i.) By PERCUSSION—When the crepitations give place to a coarser or more metalic crepitus an association with breathing of very pronounced amphoric quality, the presence of a cavity is suggested.

The third stage is called *the stage of gray hapatization* which occurs usually after the 5th day (but may recur earlier) and lasts upto the 8th or 9th days.

THE FOURTH STAGE—

The *crists* i. e., an abrupt drop in the temperature with the fall of the pulse rate. Along with the fall of temperature, which may be subnormal, there is often profuse sweating. The respiration falls in frequency and the breathing becomes free.

PHYSICAL SIGNS :—(i.) By INSPECTION—The movement of lhe affected side increases.

(ii.) By PERCUSSION—The dullness is less marked i. e., diminishing.

(iii.) By AUSCULATION—Mucous rales of all the varities may be heard. Bronchial breathing becomes broncho-vesicular. Eventually the normal vesicular murmur returns.

The fourth stage is called *the stage of resolution*, which occurs usually after the 9th to 12th days. It may also occur earlier, even after the 3rd day.

4. Give symptoms and physical signs of the Catarrhal (or Broncho) Pneumonia.

SYMPTOMS :—The symptoms are usually those of Acute Bronchitis with marked constitutional disturbances as *fever and rapid pulse* and the *involvement of the respiratory organs*, as rapid breathing, shortness of breath, *cough* (at first loose, later dry and ineffectual) *with scanty muceus or muco-purulent expectoration. Leucoponia.*

In severe cases it is usually attended with dyspnœa and cyanosis and the heart shows sings of failing.

PHYSICAL SIGNS :—Decidedly irregular,

(i.) By PERCUSSION—is detected patches of localized dullness. In severe cases *absence of marked dullness* is an important feature, when judged in conjunction with the severity of the other associated symptoms.

(ii.) By AUSCULATION—is detected numerous patches of fine rales ; tubular breathing, when the consolidated areas closely grouped.

5. Give symptoms and physical signs of Pleurisy with Effusion.

It is also known as the SEROFIBRINOUS PLEURISY.

SYMPTOMS :—The initial symptom is usually a severe pain in the side which is accompanied by moderate fever ; there may be some cough of a dry and harassing character, due to pain, there may be some embarrassment with respiration.

Effusion takes place with the progress of the disease when the pain diminishes but the dyspnœa increases. The patient is more comfortable when lying on the affected side. Weakness, loss of appetite and emaciation become prominent.

In cases with large or rapidly increasing effusion there may be aphonia, dysphagia and singultus attended with them.

PHYSICAL SIGNS :—In cases with small effusions (4 or 5 oz.) there may be no evidence of fluid in the chest.

In the first stage, the *friction murmur* becomes more marked with the increase of stethoscopic pressure, but when effusion takes place it disappears, but there is dullness on precussion over the fluid accumulation.

The affected side of the chest appears to be unduly rounded or bulging ; the despressions between the ribs are lessened and the displacement of the adjacent organs is very common. The heart in the left-sided and the liver in the right-sided Pleurisy are the organs mainly affected.

With the absorption of the effusion the percusion dullness disappears.

When the effusion is large the patient usually prefers to lie upon the affected side.

6. Give symptoms and physical signs of Acute Dry Pleurisy.

SYMPTOMS :—The symptoms are indentical with Pleurisy with effusion in its first stage.

PHYSICAL SIGNS :—In Acute Dry Pleurisy, the only physical signs detectable are the restriction of the respiratory movements on the side affected and the characteristic *pleural friction rub*. The latter often escapes observation because of its short duration.

7. Give symptoms and physical signs of Pulmonary Congestion.

There are two forms of congestions. A. ACUTE ; B. PASSIVE.

A. Active Congestion of the Lungs :—

SYMPTOMS :—Rapid rise of temperature (usually from 101° F. to 103° F.) followed by an initial chill, stinging pain in the side, dyspnœa, moderate cough with muco-purulent expectoration which may be blood-streaked.

PHYSICAL SIGNS—Seldom marked. Defective resonance with some fine rales. Feeble and hurried breathing which may be sometimes bronchial in character.

B. PASSIVE CONGESTION OF THE LUNGS—

SYMPTOMS :—*Dyspnœa*—growing progressively worse ; lying in bed becomes impossible and the patient is forced to maintain a sitting posture. *Cough*—may be loose or dry and harassing. Small or copious mucoid or bloody expectoration. Hæmoptysis—sometimes sufficiently great quantities of blood come out.

It may excite general veinous stasis, especially of the kidneys and liver when additional phenomena dependent upon the same may be associated.

PHYSICAL SIGNS :—Slight impairment of resonance. Fine moist rales are audible at the bases.

8. Give symptoms and physical signs of Œdema of Lungs.

SYMPTOMS :—Feeling of oppression and pain in the chest. Pulmonary embarrassment—rapid breathing which soon becomes dyspnœic or orthopnœic. Incessant short cough almost ineffectual ; when successful in bringing up expectoration it is copious and frothy and is sometimes blood-tinged. Face pale and covered with cold sweat. Cyanosis. Feeble pulse. Weak heart—Angina Pectoris, not infrequent.

PHYSICAL SIGNS :—Whistling and bubbling rales over the entire chest. The breath sounds are deficient and marked by fine rales. Impaired pulmonary resonance.

9. Give symptoms and physical signs of Abscess of the Lungs.

Though the abscess of the lungs is an actue lesion, it is a secondary process which may be engrafted upon Pneumonia, Broncho-pneumonia, embolic infection, perforating wounds and tuberculous destruction.

SYMPTOMS :—It has no definite symptomatology. The symptoms are those of the primary affection plus the constitutional disturbances attended upon suppuration and expectoration of a large quantity of pus. The constitutional symptoms include fever of septic type, the temperature being usually high with or without chill. The initial expectoration of pus is unexpected and is very free and is not offensive— later the fœtor may be very pronounced.

PHYSICAL SIGNS :—A localized dullness on percussion, with absence of vesicular murmur differentiated from Pleurisy with effusion, by the absence of visceral displacements, and the preservation of vocal fremitus.

10. Give symptoms and physical signs of Pulmonary Gangrene.

SYMPTOMS :—Pulmonary Gangrene is always secondary and its etiology is in many ways intertwined with that of the abscess of the lungs. As such, usually definite symptoms of local pulmonary disease precede the characteristic features of gangrene. The time of onset of the gangrene is frequently marked by a rigor, which may be repeated. The patient shows profound constitutional disturbances. e.g., prostration, remarkable elevation of temperature, rapid weak pulse and progressive emaciation. The *expectoration* is very characteristic—it is profuse, thin, greenish or brownish or black and is *horribly offensive*. Hæmorrhage is frequent.

PHYSICAL SIGNS :—Not distinctive. *Foetid sputum,* plays the most important part in its diagnosis.

11. Give symptoms and physical signs of Acute Catarrhal Bronchitis.

SYMPTOMS :—Slight fever (100° to 102°F.). Cough dry and hawking at first, later with free expectoration. Dyspnœa, usually mild. Slight acceleration of the pulse and weakness. Pain seldom present : at most a distress. The symptoms of an ordinary "cold" accompany the onset.

PHYSICAL SIGNS :—Limited to the presence of rales, which include "squeaking and piping" due to air passing through large tubes whose calibres are narrowed, and in which there are no secretions and "bubbling and crackling" due to column of air disturbing the exudate. Low pitched sounds and large bubbling rales emanate from the larger tubes ; fine crackling, from the smaller.

12. Give symptoms and physical signs of Acute Miliary Tuberculosis.

SYMPTOMS :—The initial symptoms are those of a diffuse bronchitis. *Cough*—may be dry and hacking or moist with expectoration of a muco-purulent character, sometimes attended with hæmoptysis. *Dyspnoea*—a prominent feature. Cyanosis—particularly manifested in the lips and tips of the fingers, Fever—always present, ranging around 103° F. As the case progresses to a fatal termination the typhoid state becomes manifest

PHYSICAL SIGNS :—Similar to those of a severe grade of bronchitis. Auscultation discovers numerous rales—crepitant, fine, sonorous and sibilant. In the later stages the rales become coarser.

13. Give symptoms and physical signs of Acute Pneumonic Phthisis.

SYMPTOMS :—The attack sets in with chill abruptly. The temperature rises rapidly after the chill, with pain in the chest and cough ; the sputum is tenacious and may be either rust-colored or bloody, Respiratory embarrassment is often extreme. The fever attains a high degree of temperature but is noted for its daily remissions. Emaciation and prostration are sometimes pronounced. The pulse is rapid.

After a short period, the fever assumes the well-known hectic type and is associated with rigors, night-sweats and general emaciation. The sputum at first mucoid, soon becomes muco-purulent and in turn purulent or greenish material.

PHYSICAL SIGNS :—Signs of lobar consolidation, dullness, increased fremitus, at first feeble or suppressed vesicular murmur, and subsequently well-marked bronchial breathing.

DIAGNOSIS—These cases cannot be distinguished from the pneumonic fevers in the early stage. The study of the physical signs from day to day and the careful *examination of the sputum for elastic fibres and tubercle bacilli* determine the true nature of the case.

14. Give symptoms and physical signs of Fibro-caseous Tuberculosis.

SYMPTOMS :—Divided into two classes ; (A) LOCAL, and (B.) GENERAL.

A. THE LOCAL SYMPTOMS—

Cough—with at first *mucoid*, subsequently *rust-colored expectoration* which may contain tubercle bacilli.

Pain in the chest, in the side involved.

Dyspnœa—may become extreme and the patient may have suffocative attacks.

Hæmoptysis—usually of bright red color or blood-streaked sputum.

B. GENERAL SYMPTOMS—

Chills—in cases of sudden onset. Usually mild and attended with slight shivering, goose flesh and blueness of the skin. In the third stage chills are quite common.

Fever—the most important constitutional symptom, forming the standpoint of diagnosis. In the initial stage, the temperature in the morning is usually *subnormal* ($97°-97.5°F.$), in the evening *hypernormal* ($99°$ to $100.5°F.$, in severe cases it may reach $103°$ to $104°F.$). As a rule the *maximum* is attained between 4 and 6 P.M. and the *minimum* between 2 and 4 A.M.

Night-sweat—uncommon in the early stages: pronounced in the 2nd stage; profuse and obstinate in the 3rd stage.

Blood Pressure—usually low.

Pulse—rapid.

Emaciation—common; wasting may start in before any other symptom is available,

Languor.

Palpitation of the heart.

Aphonia.

Anorexia.

Tongue—in the early stages usually normal; later, it may present sordes and fissures in the third stage—red shiny appearance.

Gastric disturbances—exceedingly common.

Constipation—in the early stage.

Diarrhœa—a late symptom and is always serious.

Caries of the teeth—more common.

Menstrual disturbances in females.

Œdema of the lower extremities—very common as a terminal symptom.

Nervous disturbances as Meningitis, Neurasthenia, and Psychoses.

PHYSICAL SIGNS :—

In the early stages—the presence of small, moist rales at the pulmonary apices, diminished elasticity of the chest, or localized and persistent cog-wheel respiration.

In the next stage—in addition to the signs noted above, more or less dullness on percussion, increased vocal resonance, broncho-vesicular and tubular breathing.

In the advanced stage—complete flatness; tactile fremitus, as evidence of consolidation and vocal fremitus becomes especially evident. Coarse rales are audible.

When cavities are formed—amphoric breathing, cracked-pot resonance and coarse, gurgling rales.

15. Give symptoms and physical signs of Fibroid Tuberculosis.

SYMPTOMS :—Cough, often paroxysmal in character and most marked in the morning. Expectoration is purulent, in some cases fœtid. Hæmoptysis is not uncommon. Dyspnœa on exertion. There is rarely any fever.

PHYSICAL SIGNS :—The chest is retracted and the shoulder lower on the affected side. Impaired resonance, weakness of the respiratory sounds or broncho-vesicular breathing and fine cracking rales which may be widely distributed. If cavities form, they are usually dry.

16. Give symptoms and physical signs of Empyema.

SYMPTOMS :—are of Pleurisy with effusion as described in Q. 5 of this chapter, all in severe forms. Septic fever, Anæmia and emaciation develop rapidly. The leucocyte count is high.

PHYSICAL SIGNS :—also are identical with "Pleurisy with effusion". Besides, the disproportion between the sides may be extreme; the greater weight of the fluid in Empyema, probably causes a greater bulging of the thoracic walls and greater displacement of the heart and liver with a given accumulation of the fluid. Not infrequently, there is œdema of the chest-walls. The network of the subcutaneous veins may be very distinct.

17. Give symptoms and physical signs of Hydrothorax.

SYMPTOMS :—As it is rarely a primary affection, occurring as a secondary process in course of such disease as general Dropsy, either, renal, cardiac or hæmic, most of its attendant symptoms are those of the primary affection, associated with those of the pulmonary compression. It may however occur alone or with only slight œdema of the feet. Cough and expectoration are often present. At first the respiration is but slightly disturbed; later, there are dyspnœa and cyanosis.

PHYSICAL SIGNS:—are those of pleural effusion.

18. Give symptoms and signs of Pulmonary Fibrosis or Chronic Interstitial Pneumonia.

SYMPTOMS:—Paroxysmal cough, with copious, muco-purulent or sero-purulent expectoration, which is sometimes fœtid. Hæmorrhage or hæmoptysis is not infrequent. Dyspnœa on exertion or when ascending upstairs.

PHYSICAL SIGNS:—The affected side of the chest is retracted and shrunken. The intercostal spaces may be obliterated and the ribs may over-lap. The shoulder lowers down on the affected side and the muscles of the shoulder-girdle wasted. The spine is bowed. The heart is displaced, towards the affected side. If the left lung is affected, a larger portion of the heart comes in contact with the thoracic walls and there may be a large area of visible impulse. Percussion shows dullness over the affected side and hyper-resonance on the opposite side. There are rales of various kinds, the breath-sounds have either a cavernous or amphoric quality at the apex, and at the base, feeble with mucous bubbling rales. Voice-sounds are usually exaggerated. Cardiac murmur is common, particularly late in the disease.

19. Give symptoms and physical signs of Atelectasis (Collapse of the Air-Vesicles).

SYMPTOMS:—The onset is sudden. At first, there is pain beneath the lower end of the sternum, quickly followed by dyspnœa and cyanosis. The temperature rises high, the pulse becomes rapid and respiration quick. The condition of the patient becomes alarming.

In congenital ones, the child presents shallow breathing and a feeble cry.

PHYSICAL SIGNS :—Early inhibition of respiratory movement and displacement of the heart towards the affected side. There is also absence or slight evidence of the respiratory murmur over the collapsed area ; impairment of the percussion-resonance, if the area is comparatively large.

20. Give symptoms and physical signs of Chronic Bronchitis.

SYMPTOMS :—*Cough* and *expectoration*. Dyspnœa if the heart or the lung is involved. Constitutional disturbances, in far advanced cases. Expectoration may be scanty or profuse and in character may be mucoid, muco-purulent or even purulent.

PHYSICAL SIGNS :—They are limited to *bronchial rales*—moist, with feeble respiratory murmur, heard over the posterior aspect of the chest, and are *diffuse*. Percussion-resonance is normal but if associated with Emphysema there is hyper-resonance, and impaired, if not actual dullness in Atelectasis or collapse of air-vesicles.

21. Give symptoms and physical signs of Emphysema.

SYMPTOMS :—The cardinal symptoms are *cough*, *expectoration* and *dyspnœa*. Cyanosis, at a later stage.

PHYSICAL SIGNS :—Rounded shoulders, barrel-shaped chest, the thin mascular form, hyper-resonance to percussion, impaired respiratory excursion, prolonged expiration, feeble inspiratory sound and prolonged respiratory murmur. Vocal fremitus is somewhat enfeebled but not lost. The breath-sounds are usually enfeebled and may be masked by bronchitic rales. The heart-sounds are usually feeble, but clear.

22. Give symptoms and physical signs of Bronchiectasis.

SYMPTOMS :—Characteristic symptom is *cough* with profuse expectoration of sputum, at long intervals. The paroxysms of cough usually occurs in the morning and the character of the expectoration is grayish or grayish-brown in color, fluid, purulent and sometimes very fetid odor. There may be hæmorrhage and Arthritis may occur. Clubbing of the fingers and toes is common. It may be associated with abscess of the brain.

PHYSICAL SIGNS :— Cracked-pot resonance, amphoric breathing, gurgling rales and bronchophony. As it is associated with various conditions, the signs may vary greatly. *Dullness on percussion is either late or absent.*

> Note :—It may be mistaken for Phthisis, but its characteristic lesions are found mostly at the base of lungs, while those of Phthisis are situated in the apex and dullness on percussion is an early phenomena of the latter.

23. Give symptoms and physical signs of Asthma.

SYMPTOMS :—The characteristic symptom is paroxysms of dyspnœa of expiratory type, continuing for a variable length of time, and terminating in the expectoration of thick glairy mucus. When severe, there are signs of defective æreation, cyanosis, with sweating, feeble pulse and cold extremities. Coughing is difficult, very light and dry at first, aud then more violent, with expectoration of the distinctive sputum.

PHYSICAL SIGNS :—Loud wheezing respiration, the inspiration is short and the expiratory movement much prolonged. Percussion may be hyper-resonant. On auscultation, there are sibilant and sonorous rales, which become moister in the end.

CHAPTER XII.

RESPIRATORY ORGANS.
(continued)

LUNGS, TRACHEA & BRONCHI.

1. In what dieseases is the Quantity of the Expectoration likely to be large ?

Empyema and Bronchiectasis.

2. What is suggested by Black Sputum ?

Anthracosis.

3. What is Hæmoptysis ?

Bloody sputum or blood-spitting.

4. In what conditions may Hæmoptysis occur ?

Tubercular lung diseases, Malignant diseases of the lungs. Congestion of the lungs. Gangrene of the lungs. Plastic Bronchitis. Ulcerations of the larynx, tarachea and bronchi. In many affections of the heart, particularly mitral lesions. Aneurysm of the Arota. Gouty Endarteritis. Vicarious menstruation. Blood changes, as in purpura, Pernicious Anæmia, Leucocythæmia and many of the acute infections. High arterial tension. Unknown causes.

5. What lesions of the Tuberculosis may be productive of Hæmoptysis ?

(i.) Collateral congestion around the infiltrated areas. (ii.) Rupture of a small aneurysm. (iii.) Erosion of a vessel.

6. What conditions characterized by Pulmonary Congestion may be productive of Hæmoptysis ?

Croupous Pneumonia. Phthisis. Hæmorrhagic infarcts.

7. What condition is suggested by a suddenly appearing Hæmoptysis, the quantity of blood being large and the patient dying by strangulation?

Aneurysm of the Aorta, rupturing into the respiratory passage.

8. What is suggested by a repeated attack of Hæmoptysis over an extended period of time?

Malignant disease of the lungs.

9. What diseases of the blood may be associated with Hæmoptysis?

Purpura. Pernicious Anæmia. Leucocythæmia.

10. What are the usual symptoms associated with Hæmoptysis?

Anxiety. Nausea, vertigo and syncope, if the quantity of blood expectorated is great. Fever, commonly present; may be high. Dyspnœa and pain in the chest may be present. Cough, induced; sometimes hacking and spasmodic. Excited pulse—sometimes weak and small.

It may be preceded by a sense of tickling in the throat and constriction or discomfort about the chest.

11. Differentiate Hæmoptysis and Hæmatemesis.

IN HÆMOPTYSIS—the blood is coughed up and is nearly always bright in color and *frothy*—usually mixed up with mucus and if clotted, it is small and air-bubbles are present in the clot and muco-pus mixed with it. It is *alkaline* in reaction.

IN HÆMATEMESIS—the blood is vomited; it is usually dark and clotted, *not frothy*, and mixed up with gastric contents. It is *acid* in reaction. It is often followed by Melæna (black vomiting) and subsequent to the attack, the patient may experience a feeling of giddiness or faintness and passes tarry stools.

12. Describe a method for the Collection of Sputum for Microscopic Examination.

The mouth should be cleansed before expectoration and the sputum brought up by coughing should be collected in a scrupulously clean vessel for microscopic examination. Sputum thus obtained, shortly after eating may contain particles of food, which should be avoided.

13. How should you examine for Elastic Fibres in the Sputum?

A small quantity of the sputum, should be pressed out between 2 glass plates, on a black background, the upper being 4" square, the lower 6" square. The elastic fibres appear as grayish-yellow spots on the black back-ground. When viewed with the microscope, they appear as branching fibres having a double outline; WHEN DERIVED FROM THE LUNGS they present an alveolar arrangement, when from the BRONCHIAL TUBES they are branched.

14. What diseases within the Chest are associated with Pain?

PLEURISY. Inter-costal *Neuralgia* and inter-costal *Rheumatism*. Early stages of *Tuberculosis* and *Croupous Pneumonia*.

15. What are the usual subjective symptoms of Bronchitis?

Sensation of burning, rawness, stuffiness, etc.

16. What are the most frequently observed causes of Pain in the Chest?

Inter-costal Neuralgia and Inter-costal Rheumatism.

17. What is Inter-costal Neuralgia?

A painful affection of the inter-costal nerves.

18. Give the diagnostic features of Inter-costal Neuralgia.

It is associated with certain tender points in the course of an inter-costal nerve. The pain is intermittent in character, and *not constant*, with absence of any physical sign pointing to the inflammation of the Pleura or some definite pathological condition.

19. What diseases of the Heart and Blood-vessels are associated with Pain?

Peri-carditis. Pneumo-pericarditis. Acute Aortitis. Sub-acute and chronic Aortitis. Aneurysm of the Aorta. Endo-carditis. Valvular diseases of the heart. Angina Pectoris. Myo-carditis. Rupture of the heart.

20. In what condition does Expectoration have an Offensive Odour?

In Pulmonary Gangrene.

21. What disease is suggested by Rust-Colored Sputum?

Croupous Pneumonia.

22. Under what circumstances may the Expectoration contain bile?

In *Jaundice* the expectoration may contain bile; if otherwise i.e., if there is no symptom of Jaundice, it is suggestive of the rapture of an abscess of the liver into the lungs.

23. Differentiate Hæmoptysis and Hæmorrhage from Mouth and Throat.

In HÆMOPTYSIS, the blood expectorated is forthy and usually mixed up with mucus. IN HÆMORRHAGE FROM THE MOUTH AND THROAT the blood expectorated is watery and bright red in colour.

24. How would you examine Sputum for Tubercle Bacilli?

Small quantity of cheesy-looking particles from the suspected sputum is to be placed between two thin cover-glasses (claned first with water, then with absolute Alcohol) and *compressed between the fingers carefully*. They are then separated, and one of them is selected for examination and the sputum on it, is to be fixed on the same, by drying it over an Alcohol flame, taking sufficient care not to clear the specimen. When dried, *Carbol-Fuchsin Solution* is dropped on the surface of the film, until the latter is covered evenly with the solution. Then holding the glass in forceps, it is to be placed over the Alcohol flame, until it is observed to steam, when it is to be removed ; and as soon as the steaming ceases, it is again replaced over the flame, continuing the procedure for 7 or 8 times. The glass is then to be washed off in a gentle stream of water. It will then be found that the *solution* has stained the specimen *red*. Now the *Acid Methylene-Blue Solution*, is to be applied drop by drop until the cover-glass is covered with the same, and allowed to remain a couple of minutes ; it is then to be washed off under the spigot.

The *Acid* in *Methylene-Blue Solution* decolorizes all the specimen excepting the Tubercle Bacilli ; the Tubercle Bacilli appear in it as *minute red rods* all other objects being stained *blue*.

25. Describe the Mechanism of Cough.

The mechanism of cough, consists in the closure of the glottis, followed by a forcible ejection of air by reason of contraction of the muscles of respiration.

26. What are the factors essential for the Production of Cough ?

Irritation of the respiratory mucous membrane. The presence of mucus or a foreign body in the respiratory passages.

27. What are the Sensations which excite Cough ?

A tickling sensation, located in any portion of the respiratory tract and a peculiar stuffiness or oppression referred to the chest.

28. What is Dry Cough ?

A dry cough is one produced by irritation of the terminal Pneumogastric fibres, without any expectoration.

29. What is Moist Cough ?

Cough with free expectoration of the pathological secretions of the air-passages is known as the moist cough.

30. From irritation of what organs may Cough be Reflex.

The terminal fibres of any of the branches of the pneumogastric nerves.

31. What variety of Cough should be suppressed by Treartment ?

Long-continued cough.

32. Why it is a bad policy to suppress a Cough ?

A moist cough should not be suppressed, as it rids the air-passages of its pathological secretions.

33. In what diseases and conditions may Dry Cough occur ?

A dry cough occurs in the early stages of all bronchial and pulmonary affections. It is also found in Pleurisy, before the stage of exudation, when it is associated with stitching pains in the chest. It also occurs from reflex irritation in vartous portions of the body, and in the course of Hysteria.

34. In what diseases and conditions may Moist Cough occur ?

It occurs in fully-developed Bronchitis, Tuberculosis, Pneumonia, Bronchorrhœa, Bronchiectasis, Emphysema, and the terminal stage of Asthma.

35. What is suggested by a Constant Cough ?

It indicates the constancy of cause. It is of pulmonary origin aud occur in conjuncticn with

Bronchitis, Phthisis, Pleurisy and pulmonary consolidations.

36. What is suggested by a Night or Evening Cough?

It may suggest bronchial catarrh or early stage of Phthisis.

37. What is suggested by a Winter Cough?

It indicates mild cases of Chronic Bronchitis.

38. In what way do Heart Diseases produce Cough?

The cough produced by heart diseases may be due to the pressure of a distended pericardium upon a bronchus or upon the left pneumogastric nerve, or to the congestion of lungs from defective cardiac action.

39. Under what circumstance is Cough absent in Pneumonia?

A cough is absent in Pneumonia, when it occurs in the aged, or in sufferers from Alcoholism and Chronic Bright's Disease.

40. What pernicious effects follow severe coughing for a long period?

Bronchiectasis, Emphysema and Hæmoptysis.

41. What is Serous Expectoration?

Albuminous sputum is known as serous expectoration. It presents a clear or frothy appearance and is of thin consistence.

42. In what conditions does Serous Expectoration occur?

It occurs mainly in Œdema of the Lungs; also observed after paracentesis for pleural effusion.

43. What is Mucous Expectoration?

Clear and glairy or viscid sputum is known as mucous expectoration.

44. In what conditions may Mucous Expectorations be observed?

It is observed in the early stages of Acute Catarrhal Bronchitis, and in Asthma.

45. What is the appearance of Muco-Purulent Expectoration?

It presents a thick consistence and a yellow color

46. In what conditions may Muco-Purulent Expectoration occur?

It occurs in fully developed Acute Bronchitis, Catarrhal Pneumonia, and in Pulmonary Tuberculosis before there is any disintegration of lung-tissues.

47. What is the appearance of Purulent Sputum?

It presents a green or yellowish-green color.

48. In what conditions may Purulent Sputum be observed?

It is indicative of suppurative conditions and is observed in Empyema, Pulmonary Abscess, Bronchiectasis, and cavity formation in the course of Tuberculosis.

49. What disease is suggested by the expectoration of large quantities at long intervals?

Bronchiectasis.

50. Give the method of preparation of Sputum for Examination.

After collection of the sputum as described in Q. 12 of this Chapter, a portion of the same is placed on a cover-glass and carefully spread out in as thin and as even a layer as possible. In many examinations, this may be all that is necessary, while in others, special preparation and staining methods are necessary,

51. Describe the appearance of Elastic Fibres in the Sputum.

See Ans. to Q. 13 of this Chapter.

52. Describe the appearance of Spirals in the Sputum.

The spirals are found in gelatinous sputum, having a central thread known as *the central fibre* with spiral mass about it, known as the MANTEL. In the naked eye they appear as spiral fibres with a wavy shining stripe within; under the microscope, the mantel can be seen to consist of loose, cork-screw like fibres wound about the shining central thread. Some of the spirals are consisted of mantels alone, while others are limited to the nude central fibres, wavy in outline.

53. Describe the appearance of Fibrinous Coagula in the Sputum.

They appear in the sputum as small lumps mixed with mucus. When shaken gently in water, they are found to be grayish-white in color, and hollow. A transverse section usually appears as made up of several layers.

54. Describe the appearance of the Charcot-Leyden Crystals in the Sputum.

They appear as shining blue elongated octahedra of various sizes. The points where these crystals are found appear to the naked eye as dry crumbs. They are intimately associated with the spirals,

55. Describe the appearance of Tubercle Bacilli in the Sputum.

See Ans. to Q. 24 of this Chapter.

56. Describe the appearance of the Pneumococcus in the Sputum.

There are two varieties of Pneumococcus: (i.) Friedlander's Pneumococcus, and (ii.) Frankel's Pneumococcus.

(i.) FRIEDLANDER'S PNEUMOCOCCUS is a oval body 1 μ in length occurring in pairs or in chains, and enclosed in a capsule. In the microscope they appear as capsulated micrococci.

(ii.) FRANKEL'S PNEUMOCOCCUS, also occurs in pairs and had a capsule. It is oval or lancet-shaped.

57. Describe the appearance of Bacillus of Influenza in the Sputum.

The bacillus of Influenza has rounded extremities, staining more deeply at the ends than at the middle. It is also known as Pleffer's Bacillus and found in large numbers in the sputum of Influenza.

58. Outline the cardinal symptoms of Whooping Cough.

The *cardinal symptoms of* WHOOPING COUGH are:—

Cough—in the preliminary stage, becomes more and more annoying and exhibits *remarkable nocturnal exacerbations.*

A long-drawn *crowing inspiration,* succeeding a number of violent expulsive coughing acts.

CHAPTER XIII.

CIRCULATORY SYSTEM.

THE HEART.

1. Mention two lesions affecting the Aortic Valve and tell of the Murmurs associated with each.

(i.) *Aortic Regurgitation*—It is associated with a pre-systolic murmur known as "the *Austin Flint Murmur*" audible in the mitral area and also a diastolic murmur audible in the aortic area, on the left side of the sternum at about the level of the fourth costal cartilage and in the left third interspace, exactly over the pulmonary valves and artery. It is usually soft and aspirating in character and may be short or long

(ii.) *Aortic Stenosis*—It is associated with a *systolic murmur* most pronounced in the second intercostal space, to the right of the sternum. It is a long murmur continuing to the end of the ventricular systole. Its area of transmission is extensive, especially along the line of the great blood-vessels. Hence it is audible in the axillary and carotid arteries. In character, it is harsh and loud, though it may be musical. Its intensity will vary from time to time according to the strength or the ventricular systole. When the latter weakens, tho murmur becomes weaker and may be softer.

2. Name in general some symptoms which would lead you to suspect Heart Disease.

Palpitation, dyspnœa, Dropsy, diminished secretion of urine, albuminuria, indigestion, mental sluggishness, etc.

3. What is Hypertrophy of the Heart?

Enlargement of the heart brought about by extra work, either *general*, as in the strain of athletes or *special* to combat a deficiency of cardiac structure, such as a damaged valve.

4. What are some of its causes?

Obstructive valvular disease of thr heart, high blood pressure, narrowing of the aorta, pericardial adhesions, sclerotic Myocarditis, Arterio-sclerosis, etc.

5. Mention some changes in the Heart-Sounds consequent upon a diseased Muscle.

Diminished intensity of all the cardiac sounds.

6. Describe the physical signs of Pericardial Inflammation.

The friction or rubbing sound synchronous with the cardiac pulsations, audible only in the space over the heart and its points of great distinctness are generally in the third and fourth interspaces on the left side. This disappears with the advent of pericardial effusion and reappears when the effusion has been absorbed. Daily or repeated examinations are necessary for its discovery.

7. Describe the physical signs of Endocardial Inflammation.

The first evidence is a muffling, with prolongation of the first sound, which may gradually increase to a distinct murmur,—in the majority of cases, mitral systolic. In the beginning accentuation of pulmonic sound is not noted, which is of relatively late occurrence. Reduplication and accentuation of the pulmonic second sound are frequently present.

8. What is the cause of the First Heart-Sound?

The first or the long heart-sound, is caused by the *blood forcing onwards* through the aortic and pulmonary orifices, *at the moment* when the ventricles contract and the auriculo-ventricular valves close, in their normal function.

9. What is the cause of the Second Heart-Sound?

The second or short heart-sound, is caused by the closure of the aortic and pulmonary valves.

10. In listening to the normal Heart-Sounds to what point you should pay your attention?

It is important always to have an appreciation of the particular period of the cardiac cycle at which they occur.

11. What is the significance of Accentuation of the Aortic Second Sound?

It is significant of *high arterial tension* and as such it may be noted in Chronic Interstitial Nephritis, Arterio-Sclerosis, Hypertrophy of the Heart, and Aneurysm or Dilatation of the Arch of the Aorta; or of *increase of the intravascular tension* which may be observed in rigors, Epilepsy and other convulsive disorders, sometimes in Hysteria, and in the Toxæmia of certain acute infectious diseases, as Scarlatina.

12. What is the significance of the Accentuation of the Pulmonary Second Sound?

It is significant of the increase in pressure in the pulmonary artery and as such it may be observed frequently in all conditions which induce pulmonary congestion, including acute inflammatory diseases of the lungs, Emphysema, Chronic Bronchitis, and Phthisis; it also occurs in the mitral diseases, whether obstructive or regurgitant.

13. What is the Mitral Area?

The area covered by the Mitral Valve is known as the mitral area. It is over the apex of the heart in the fifth interspace, slightly within the nipple line.

14. What is the Aortic Area?

The area covered by the Aortic Valve is known as the aortic area. It is in the second right intercostal space near the edge of the sternum.

15. What is the Tricuspid Area?

The area covered by the Tricuspid Valve is known as the tricuspid area. It is at the lower end of the sternum, near the ensiform cartilage.

16. What is the Pulmonary Area?

The area covered by the pulmonary valve is known as the pulmonary area. It is at the second intercostal space on the left side, near the sternal edge.

17. What are the reasons for Percussing the Heart?

The reasons for percussing the heart are to interpret the sounds elicited from percussion and to detect their differences with the normal sounds, to enable one to delimit areas of relative dullness.

18. How is the Heart to be Percussed?

The same attention to details as is advised in case of the physical examination of chest, in answering Q. 54 of Chapter IX., should be taken. Instead of unaided fingers, a pleximeter (preferably a Sansom Pleximeter) should be used for detection of the fine differences in percussion sounds. The instrument is to be held by the fore and middle fingers of the left hand applied on each side of the vertical column, the sensitive tips of the fingers resting on the upper surface of the horizontal plate; the lower surface of the latter being applied closely to the wall of the chest. Percussion is to be made by one or two fingers of the right hand, with an even stroke, upon the upper plate. The real nature of the sounds or vibrations, will be obtained through the tips of fingers, resting on the upper surface of the larger horizontal plate.

19. Name the two Cardiac Areas.

(i.) The area of *absolute or superficial dullness*, and (ii.) the area of *relative or deep cardiac dullness*.

20. What do you understand by the Area of Superficial Dullness?

THE AREA OF SUPERFICIAL DULLNESS, is ascribed to that portion of the chest under which a portion of the heart lies in direct contact with its anterior wall constituting a triangular space bounded by lines connecting one point at the mid-sternal line opposite the fourth costal articulation, a second in the mid-sternal line opposite the sixth costal articulation and a third over the apex-beat.

21. What do you understand by the Area of Comparative Dullness?

The area of comparative or the relative dullness is ascribed to that portion of the chest, under which the remainder of the heart lies overlapped by the projecting portion of the lungs. Its upper boundary will be found at about the third cartilage; its left at the middle line; its right projects slightly beyond the line of absolute dullness—to the right margin of the sternum; while its lower boundary cannot be delimited by percussion because it is continuous with the dullness of the liver, with which organ the heart is in close contact. Its limit is greater than those of superficial dullness.

22. Describe the Percussion Note in the Area of Superficial Dullness.

IN THE AREA OF SUPERFICIAL DULLNESS the percussion-note is of high pitch, low intensity and short duration.

23. Give the upper Border of the Heart in the Median Line.

The upper border of the heart in the median line is about two inches below the left nipple and one inch in the sternal side,—between the fifth and sixth ribs.

24. Give the Right Border of the Heart.

The right border of the heart is formed by the right auricle. It is long, thin and sharp.

25. Give the Left Border of the Heart.

The left border of the heart is formed by the left auricle. It is short, but thick and round.

26. What may you learn by Auscultation?

From AUSCULTATION OF THE HEART one is able to determine the condition of the heart-sounds as a whole and also the correct appreciation of their individual elements.

27. Give the causes of Increased Intensity of all the Cardiac Sounds.

They may result from —
(i.) Thinness of the chest-walls. (ii.) Conditions of the lungs favoring the conduction of sound. (iii.) Pericardial adhesions. (iv.) Hypertrophy of the heart. (v.) Over-action of the heart from nervous causes.

28. Give the causes of the increased Intensity of all the Cardiac Sounds.

They may result from—
(i.) General exhaustion. (ii.) Thickness of the chest-walls. (iii.) Emphysema of the lungs. (iv.) Fluid or air in the pericardial sac. (v.) Degenerative changes of the heat-muscles.

29. Describe the Heart-Sounds as heard at the Apex.

The first or systolic sounds of the heart are heard most distinctly at the apex beat in the fifth interspace. They are dull and prolonged and their commencement coincides with the impulse of the heart against the chest-wall, and just precede the pulse at the wrist. Due to pathological conditions, they are altered in quality or force.

30. What do you understand by the term "Murmur" as applied to the Heart-Sounds?

The sounds of vibration produced by blood, when flowing through a vessel, enter a dilated portion of the heart are known as MURMURS.

31. How do you determine the origin of a given Murmur in the Cardiac Region?

By determining (i.) its point of maximum intensity, (ii.) its place in the cardiac cycle, (iii.) whether transmitted or not; and, if transmitted, the direction in which it is heard; and (iv.) the way in which it is influenced by exertion, respiration and position.

32. Name the varities of Murmurs as to Time.

Systolic murmurs and diastolic murmurs.

33. Name the varities of Murmurs as to Quality.

They are—Mitral systolic, Mitral presystolic, Aortic diastolic, Tricuspid systolic, Tricuspid presystolic, Pulmonary systolic, and Pulmonary diastolic murmurs.

34. Name the varities of Murmur as to the Mechanism of the Valves.

They are—Mitral, Aortic, Tricuspid and Pulmonary Murmurs.

35. How will you distinguish the Character of a Murmur?

If the murmur takes place at the same time as the apex-beat, it is a SYSTOLIC MURMUR; if otherwise, it is DIASTOLIC.

36. What do you understand by the term "Stenosis"?

The narrowing or stricture of a valve, whereby the normal outflow is retarded and there is difficulty in the expulsion of the contents of the chamber through the narrowed orifice, is known as "STENOSIS."

37. What do you understand by the term "Insufficiency"?

It indicates the incompetency of a normal valve to effect a *complete* closure, either from changes in its segments or muscular walls.

38. Describe the Murmurs of Mitral Regurgitation.

The murmurs of mitral regurgitation, are systolic in time, and heard with maximum intensity over the mitral area, i. e., *at the apex*. They are transmitted from the apex to the left into the axilla, and may be heard even at the angle of the scapula.

39. Describe the Murmurs of Mitral Stenosis.

The murmurs of mitral stenosis is diastolic in time. Their area of maximum intensity is limited—almost always to the apex or a little to the inside of the apex. They are transmitted not usually but exceptionally to the axilla and angle of the left scapula.

40. Differentiate a Peri-cardial Murmur from an Endo-cardial One.

A peri-cardial murmur is differentiated from an endo-cardial one, by the nature of the sound produced in the former, which has aptly been compared with the sound produced by the creaking of new leather—when softer, it resembles the sound produced by gently rubbing together the palms of the hands and audible only in the space over the heart.

41. Differentiate Regurgitant and Stenotic Murmurs.

REGURGITANT MURMURS are produced by the inability of the valves to close at the proper time.

STENOTIC MURMURS are due to orificial obstruction.

42. What changes do the Heart-Sounds undergo during Dilatation?

The cardiac impulse is feeble or flapping and and diffused over a wide area of the chest-wall. The first sound is short and sharp. If the left auriculo-ventricular orifice is dilated a mitral systolic murmur will be audible. If the right ventricle is involved, the second pulmonic sound will be feeble. Apex-beat may be heard over an increased area.

43. Describe the phenomenon of the Revolution of the Circulation.

The blood is conveyed away from the *left ventricle* of the heart by the aorta, through the *semilunar valves* (guarding the orifice of the aorta) to the arteries and returned to the *right auricle* by the veins. From the *right auricle* the blood passes to the *right ventricle* through the *tricuspid valve* and then to the *pulmonary arteries*, through the *semilunar valves* guarding the orifice of the pulmonary arteries (which divides into two, one for each lung), then through the *pulmonary veins* (two from each lung) to the heart into the *left auricle*, and enters into the *left ventricle* through the *mitral valve* and completes a revolution.

44. Give in general some of the Displacements of the Apex-beat.

(i.) DISPLACEMENT OF THE APEX-BEAT TO THE RIGHT SIDE OF THE CHEST—may result from accumulation of the air in the left pleural sac, tumors, enlargement of the left lung and retraction of the lung.

(ii.) DISPLACEMENT OF THE APEX-BEAT TO THE LEFT—may result from pleural effusion, right pneumothorax, right pleural tumors, tumors of the right lung and retraction of the left lung.

(iii.) UPWARD DISPLACEMENT—may result from abdominal tympanites, ascites, enlargements of the liver (upwards to the left) for spleen (upwards to the right), and abdominal tumors generally.

(iv.) DOWNWARD DISPLACEMENT—may result from hypertrophy or dilatation of the heart.

45. Describe Tracheal Tugging and tell of what it is suggestive.

Tracheal tugging is a tugging by the trachea in response to the pulsatile retractions of aneurysmal walls, detected at the trachea, by grasping the cricoid cartilage between the finger and thumb and exerting gentle upward pressure. The pulsations it presents, are distinctly transmitted through the trachea to the fingers. It is suggestive of *Aneurysm of the Aorta*.

46. Describe the term "Thrill."

THRILL is a sort of quiver or shiver of the cervical arteries, in certain cases of cardiac diseases.

They are felt best with the patient sitting upright or bent slightly forward.

47. Mention some of the varieties of the Cardiac Thrills and tell their significance.

FRICTION FREMITUS—peri-cardial thrills are so called. They are suggestives of Peritonitis.

ENDOCARDIAL THRILLS—

(i.) SYSTOLIC THRILLS—when felt in the *second right intercostal interspace* near the border of the sternum, suggest Aortic Aneurysm or Stenosis of the aortic orifice; over the *pulmonary area*—obstruction at the pulmonary orifice; *at the apex*—Mitral Regurgitation; and *at the lower end of the sternum*—Tricuspid Regurgitation.

(ii) DIASTOLIC THRILLS—felt over *the pulmonary area*, nearly always indicate Aortic Regurgitation.

(iii) PRESYSTOLIC THRILLS felt *at the apex* suggest Mitral Stenosis.

48. What may increase the Area of Cardiac Dulness?

THE AREA OF CARDIAC DULLNESS may be increased by the increase in the size of the heart, i. e., in hypertrophy and dilatation, pericardial effusion, by fibroid (pulmonary) changes, by pleuritic adhesions and in Pneumonia, Aneurysm, Pleural Effusions, Mediastinal Tumors and local enlargement of the liver.

49. What essential details are necessary to learn in connection with any Adventitious Sound of the Heart?

(i.) Its point of maximum intensity; (ii.) its place in the cardiac cycle; (iii.) whether transmitted or not, and if transmitted, the direction of its transmission; and (iv.) the way in which it is influenced by exertion, respiration and position.

50. Name the Endocardial Causes of a Mitral Systolic Murmur.

(i.) Damage of the mitral valves by acute, simple, ulcerative or malignant Endocarditis; and (ii.) stretching of the left auriculo-ventricular orifice from dilatation of the left ventricle.

51. Give the causes of an Aortic Systolic Murmur.

(i.) Roughening, stiffening or malformation of the aortic orifice; (ii.) Stenosis of the aortic orifice; (iii.) roughening or dilatation of the arch of aorta; (iv.) pulmonary stenosis; (v.) open ductus arteriosus; (vi.) Mitral Regurgitation; and (vii.) blood-conditions (anæmias).

52. Describe one of the so-called Functional Murmurs of the Heart.

Murmurs originating in anæmia are heard less frequently over the aortic, than any other valvular area. They are soft in character and systolic in time. They are not transmitted in any definite direction and are liable to be confounded with the soft murmur produced by slight rheumatic changes of aortic valves or to papillomata.

53. Describe the Pain in Pericarditis.

Though the pain may be of agonizing severity and radiate all over the chest, even extending down the arms, especially the left, in the majority of cases it is dull or very slight, scarcely more than annoying. It is aggravated by pressure or movements. It is *a most prominent symptom* of Pericarditis.

54. Describe the Pain in Aortitis.

The pain is most agonizing, sometimes radiating all over the chest and down one or both arms. It originates in the aorta and is referred to beneath the sternum and along the vertebral column posteriorly. It is associated with great anxiety and distress.

55. Describe the Pain in Aneurysm of the Aorta.

Pain due *strictly to the aneurysm* is of a dull, aching character, and is aggravated by any movement.

Pressure of the tumor upon bony streutures, exerts a constant boring or gnawing pain, more or less sharply localized.

Pressure of the tumor upon the sensory nerves, exerts most severe pains. They are acute, come in paroxysms and extend over an wide area and may be manifest in the neck, shoulders, both arms and even in the face. They closely simulate the pains of Angina Pectoris.

56. Describe the Pain in Endo-carditis.

Pain about the heart in the initial attacks is rarely experienced beyond some præcordial discomfort. With repeated attacks and in the ulcerative varieties, it is sometimes experienced and may even be anginal in severity and character.

57. Describe the Pain in Anginá Pectoris.

The pains in the Angina Pectoris are usually pectoral and paroxysmal in character, lasting from several seconds to a minute or two. They are always associated with well-marked clinical phenomena of cardiac origin.

IN THE MILDEST FORM of the disease—they appear as substernal oppression, tension, uneasiness or discomfort, rising at times to positive pain of short duration.

IN THE MILD FORM, the pain is of moderate severity and may be sharp and shooting.

IN THE SEVERE FORM the pain is atrocious, radiating over the ehest to the neck, down the arm.

58. Describe the Pain in the Rupture of the Heart.

Sudden sharp pain about the heart, with præcordial anguish, in association with pallor, prostration and collapse.

59. What do you understand by the term Palpitation?

Irregular or forcible action of the heart producing cardiac pulsations, perceptible to the individual is known as PALPITATION. It is associated with distress and suffering.

60. Give some of its Causes.

Increased excitability of the nervons system.

Emotions, especially those of a depressing character, such as fright, are common causes of palpitation.

It may occur as a sequence of some acute fevers or as a reflex disturbance by reason of diseases in some other organs.

It is common in Hysteria and Neurasthenia.

It may result from the action upon the heart of certain substances, such as tobacco, coffee, tea and Alcohol.

61. What diseases, particularly of the Heart are accompanied by Sudden Death?

Diseases of the aortic orifice; Angina Pectoris; fatty degeneration of the heart-muscle; chronic and myocardial degenerations and the acute nervous and myocardial lesions complicating the infections diseases e.g., Diphtheria and Typhoid Fever and obstruction of the coronary arteries.

62. Give some of the symptoms and diagnosis of Aneurysm of the Aorta.

SYMPTOMS:—The clinical picture of Aneurysm of the Aorta is extremely varied. Aneurysms of the last portion of the arch and descending aorta present characteristic symptoms but no physical signs, while Aneurysms of the ascending aorta have well-marked physical signs and few or no symptoms. The symptoms of the first are—

Pain—an early feature. *Dyspnœa*—stridulous breathing. *Dysphagia. Tracheal tugging.* Cough. Laryngeal symptoms—loss of voice, hoarseness.

DIAGNOSIS—depends upon the recognition of a *pulsating tumor* in the area of the chest occupied by the aorta. Dullness on percussion, with pulsation within that area of dullness, is evident when the Aneurysm is not deep-seated. A thrill, systolic in time and vibratile in character, is detected, in probably less than 50% cases. Tracheal tugging. In addition to the above there may appear any of the following, viz., inequality of the pupils, inequality in the radial pulses, severe pain in the pericardium, radiating into the left arm or neck, and œdema of one arm. X'ray examination should be made in doubtful cases. The diagnosis may rest on it alone in cases in which a physical sign is scarcely present.

63. Give some of the symptoms and diagnosis of Angina Pectoris.

SYMPTOMS :—*Præcordial pain* (as described in Ans. to Q. 57 of this Chapter) is the most prominent symptom and is associated with coldness and numbness of the extremities, feeling of faintness and palpitation. The next prominent feature is the sense of great anxiety depicted on the patient's countenance with restlessness. The face becomes pallid, often a grayish hue.

> Notes :—Males are especially liable in the degenerative period of life or early middle age.

DIAGNOSIS :—The *paroxysmal nature* of Angina Pectoris, the *situation of the pains* and *severity* and *short duration*, and the *age* and *sex* of the patients are determining factors.

> Note :—It must not be confused with pesudo-angina, which is neurotic or hysterical and must not be mistaken for acute indigestion.

64. Give some of the symptoms and diagnosis of Myocarditis.

SYMPTOMS :—*Cardiac weakness* is the characteristic feature. *Restlessness* and *apathy* are important. There may be dyspnœa on slight exertion, præcordial distress of any kind, anginoid pains, vomiting, venous distensions and cyanosis.

Diagnosis :—Uncertain.

65. Give some of the symptoms and diagnosis of Fatty-Degeneration of the Heart-Muscle.

SYMPTOMS :—*Caridac weakness* is the characteristic feature. The patients may for many years present a feeble but regular pulse ; the heart-sounds are weak and muffled and a murmur may be heard at the apex. Attacks of dyspnœa are common and the patient may suffer from Bronchitis.

DIAGNOSIS—Uncertain.

66. Give some of the symptoms and diagnosis of Pericarditis.

SYMPTOMS :—Pain is a decidedly variable factor ; (See Ans. to Q. 53 of this Chapter) ; fever—moderate ; pulse—rapid ; dyspnœa ; palpitation.

DIAGNOSIS—Depends exclusively upon the presence of its characteristic *friction-murmur* (See Ans. to Q. 40 of this Chapter.)

67. Give some of the symptoms and diagnosis of Acute Endo-carditis.

SYMPTOMS :—As a rule, the subjective phenomenon is of a mild grade consisting of some præcordial discomfort or actual pain about the heart, palpitation and slightly distressed respiration. Many cases are latent. There may be fever and the pulse-rate is always increased.

DIAGNOSIS :—*Rests upon physical signs.* The first evidence is usually found in a muffling, with prolongation of the first sound of the heart. A mitral systolic murmur indicates the damage has been done.

68. Give some of the symptoms and diagnosis of Malignant Endocarditis.

SYMPTOMS :—Constitutional symptoms are pronounced almost from the beginning. *Anæmia* is a prominent feature. Temperature is irregular and is usually high. The pulse is rapid.

DIAGNOSIS—is based upon the general constitutional state, together with the condition of the heart, early leucocytosis, septic temperature-curve, embolic phenomena, purpura and hæmorrhages and cardiac disturbances. Murmurs usually appear early and they are pronounced from day to day.

CHAPTER XIV.

THE URINE.

1. What is the true criterion of Kidney Action?

The true criterion of the kidney action is to excrete the urine from the blood and eliminate the same from the body.

2. What is the Normal Daily Quantity?

The normal daily quantity of urine is fifty fluid ounces or 1500 cubic centimeters.

3. What is the Normal Daily Quantity in Infants?

From 8 to 12 ounces.

4. What are the Physiological Variations in the Quantity?

The urine may be *increased* or *decreased* due to diet, drink, temperature, exercise, mental emotions and age.

5. What is Polyuria?

When the quantity of urine passed is greater than the normal, it is known as POLYURIA.

6. What is Oliguria?

When the quantity of urine passed is decreased or suppressed, the condition is known as Oliguria.

7. What are the pathological causes of Increased Urination?

(i.) Diabetes insipidus or mellitus. (ii.) Phosphatic Diabetes. (iii.) Increased arterial tension. (iv.) In the early stage of waxy kidney.

(v.) During the stage of convalescence from many acute diseases. (vi.) In dropsy. (vii.) In Hysterical seizures. (viii.) After anger or emotional disturbances. (ix.) After Epileptic seizures. (x.) After taking food containing large quantities of sugar.

8. What are the Pathological Causes of Deficient Urination ?

(i.) Various acute diseases of the kidneys. (ii.) Chronic Bright's Disease. (iii.) Diseases attended by marked dehydration of the tissues. (v.) Mechanical mpediments to the escape of urine from one or both kidneys. (vi.) Cirrhosis of the Liver. (vii.) Diminished arterial pressure. (viii.) Febrile affections.

9. What is the Normal Color of the Urine ?

A pale-yellow or amber.

10. Give the Causes of Pale Urine.

(i.) Diabetes Mellitus or Insipidus. (ii.) Chronic Bright's Disease. (iii.) Hysteria. (iv.) Anæmia. (v.) In the convalescent stage of the acute diseases. (vi.) After taking diuretic medicines.

11. Give the causes of a Pale Yellowish-Green Urine.

(i.) In some cases of Diabetes with a great quantity of sugar. (ii.) Jaundice. (iii.) Poisoning by Carbolic Acid, Hydrochinon, Resorcin and Pyrocatechin. (iv.) Salol and Salicylic Acid derivatives. (v.) Hæmoglobinuria.

12. Give the causes of Blue Urine.

(i.) The ingestion of Methylene Blue (medicinal). (ii.) Taking of Indigo.

13. Name some of the causes of Cloudy Urine.

(i.) Cholera Asiatica. (ii.) Typhus. (iii.) The presence of *Urates* or *Phosphates* in the urine.

14. What constitutes a complete Urinary Analysis?

A complete urinary analysis constitutes: the finding out of the component parts of the urine both *chemically* and *microscopically*.

15. To what points you should pay your attention in an Analysis of the Urine?

(i.) To determine the presence of abnormal constituents, and (ii.) to determine the proportion in which the normal constituents may be found.

16. What disease is suggested by a Pale Urine of High Specific Gravity?

Diabetes Mellitus.

17. What is suggested by Whitish Urine?

Phosphates or Urates in the urine.

18. What is suggested by Cloudy Urine, clearing on the application of Heat?

Excessive quantity of *urates* in the urine.

19. What is suggested by Cloudy Urine, clearing on the addition of an Acid?

The presence of *phosphates* in the urine.

20. What is the clinical significance of Yellowish and Milky Color of the Urine?

Pyuria.

21. What conditions may produce Greenish-Yellow or Black Urine?

For production of greenish-yellow urine, see Ans. to Q. 11 of this Chapter. BLACK URINE is produced in Multiple Melanotic Sarcoma or after poisoning by Arseniuretted Hydrogen inhalations.

22. What conditions may produce Concentrated Urine?

(l.) Violent exercise. (ii.) Profuse sweating. (iii.) Fevers. (iv.) Renal congestion. (v.) Hepatic disorders. (vi.) Intestinal obstruction. (vii.) Dehydration of the body. (viii.) The ingestion of a full meal.

23. What produces Milky Urine?

Chyluria, Pyuria or bacterial changes.

24. What is the significance of Smoky Urine in Scarlatina?

Scarlatinal Nephritis.

25. What is the clinical significance of Ammoniacal Urine?

Cystitis.

26. What is the clinical significance of Sugary or Sweet Odor in the Urine?

Diabetes Mellitus.

27. What is the clinical significance of Urine having a Fæcal Odor?

Fistulous communication between the urinary and the intestinal tracts.

28. When is the urinary cloudness appearing in clear urines after standing sometimes, not changed by the addition of Alkalis or Mineral Acids?

When due to mucus.

29. What is suggested by a urinary cloudiness disappearing on the addition of an Acid?

Indicates *earthy phosphates* in the urine.

30. What is the indication of cloudiness of the urine appearing on cooling?

Indicates *urates* in the urine.

31. Describe a Waxy Cast.

Waxy casts are transparent cylindrical bodies, found in the urinary sediment, being marked by numerous indentations, suggesting segmentation. They are tinted somewhat yellow and are highly refractive. They are not dissolved by *Acetic Acid*. Sometimes they present a cloudy appearance, due to bacterial contamination. They may be found in acute and chronic Nephritis, and in contracted and amyloid kidneys. Their presence always means chronicity; hence they are indicative of serious lesions.

32. Describe the microscopic appearance of Tripple Phosphates.

Through the microscope they appear as white deposits in abundance.

33. Describe the microscopic appearance of Oxalate of Lime Crystals.

They appear in octehedra shapes of various sizes, with highly refracting edges. Rarely they are of dumb-bell, hour-glass, hatchet and biscuit shapes. Modifications of octehedral forms also may occur, appearing as quadratic prisms surmounted at each end by a pyramid. May also appear as numbers needles.

34. What is Pyuria ?

Pus in the urine.

35. Describe the Chemical Test for Pus in the Urine.

By adding a small piece of *Caustic Soda* to the suspected urine, there will appear *a thick gelatinous deposit*; adhering to the bottom of the tube, if there is pus in the urine.

36. Under what circumstances is the discovery of Pus impossible by the Microoscope ?

Pus-cells cannot be discovered microscopically, when the urine is strongly *alkaline*, in consequence of which there is a thick glairy mass in the urine.

37. Name the diseases of Kidneys which may produce Pyuria.

(i.) Acute and Chronic Pyelitis. (ii.) Primary and secondary Pyelitis. (iii.) Pyelo-nephritis.

38. Describe the characteristics of Vesical Pyuria.

The characteristics of vesical pyuria are that, it is attended with an alkaline reaction of the urine, which is usually found to have undergone ammoniacal decomposition and that microscopical examination discovers tripple phosphate in the urinary sediment in abundance.

39. What is the clinical significance of an Intermittent Pyuria ?

It suggests an intermittent cause, which is usually found in renal suppuration with urethral obstruction, which is relieved from time to time. It also suggests an extra-urinary suppuration, the fistulous communication with which becomes closed from time to time.

40. What is the clinical significance of appearance of Flakes of Pus in the Urine ?

They indicate an urethral source.

41. From what portions of the Urinary Tract may Pyuria proceed ?

Pyuria may originate in (i.) Urethera, (ii.) Bladder, (iii.) Ureters or (iv.) the kidneys.

42. Of what value is the Chemical Reaction of Urine in determining whether a given case of Pyuria has a Renal or Vesical Origin ?

It offers a rough guide.

43. Describe the 3 or 4 Glass Tests for determining the Origin of Pyuria.

FIRST the urethra is washed out with a weak solution of *Boric Acid* and a portion of the washing is collected in a glass. If it contains pus-cells, it is evident that some of the pus comes from the urethra. A portion of the urine is then passed into a SECOND GLASS and if this is free of pus-cells, it proves that the pyuria is urethral. If it contains pus then the pyuria must be either vesical or renal.

Insert the finger into the rectum and massage the prostate forwards; the contents of the ducts of this gland and seminal vesicles will be forced out, in the urethra, whence they may be collected into a THIRD GLASS by urination. If pus is found in the urine, it originates in the accessory glands of the deep urethra.

44. Name the Diseases of the Bladder which may produce Pyuria.

Cystitis. Secondary Pyelitis.

45. What is Hæmaturia?

BY HAEMATURIA is meant *blood in the urine*.

46. Give a Chemical Test for the presence of Blood in the Urine.

To 10 c.c. of the suspected urine add a mixture of *Tinct. of Guaiacum* and old *Oil of Turpentine*. At the point of junction of the two there will appear a white line, changing to blue, if blood-coloring matters are present in the urine.

47. What is the best Test ordinarily for the Discovery of Blood in the Urine?

Add with a mixture of *Tinct. of Guaiacum* and old *Oil of Turpentine*, 10 c.c, of the suspected urine. If blood-coloring matters are present there will appear a white line, changing to *blue*, at the point of junction of the two liquids.

48. How is the color of the Urine affected by reason of the Source of the Hæmorrhage in Hæmaturia?

The brighter and the more arterial the color of the bloody urine, the nearer is the source of the hæmorrhage to the meatus-urinarius.

49. What conditions of the Bladder may produce Hæmaturia?

(i.) Stone in the bladder. (ii.) Malignant ulceration. (iii.) Traumatism. (iv.) Parasites. (v.) Varicose veins. (vi.) Diphtheritic Cystitis. (vii.) Villous Tumors. (viii.) Tuberculosis.

50. What is suggested by a Hæmaturia excited by slight Injury?

Strongly suggestive of calculus or malignant disease.

51. What is suggested by the appearance in the Urine of long Earthworm-like Clots?

Suggestive of blood passing through the ureters and that the hæmorrhage must be either renal or ureteral,—usually the former.

52. What is the significance of Cloudiness in the freshly-passed Urine?

Indicates *phosphates* or *pus* in the urine.

53. What is the Normal Specific Gravity of the Urine?

Normal specific gravity of urine ranges from 1016 to 1020.

54. What precautions should be adopted to avoid inaccuracies when determining the Specific Gravity of Urine?

IN THE FIRST PLACE, any froth or bubbles on the surface of the urine should be removed by blotting-paper or a pipette, as they act as floats, preventing the instrument from sinking to the proper point. Care must be taken that the urinometer does not adhere to the side of the vessel in which It is floated and also there is sufficient urine in the jar to float the instrument. When taking the reading, the eye should be on a level with the apparatus, and the figure opposite the lowest portion of the surface of the urine taken as the correct one. Attention should also be paid to the temperature of the urine under examination (See also Ans. to the next Q.)

55. What allowances should be made for the Temperature of the Urine when taking its Specific Gravity when freshly passed ?

Add one degree of specific gravity, for every seven degrees of temperature of the urine, above that for which the urimometer is standardized.

56. Describe the method for determining the Chemical Reaction of the Urine.

It should be determined by means of *litmus paper*. Blue litmus paper is changed red by acid urine, and red paper blue by alkaline urine. In some cases, the blue litmus is changed into red and red litmus blue by the same urine, due to the presence of acid and neutral *Sodium Phosphate* in the urine.

57. Describe the method for the approximate estimation of the total Urinary Solids.

Multiply the last two figures of the specific gravity by 2·33, which gives the solids in 1000 c.c. of urine. By simple rule of three, the daily excretion of solids in the total quantity of urine passed may be calculated.

58. What proportion of the Urinary Solids consists of Urea ?

In health, 50 per cent of the solids consist of *urea*. It is different in pathological conditions.

59. What is the Normal Chemical Reaction of Urine?

Acid.

60. To what causes may increased Urinary Acidity be due?

Normally the increased acidity is due to diet consisting very largely or entirely of animal food, muscular exercise, taking of acids and saccharine. It is also observed in Diabetes, Leucocythæmia, Scurvy and Gout.

61. To what may Alkalinity of the Urine be due?

Alkalinity of the urine may be due to diet consisting almost entirely of vegetable food, loss of gastric juice and by the administration of alkalies. It may also occur in debility and Anæmia.

62. What is suggested by an Abundant white Deposits in the Urine?

It suggests *pus* or *phosphates* in the urine, when the former, the sediment is creamy.

63. Describe Two Tests for the detection of Albumin in the Urine.

(i.) HEAT AND ACID TEST—A small quantity of the suspected urine (filtered) is boiled in a test tube. Then a drop of *Nitric Acid* is added to the same. If albumin is present, a cloudiness will appear.

(ii.) PICRIC ACID TEST—First, a solution of cane sugar of sp. gr. 1060 is prepared and with this a saturated solution of *Picric Acid* is made. Pour some quantity of the suspected urine in the same; if albumin is present, *a white ring* will appear at the line of contact of the two fluids.

64. What is Albuminuria?

Albumin in the urine.

65. Name some of the conditions which may produce Albuminuria.

Acute and chronic renal diseases. Renal congestion, with heart diseases and Emphysema. During pregnancy and puerperal state. Obstruction of the ureters. Digestive disturbances. Dyspepsia. Certain nervous affections. Functional Albuminuria. In the essential Anæmias, including Leukæmia and Exophthalmic Goitre. Lead-poisonings.

66. What is the probable status of the so-called Physiological Albuminuria?

It is either the terminal urinary condition of a convalescing disorder or it is the beginning of a chronic renal disease.

67. What are the probable factors in the production of Albuminuria in the course of Fevers?

In the early stage—Anæmia of the kidneys; *in the later stage* due to congestion of the kidneys.

68. Which of the varieties of Nephritis is apt to exhibit the most marked Albuminuria?

Acute Parenchymatous Nephritis.

69. Which variety of Chronic Nephritis is attended with but slight Albuminnria as a rule?

Chronic Interstitial Nephritis.

70. What is False Albuminuria?

When the albumin present in the urine is due to mixture of an albuminous fluid like *pus* or *blood*, it is called false or accidental albuminuria.

71. What is the appearance of the Urine in Renal Hæmaturia?

In renal Hæmaturia the urine may be bright red in colour to dark-brown, or even black or smoky.

72. Name some diseases of the Kidneys which may produce Hæmaturia.

Acute Nephritis, Chronic Interstitial and Parenchymatous Nephritis. Active congestion of the kidneys. Malignant diseases of the kidneys. Embolism of the kidneys. Tuberculous disease. General diseases in which the kidneys are affected, such as, Scurvy, Hæmophilia, Leucocythæmia, Purpura Hæmorrhagica, Yellow Fever, Pernicious Malarial Fevers, Relapsing Fever, Typhoid and Typhus Fevers.

73. Describe Test for Bile in the Urine.

An alcoholic dilution of *Tinct. of Iodine* 1 to 10 is applied to the suspected urine by the contact method. A *green ring* will appear at the point of contact, if bile is present.

74. What is the clinical significance of Bile in the Urine?

It signifies Jaundice or obstruction of the biliary ducts.

75. Describe a method for determining the Percentage of Urea.

Fill the long arm of an urinometer with *Hypobromite solution*, then insert 1 c. c. of the urine by means of the pipette attached to the urinometer graduated to measure the urine. The decomposition of the urine begins at once, and *Nitrogen* being evolved, takes the place of the liquid in the long arm of the instrument. The process is continued for about 15 minutes, when the extent of the displacement indicates the percentage of urea in the urine.

76. In what conditions are the Urea Percentage increased?

The urea percentage is increased in febrile disorders and in Diabetes.

77. In what conditions are the Urea Percentage decreased?

IN NORMAL CONDITIONS—by an indolent life, by a vegetable diet, by prolonged fast, or by excessive use of alcoholic beverages.

IN PATHOLOGICAL CONDITIONS—disorders of the liver (particularly Acute Yellow Atrophy of the Liver) and the spleen, in renal disorders and in nerve-prostration attended by defective metabolism.

78. What is the appearance of the Uric Acid Crystals under the Microscope?

They usually appear in whetstone-shape, either singly or in groups. They may also appear as large rosettes, tube-shaped or long, pointed crystals, rhombic plates with rounded edges and as dumb-bells. Usually they are of a orange-red color, though they may also appear as colorless.

79. What is the clinical significance of Glycosuria?

Occurring as a persistent symptom, it is to be regarded as diagnostic of Diabetes Mellitus.

80. Describe a Test for Sugar in the Urine.

Equal parts of the suspected urine and saturated solution of *Picric Acid* are mixed in a test tube, and half a fluid drachm of *Liq. Potassæ* is added. The mixture becomes orange-red in color. If sugar is present in the urine, it will change into a dark *mahogany color*, when the contents of the tube are *heated*.

81. What is Glycosuria?

When sugar is present in the urine in abnormal quantity, the condition is known as Glycosuria.

82. Describe the Fermentation Test for Glycosuria.

Four ounces of the urine are placed in a bottle along with a piece of compressed yeast. The cork of the bottle is nicked, to permit the escape of the *Carbonic Acid Gas* evolved in the process. Another bottle containing the urine, but without yeast, and well-corked is also prepared. Both the bottles are placed in a warm space from 12 to 24 hours, after which specific gravities of the two specimens are taken and the difference noted. For each degree of specific gravity lost, one grain to the fluid ounce of urine is estimated. If this figure be multiplied by 0·23, we obtain the *percentage of sugar*.

83. In what conditions may the Chlorides be absent from the Urine?

In diseases characterised by exudation—hence in Croupous Pneumonia and Pleurisy with effusion.

84. What is the significance of Acetonuria and Diaceturia in Diabetes?

They are prominent features of Diabetes and their presence may be regarded as unfavourable, as they are present only in worst cases.

85. How would you prepare a specimen of Urine for Microscopic Examination?

Sedimentation of urine is necessary in all cases, except where the urine contains large quantities of solids held in suspension. For this purpose, two methods, (i.) by permitting the urine to deposit its sediment in a conical glass, whence it may be removed by means of a pipette or (ii.) by sedimentation by the Centrifuge, may be employed. As the former method takes much time, during which chemical changes and disintegration of the tube-casts, etc., may take place, the latter method is the best, as it enables one to prepare the specimen while the patient is still in the consulting room and as such makes it possible to examine the urine before any change has taken place.

86. What varieties of Epithelium may be found in the Urine?

The URINARY EPITHELIUM may be divided into 3 classes, viz.. (i.) ROUND, (ii.) CAUDATE and (iii.) FLAT.

87. Describe the Composition of a Tube-Cast.

It is composed of the coagulable elements of the blood which have been transuded into the urinary tubules, by reason of patholgical changes in the renal structure, and have become moulded. It is either straight or convoluted, and exceedingly variable in diameter and length.

88. Describe a Hyaline Cast.

It is one of the varieties of tube-casts found in the urine. In color, it may vary from yellowish-white to brownish-red crystals. It may occur in renal Anæmia and hyperæmia, Diffuse Nephritis and Interstitial Nephritis.

89. Describe a Granular Cast.

It is found in Acute Nephritis and Chronic Diffuse Nephritis indicating granular degeneration of the epithelium and blood-cells. When numerous they indicate an inflammatory condition.

90. Describe an Epithelial Cast.

It consists of the epithelium of the tubules imbedded in hyaline matrix. It is found in a state of granular degeneration and liable to occur in Acute Desquamative Nephritis and Chronic Parenchymatous Nephritis.

81. Describe a Fatty Cast.

It is characterized by the percentage of flat globules of various sizes adhering to the basement structure. It may occur in cases of Nephritis running a protracted course.

92. What is the clinical significance of Pale Urine?

Deficiency of solids in the urine.

93. Name some diseases in which the Urine is abnormally Pale.

Diabetes Mellitus and Insipidus. Chronic Bright's Disease. Hysteria. Anæmia.

94. What are Pseudo-Casts?

They bear a strong resemblance to true casts, but differ from them in that they have no basement-structure. They may consist of epithelium, red blood-corpuscles or leucoytes derived from the uriniferous tubules and thrown off *en masse*. Those composed of epithelium are hollow, while the blood-casts are consisted of fibrin and red corpuscles. They appear in the urine *as hollow moulds*.

95. What are Cylindroids?

They are long, ribbon-like bodies, presenting an uniform breadth, and like the hyalin casts, may entangle certain cellular and crystalline elements. They are formed in the kidneys and closely related to the hyaline casts.

96. Give the method of Staining for Tubercle Bacilli.

The specimen is to be covered with *Carbol-Fuchsin* fluid, placed over a flame of the Bunsen burner, and permitted to simmer gently for two minutes. Next, pour off the *Fuchsin* and immerse the slide in the *Nitric-Acid* solution, for 20 to 30 seconds, when it loses all its red color. Immerse again in water to wash off the excess of the *Acid*, and cover the slide with absolute Alcohol, for three times, one-half minute each. This will decolorise Smegma Bacilli, which often occurs in the urine. Immerse again in water to wash off the Alcohol. Next, cover the slide with the *Methylene Blue* for one minute. Then wash off the *Blue* and dry the slide; place a drop of immersion oil on the dried film. It is now ready for examination.

97. Give the method of Staining for Gono-Cocci.

The suspected discharge is placed on a cover-slip, fixed by heat, and stained with *Methylene Blue*. This stains the Gono-Cocci and the nuclei of the pus-cells *blue*. The former appear as biscuit or kidney-shaped bodies in the pus-corpuscles.

98. Name the causes of the increased Irritability of the Bladder.

NERVOUS CAUSES such as mental strain or excitement.

GASTRO-INTESTINAL CAUSES, due to overloading of the large intestines, lesions of the rectum and anus, and seat-worms.

LESIONS OF THE EXTERNAL GENITAL, such as strictured urethra, retention of Smegma and Phimosis in the male, and papillomata and other tumors of urethra and various vaginal lesions in the female.

DISEASES OF THE BLADDER.

99. Name some of the causes of Painful Micturition.

Lesions of the bladder and urethra, such as, Cystitis, stone in the bladder, tumors and ulcerations of the bladder, disease of the prostatic urethra, Gonorrhœa, urethral stricture, urethral caruncle and urethral chancre.

Tenesmus vesicæ or Strangury also causes urinary pain.

100. Describe the causes of Retention of the Urine.

Obstructive Causes—due to stricture of the urethra, enlarged prostate, and calculus impacted in the urethra.

Paralytic Casues—due to Myelitis, Loco-motor Ataxia and Meningitis.

Spasmodic Causes—due to Cystitis, and Dysentery.

101. Give some causes of Difficult Micturition.

Weakness of the expulsive force of the bladder and partial obstruction in the lower urinary tract.

102. Name the Spinal Affections causing Incontinence of Urine.

Loco-motor Ataxia. Ataxic Paraplegia. Acute and chronic transverse Myelitis. Disseminated Sclerosis. Spinal Meningitis. General Paralysis of the Insane. Meningeal and intra-spiral hæmorrhage.

103. Name some Reflex Irritations causing Incotinence of Urine.

Ascarides. Phimosis.

104. Name the Urinary Causes of Incontinence of Urine.

Hyper-acidity. Presence of crystalline sediments.

105. What local weaknesses may cause Incontinence of Urine ?

(i.) Local weakness of the vesical sphincter from sexual excesses and (ii.) Prostatitis.

106. What condition throwing unusual strain upon the Vesical Sphincter may cause Incontinence of Urine ?

(i.) Vomiting, (ii.) Coughing.

CHAPTER XV.

THE KIDNEYS.

1. Give the Position of the Kidneys.

The kidneys are situated in the posterior section of the abdominal cavity in either side of the median line, and on a level with the last dorsal and the upper two or three lumbar vertebræ. Their upper extremities are beneath the 11th. and 12th. ribs. The upper extremity of the right kidney is in relation in front with the duodenum and the commencement of the transverse colon; that of the left with the descending colon. The right kidney is connected with the lever, while the left, with the spleen.

2. Give some general symptoms of Kidney Disease.

Headache. Uræmia—convulsions and coma. Retinitis. Dropsy. Paroxysmal dyspnœa. Cardio-vascular disorders.

3. Give some of the causes of the Kidney Disease.

Urinary changes. Calculus. Displacement and enlargement of the kidneys. Irritation of poisons introduced from without. Exposure to cold. Poisons of the acute infectious fevers. Extensive lesions of the skin. Syphilis. Tuberculosis. Traumatism. Sarcomata. Carcinomata. Etc.

4. What may be learned by Inspection in Kidney Diseases?

Nothing, except unusually great enlargements.

5. What may be learned by Palpation?

It enables us to discover the presence of renal displacements and renal enlargements.

Chap. XV.] THE KIDNEYS 219

6. Give the diagnostic features of the Floating Kidney.

It is readily discernible by palpation as a *movable slippery tumor* presenting the characteristic kidney-shape, far or near the position it normally held, which by *inspection* is found to be less full and on *palpation* less resistant than the other side—from behind it may show a distinct flattening in the lumbar region on the side in which the kidney is movable. Pressure upon it gives rise to a peculiar *pain* or *sickening sensation*.

7. Name the varieties of Renal Enlargements.

Renal abscess. Hæmorrhagic infarcts. Malignant tumors. Renal hypertrophy. Pyonephrosis. Hydro-nephrosis. Cysts.

8. Diagnose the Abscess of the Kidneys.

It presents a rounded enlargement, associated with some fullness of the loins. The affected kidney is tender and may be painful. Microscopical examination usually discovers pus and blood in the urine. If of tuberculous origin, tubercle bacilli also is present in the urine.

9. Diagnose Hydro-nephrosis.

It appears in palpation as a tense, smooth, globular tumor of variable size, soft one day and tense another, usually disappearing following a free flow of urine, to appear again. Its situation usually identifies it with the kidney. It increases gradually in size. In doubtful cases, the tumor is aspirated, and out of it is drawn a turbid fluid containing epithelial cells.

10. Give the causes of Renal Pain.

Lesions causing rapid distension of the capsules of the kidneys or irritating the lining membrane of the renal pelvis, are usually the causes of the production of renal pain. Certain other conditions, such as calculus, malignant disease. Tuberculosis and the so-called Neuralgia of the kidneys also produce renal pains.

11. Describe the Active Congestion of the Kidneys.

It is not a primary affection, but met with in the initial stages of Nephritis. The causes include, cold, the action of poisons and severe irritants, the elimination of the toxic substances formed within the body and irritation of the lower urinary tract. Symptoms in the majority of cases are most indefinite, excepting the urinary changes,—sometimes the patient complains of discomfort in the back. The urine is diminished (not to an alarming extent) in amount, and always contains more or less blood, albumin and tube-casts. Etiological factors afford an important diagnostic clue and differentiated from Acute Nephritis, by the absence of Dropsy in the congestion.

12. Give the cardinal symptoms of Chronic Parenchymatous Nephritis.

The cardinal symptoms are—(i.) *the urinary changes*—the urine is diminished in quantity; has a dirty yellow, sometimes smoky color and turbid; leucocytes and albumin abundant; tube-casts of various forms and sizes; and the urea is always reduced in quantity. (ii.) *Dropsy*—general; the face, pasty in complexion, with marked pallor, and puffy and the eyelids are œdematous; the œdema beginning as a slight puffiness, increases in severiy, finally invading the extremities and the serous sacs. (iii.) *Anæmia*—the skin presents a peculiar waxy color. (iv.) Tendency to digestive and respiratory disturbances. The diagnosis is based upon the urinary conditions.

13. Give the cardinal symptoms of Acute Nephritis.

The cardinal symptoms of Acute Nephritis are the *œdema* and *the urinary changes* in association with some general phenomenon such as fever, chilliness, pains in the back, nausea and vomiting. In children there may be convulsions at the outset.

The *urinary symptoms* are the most characteristic, and important diagnostically. At first there may be suppression ; more commonly the urine is scanty, high colored containing blood, albumin and tube-casts. *Œdema* about the face and eyes—generally it may be pronounced.

14. Give the cardinal symptoms of Chronic Interstitial Nephritis.

Out of the diversified symptomatology of chronic Interstitial Nephritis, its diagnosis is based upon the *urinary findings*, the increased blood-pressure and the condition of the heart and arteries. In a patient with increased pulse tension, with the apex beat of the heart dislocated to the left, the second aortic sound ringing and accentuated, high blood pressure, the urine abundant and of low specific gravity— with a trace of albumin and occasional tube-easts, the diagnosis may be safely made.

15. Give the cardinal symptoms of Amyloid Kidney.

Polyuria with low specific gravity and a large amount of albumin and few casts. Dropsy is present in many cases, particularly when there is much Anæmia and profound cachexia. When occurs in association with such constitutional affections, as Syphilis, disease of the bones, prolonged suppuration or Tuberculosis—a large quantity of clear pale urine is passed, even without the presence of albumin.

16. Give the cardinal symptoms of Pyelitis.

The symptoms include the constitutional phenomena of suppuration, the local subjective manifestations of a suppurative inflammation such as pain with sensitivenes on deep pressure over the region of the kidneys, backache, and the *urinary changes*—the urine is of acid reaction and contains pus.

17. Give the cardinal symptoms of Nephrolithiasis.

Dull pain in the small of the back over the affected kidney, paroxysms of renal colic, Hæmaturia, the vesical irritation, the retraction and tenderness of the testicles and the turbid and smoky *urine* containing blood and abundant epithelium from the pelvis, are the distinctive features of Nephrolithiasis.

18. Give the cardinal symptoms of Perinephritic Abscess.

Severe pain in the lumbar region, on the side of the affected kidney is the prominent symptom. It is greatly aggravated by pressure and motion, the patient flexes the knee and the thigh of the affected side for relief. Next, a swelling appears in the region of the kidneys, the cutaneous surface over which is unduly red, and is doughy to palpation. The skin becomes œdematous and finally fluctuation is plainly discernible, Constitutional symptoms of suppuration such as rigors, remittent fever, profuse sweating and prostration are present. In the initial stage it may be confounded with Lumbago.

19. Give the cardinal symptoms of Diabetes Mellitus.

The cardinal symptoms are *thirst, polyuria, polyphagia* i.e., *increased appetite* or *abnormal hunger, glycosuria* and *emaciation.* As a rule, the quantity of sugar in the urine and the severity of the case run parallel with urinary quantity.

20. Give the cardinal symptoms of Tuberculosis of the Kidney.

It presents the characteristic features of Pyelitis. The diagnosis rests upon the discovery of tuberculous lesions in other portions of the body or upon the presence of tubercle bacilli in the urine.

21. Describe the method of Palpating the Kidneys.

Bimanual manipulation is necessary for palpating the kidneys and the examination should be made when the stomach and colon are empty. The patient should stand leaning over the back of a chair, with the hands resting upon the seat of the same, supporting the trunk. The examiner will now place one of his hands upon the back below the last rib and outside the lumbar muscles. The other hand will be placed on the abdomen, opposite the former one. With simultaneous pressure and manipulation by both the hands, the kidney sought for will be readily brought under the touch of the examining fingers.

22. Name some symptoms which should suggest the presence of Renal Disease.

See Ans. to Q. 3 of this Chapter.

23. What is Nephroptosis?

The displacement of the kidney from its normal position is known as NEPHROPTOSIS.

24. Name some of the conditions capable of producing Renal Enlargement.

Tuberculosis, Malignant Endocarditis, Malignant tumors, renal hypertrophy, abscess, obstruction of the ureters, etc.

25. What are the special features of Renal Enlargement?

Renal enlargement in general starts in the lumbar region and extends upwards into the hypochondrium, backwards towards the spinal column, forwards to the umbilicus and downwards to the iliac crest. It is always behind the colon.

It presents a rounded anterior margin and a hollow can usually be felt between the upper margin of the enlargement and the costal margin. These are the special features of the renal enlargement.

26. What are the diagnostic features of Hydronephrosis?

See Ans. to Q. 9 of this Chapter.

27. What is the characteristic Pain produced by Renal Calculus?

The characteristic pain of the renal calculus is *renal colic*. It usually comes on suddenly, attaining its maximum intensity almost at once. It is usually on the side affected, but may be referred to the opposite kidney and radiates in the direction of the ureter, and in svere cases may be felt in the scrotum or even in the penis. It is paroxysmal in character and is due to the irritation of the passage of calculus and damning back of the urine. As a rule, the suffering is atrocious and is frequently associated with pronounced nausea and persistent vomiting.

CHAPTER XVI.

THE BLOOD.

1. What constitutes a Blood Examination?

For the examination of the blood, the determination of the following points is necessary.
1. Determination of its *specific gravity*. 2. Determination of its *alkalinity*. 3. Estimation of the percentage of hæmoglobin. 4. Determination of its coagulability. 5. Determination of the number of *red corpuscles* per C. C. M. 6. Determination of the number of white corpuscles per C. C. M. 7. Determination of the presence of abnormalities by examination of dried and stained blood-specimens. 8. Examination for parasites.

2. Describe the method of preparation of the skin surface for taking the Blood.

It should be thoroughly cleansed with a wet-cloth first, and then dried with gentle friction.

3. Describe the Process of making the Smear.

After wiping off the first few drops of blood from the puncture made for extracting the blood, a piece of the cover-glass is to be applied very carefully to *the apex* of the drop of blood appearing in the puncture, taking particular care *not to permit the glass to come in contact with the skin*. It will then be brought in contact with another cover-glass and the blood permitted to spread itself in a *thin layer* by the weight of that glass alone. No outside pressure should be exerted to hasten the spreading process, as such a procedure must cause distortions of the corpuscular elements of the blood. After a few seconds, they should be separated, by sliding them apart horizontally. To secure a thin and even layer this separation of the cover-glasses must be done with *great rapidity*. They should then be permitted to dry in the air and made ready for examination.

4. Describe Dare's Hæmometer.

The essential parts of Dare's Hæmometer are an automatic pipette for collecting the blood and a graduated color-comparison scale to measure the percentage of hæmoglobin.

5. Give in detail the preparation for counting Red Cells.

The counting is made with the aid of a hæmato-cytometer, of which the Thoma-Zeiss hæmato-cytometer is most convenient. It consists of *capillary pipette* or mixing tube and a *counting-chamber*.

The pipette is to be filled with blood to figure 0.5 or 1.0 marked in it. Then a solution of common *salt* (3%) is to be added up to the mark 101 in it, making the proportion of the blood and the mixture 1 to 200 or 1 to 100, according as the pipette is filled with blood to 0·5 or 1·0 respectively. The pipette is then shaken carefully to dilute the blood in the solution thoroughly. A drop of the mixture is then carefully deposited in the counting-chamber. The cover-glass is next adjusted, care being taken that no bubbles of air shall enter. The instrument is then set aside for a few minutes to permit the corpuscles to settle; after which it is placed under the microscope—an objective of low power being used, and to count the number of red corpuscles from 80 to 160 squares of the counting chamber. From the result thus obtained, the number of red corpuscles in a cubic millimeter of blood are counted, which is based upon the fact that each square of the counting chamber has overlying it $\frac{1}{4000}$ of a cubic millimeter, and the blood mixture is in the proportion of 1 to 100 or 1 to 200 as the case may be.

For example, if we find in 100 squares 200 corpuscles, and the degree of dilution is 1 to 200, we multiply $200 \times 200 \times 4000$ which gives 160,000,000. Dividing it by 100, the number of squares counted, we have 1,600,000 which is the number of red corpuscles per cubic millimeter of blood.

6. Describe the preparation for counting the White Cells.

For this purpose also a Thoma-Zeiss apparatus, with a special *leucocyte pipette* is used. The pipette has a much larger bore than the one used for red corpuscles, as also the quantity of blood required is much larger. It should be diluted with a one-third of one per cent solution of glacial *Acetic Acid* in the proportion of 1 to 10 or 1 to 20. 'As the *Acetic Acid solution* destroys the red cells, the white cells alone are visible. The count is made on exactly the same principle as the red cells, keeping in mind that the degree of dilution is 1 to 10 or 1 to 20 as the case may be. Owing however, to the small number present, a very large number of squares are counted.

7. Give the varieties of Leucocytes.

Varieties of leucocytes with their relative proportion in the normal blood are—

(i.) SMALL MONONUCLEAR LEUCOCYTES (15 to 20%). (ii.) LARGE MONONUCLEAR LEUCOCYTES (6 to 8%). (iii.) TRANSITIONAL and (iv.) POLYMORPHO-NUCLEAR LEUCOCYTES (64 to 70%). (v.) EOSINOPHILES (2%). (vi.) BASOPHILIC LEUCOCYTES (0.5%). (vii.) MYELOCYTES (not present in the normal blood).

8. How do you make a Differential Count of White Cells?

(i.) By the character of their nuclei. (ii.) By the manner in which their protoplasm reacts to acid, basic and neutral stains.

9. Give symptoms and hæmic changes in Leukæmia.

SYMPTOMS.—Progressive enlargement of the abdomen, dyspnœa, or pallor, palpitation and other symptoms of Anæmia at the onset. Gradual enlargement of the spleen is the most prominent feature in the majority of cases. The pulse is usually rapid, soft, and compressible, but often full in volume. Priapism—may be the first symptom. *Leucocytosis.* Diagnosis rests on the blood count.

HAEMIC CHANGES.—Remarkable *increase of leucoytes.* Counts over 500,000 per c. m. m. are common, may rise above 1,000,000 per c. m. m. with the *presence of myelocytes from 20 to 50%.* The proportion of white and red cells may be 1 to 5, or may even reach 1 to 1. * The color index is unusually low. The blood platelets are increased. * The hœmoglobin percentage is generally disproportionately low to the erythrocyte count and shows a remarkable tendency to crystallise.

10. **Give symptoms and hæmic changes in Splenic Anæmia.**

SYMPTOMS.—*Splenomegaly* or the great enlargement of the spleen is smooth, and usually spreads upto the navel very often to the anterior superior spine, and the organ may occupy the whole of the left half of the abdomen ; there may be pain following an infarct. *Anæmia*—progressively worse. *Hæmorrhage* from different parts of the body—usually Hæmatemesis. *Ascites*—usually a terminal event.

HAEMIC CHANGES.—Marked Leucopenia—red corpuscles may fall as low as two million. There is however little or no leucocytosis. The color index is low and the hœmoglobin percentage is disproportionately low to the erythrocyte count.

11. **Give symptoms and hæmic changes in Secondary Anæmia.**

SYMPTOMS.—Marked signs of Anæmia such as prostration, anorexia, palpitation, feeling of faintness with loss of bodily and mental vigor and loss of weight are the important features. As the Anæmia progresses, there is swelling of the feet.

HAEMIC CHANGES.—The blood picture is distinctive. The red corpuscles are reduced, but rarely below 2 millions per C. M. M. The hæmoglobin is relatively lower than the red cells with a low color index. Leucocytes are usually increased in number.

12. Give symptoms and hæmic changes in Pseudo Leukæmia.

SYMPTOMS.—The initial symptoms are pallor and weakness in children with a history of Rachitis or Syphilis behind. Afterwards the general symptoms of Anæmia with *enlargement and hardness of the spleen* sometimes associated with enlargement of the liver and lymphatic glands.

HAEMIC CHANGES.—Marked diminution of the red corpuscles, sometimes as low as one million per C. M. M. Increased leucocyte count due to increase of the polymorphonuclear neutrophiles, from 30 to 50 thousands per C. M. M.

13. Give symptoms and hæmic changes in Hæmophilia.

SYMPTOMS.—The cardinal features are, persistent bleeding from slight wounds, limitation of the victims to the male sex, an inheritendency and Hæmarthrosis.

HAEMIC CHANGES.—The blood shows no abnormality excepting a delayed coagulation.

14. Give symptoms and hæmic changes in Scurvy.

SYMPTOMS.—Insidious onset. Debility and emaciation early features. Special early and distinctive symptom is swelling and sponginess of the gums, which bleed on slight cause; teeth loosen and lost. Subcutaneous swellings—particularly marked in ankles and cough and hæmorrhages; petechiæ. Profound Anæmia.

HAEMIC CHANGES.—Ordinarily the red count does not fall below 3,500,000; in severe cases it may fall to 1 to 2 millions. The leucocytes are normal or moderately increased.

15. Give symptoms and hæmic changes in Purpura.

SYMPTOMS :—Hæmorrhagic effusions, associated with evidences of Anæmia, are the essential features of Purpura.

HAEMIC CHANGES.—Marked reduction in blood platelets.

16. Name some of the Pathological Conditions attended with a Leucocytosis.

The pathological conditions attended with LEUCOCYTOSIS are :—

(i.) Inflammations and infections. (ii.) Malignant diseases. (iii.) Severe hæmorrhages. (iv.) Coal-gas and ptomaine poisoning, ether narcosis, cholæmia and uræmia. (v.) Leukæmia, Leucocythæmia.

17. Name the different Malarial Parasites and the Types of Fever they produce.

The different malarial parasites, so far recognised are—(i.) *Tertian* parasites, producing fever on alternate days known as the *tertian fever*—a double set, producing a double tertian or *quotidian fever* occurring daily. (ii.) *Quartan parasites* producing fever every third day known as the *quartan fever* and (iii.) *astivo-autumal parasites* producing *pernicious malarial fevers*.

18. Give the general forms of the Malarial Parasites.

(i.) Intracellular hyaline forms. (ii.) Intracellular pigmented forms. (iii.) Extracellular pigmented forms. (iv.) The segmenting forms. (v.) The flagellate forms.

19. Describe the Tertian Malarial Parasites.

(i.) INTRACELLULAR HYALINE FORMS.— Observed in the red blood cells immediately or shortly after the paroxysm as small transparent bodies of frequent and varied changes in shape. They possess active amœboid movements.

(ii.) INTRACELLULAR PIGMENTED FORMS.—Observed in about 24 hours after the paroxysm, as a mass of pigment granules, yellowish-brown in color, deposited about the peripheral portion of the parasite, possessing active motions with tongue-like protrusions. The pigment increases in amount and the corpuscle becomes larger and paler, owing to progressive diminution of its hæmoglobin. With progressive development, the parasite increases in size and the amœboid movements disappear gradually. In these forms they are known as full-grown parasites.

(iii.) SEGMENTING FORMS.—In about 48 hours, many of the parasites undergo the change known as segmentation in which the pigment becomes collected into a single mass or block and the protoplasm divided into a series of 15 to 20 spores. At this stage the organism is enclosed in a thin layer of erythrocyte, which however is scarcely visible on account of its transparency. Now the corpuscles rupture and the spores or segments escape into the surrounding blood and disappear from view. Certain full-grown parasites do not undergo segmentation; they are larger than the sporulating bodies, and contain very actively dancing pigment granules and are known ae *gametocytes*—a sexually differentiated form of the parasites.

(iv.) EXTRACELLULAR PIGMENTED FORMS.— With the development of pigmentation as described above in section (ii.) of this Q., the parasite may escape from its host when it is immediately dwarfed and loses its amœboid motion. These forms are known as the Extracellular Pigmented Forms. They may become fragmented. Their outlines are obscured.

(v.) FLAGELLATE FORMS.—They develop from Extracellular Pigmented Forms which do not escape from the corpuscle until approaching the stage of fragmentation. The appearance of flagellation is preceded by a period of great activity of the pigmented granules, which finally accumulate at or near the centre of the parasite, and one or more long tentacular arms are thrust forth from the main body. They exhibit one or more bulbous enlargements, situated usually at their distal extremities.

20. Describe the Quartan Malarial Parasite as far as it differs from the Tertian.

The Quartan parasites are smaller, less motile and more refractive than the Tertian. Pigmentation is more rapid and is in larger granules, of dark-brown, almost black color, and early in their course cluster in one portion of the organism. The blood corpuscle is normal in size or shrunken and of a dark color. Their segments arrange themselves in a perfectly symmetrical manner.

21. Give the special features of the Æstivo-Autumnal Parasite.

This parasite is considerably smaller than the other varieties; at full development it is often less than one-half the size of a red blood corpuscle. The pigment is much scantier, often consisting of a few minute granules. In the hyaline form its characteristic feature, by which, it may be recognized with certainty, lies in the formation of ring-like bodies, which by reason of the amœboid movements, changes into a flattened disk; later, it returns again to the ring-like form. At first only in the earlier stages of development, small, hyaline bodies, sometimes with one or two pigment granules, are to be found in the peripheral circulation; in the later stages, they are discovered in the blood of certain organs—the spleen and bone marrow particularly.

22. What is Widal Reaction?

Widal Reaction is a test for determining the presence of Typhoid bacilli in the blood of a patient.

It is based upon the property possessed by blood from Typhoid patients, of causing clumping of the Typhoid bacilli, in young cultures in bouillon.

23. What is the clinical value of the Widal Reaction?

It is of great value when the indication is *positive*—the only doubt then to be cast upon it, is in those exceptional cases in which the patients have had previous attacks of Typhoid Fever.

Negative results also must be accepted with caution, as there may not have been sufficient time to elapse for its development in the case at hand.

24. Describe the method of preparing Blood for the Widal Reaction.

(i.) In the DRIED-BLOOD METHOD—a few drops of blood from the suspected case are deposited upon a piece of glazed non-absorbent paper or upon a glass-slide, and permitted to dry. When making the test, if the specimen is on the *glass-slide*, it is moistened with a drop of sterile water and thoroughly mixed, with the aid of a platinum loop; next it is diluted with nine drops of Typhoid bouillon culture; if the specimen, is on paper, the portion covered by the blood is carefully cut out, and soaked thoroughly face downwards, in 10 drops of bouillon culture. It is then ready for examination.

(ii.) The FRESH-BLOOD METHOD—few drops of fresh blood is mixed at the patients' bedside with 10 times its bulk of Typhoid bouillon in a test-tube. It is then ready for examination.

(iii.) The SERUM METHOD—15 to 20 drops of blood is collected in a test-tube and allowed to coagulate. The fluid serum is drained off, and the residue is diluted with ten times its milk of typhoid bouillon. It is then ready for examination.

25. How is the Specific Gravity of the Blood determined?

A mixture of equal parts of *Chloroform* (heavier than blood) and *Benzol* (lighter than blood) is made in urinometer glass. A drop of blood, whose specific gravity is to be determined, is placed on the solution, (care being taken that it does not adhere to the walls of the glass). It will not incorporate itself with the mixture, but will rise or fall according to its relative density with the fluid. The specific gravity of the mixture may be increased or decreased by adding *Chloroform* or *Benzol*, respectively, until a point is reached when the blood-drop remains suspended. Then the specific gravity of the mixture is taken with an accurate urinometer, and the result indicates the specific gravity of the blood in the glass.

26. How is the Hæmoblobin Percentage obtained?

It can be determined in a Tallquist Hæmoglobin Scale—which consists of a series of plates colored to correspond with that of various blood-specimens containing from 10 to 100 per cent of Hæmoglobin. The scale is accompanied by a book of white filter-paper. A piece of the latter is dipped into the blood, and as soon as the glass has disappeared, but before drying, it is compared with the color-scale, and the one to which it corresponds most closely in color, represents the percentage of the Hæmoglobin.

27. Describe Fleischle's Hæmometer.

It consists of the following parts:—

A stand on which is carried a movable stage, consisting of a steel frame, in which is mounted a long glass wedge, stained with cassian purple. Opposite to the wedge, the side of the frame is graduated from 0 to 100 p. c. to indicate the quantity of hæmoglobin corresponding to the shade of

Chap. XVI.]   THE BLOOD   235

color opposite to the figure. The wedge, with its carriage is moved by means of a ratchet-screw.

Immediately over the line travelled by the wedge is placed a small reservoir having two compartments, so arranged that one is immediately over the wedge, while the other is not. The former is filled with plain water and the latter with blood-mixture. Beneath the stand is a reflector of plaster-of-Paris.

In addition to the above, which constitutes the Hæmometer proper, there are a number of capillary pipettes and one of a moderately large size.

28. Describe the method for counting Red Blood-Cells.

See Ans. to Q. 5 of this Chapter.

29. Describe the method for counting the Leucocytes.

See Ans. to Q. 6 of this Chapter.

30. Describe the method for Preparing a Blood-film.

See Ans. to Q. 3 of this Chapter.

31. Describe a method for Staining Blood-films.

The specimens are stained from 3 to 5 minutes by thoroughly covering the slides in a staining solution preferably (a 0·5 p. c. solution of *Eosinate* of *Methylene Blue* in pure Methyl Alcohol). The stain is then washed off and allowed to be *well-dried in air.* It is then ready for examination.

32. What is the Color-Index of the Blood and how is it obtained?

The relation between the hæmoglobin percentage and the number of red blood-cells in a C. M. M. is known as the COLOR-INDEX OF THE BLOOD. *Normally*, the color-index is taken as 1, and number of red cells in a cubic millimetre is 5,000,000. To determine the color-index of a specimen the percentage of its hæmoglobin is to be divided by the percentage of red cells present in the specimen (calculated with the normal count). The result thus obtained is the color-index of the blood in the specimen, Thus, in a given specimen if the blood-count is, say 4,000,000 and the hæmoglobin percentage is 40 per cent, the color-index is $\frac{40}{80}$ i.e., 0·5.

33. What disease of the blood is characterized by a remarkably Low Percentage of Hæmoglobin?

Chlorosis.

34. Which of the Anæmias is especially liable to exhibit Low Red Blood-count?

Pernicious Anæmia.

35. What is Leucocytosis?

An increase in the number of *leucocytes* or the white corpuscles in the blood over the normal is called Leucocytosis. The normal count being 5 to 7 thousands per cubic millimetre.

36. Name the different Varieties of Leucocytes.

See Ans. to Q. 7 of this Chapter.

37. Which of the forms of Leucocytes is increased relatively in the Symptomatic Anæmias?

Small Mononuclear Leucocytes and the Myelocytes.

38. Which of the forms of Leucocytes is increased in the Spleno-Medullary Lukæmia?

Myelocytes.

39. Which of the forms of Leucocytes is increased in Lymphatic Leukæmia?

Small Mononuclear Leucocytes.

40. What are the Physiological causes of Leucocytosis?

The physiological causes of Leucocytosis are:—
(i.) *Digestion*, (ii.) *pregnancy* and (iii.) *infancy*.

41. What is Poikilocytosis?

Pathological change in the *shape* of the red blood-cells is known as POIKILOCYTOSIS.

42. What is the clinical significance of Poikilocytosis?

It is especially characteristic of Pernicious Anæmia. It occurs also in chlorosis and other forms of Anæmias in a lesser degree.

43. What is an Erythrocyte?

Erythrocyte is one of two kinds of Leucocytes, which is transformed into colored blood corpuscle in the spleen and bone marrow.

44. What is a Normoblast?

A normoblast is an immature red corpuscle of normal size.

45. What is a Megaloblast?

A megaloblast is a nucleated red corpuscle of larger than normal size.

46. What is the clinical significance of the Megaloblasts?

Their presence is to be regarded as evidence of serious changes. Their persistent presence is strongly suggestive of *Pernicious Anæmia*.

47. What is Eosinophilia?

Inerease of the eosinophile percentage in the constitution of white blood-cell is known os EOSINOPHILIA.

48. What condition is attended with a marked Eosinophilia ?

Trichinosis.

49. What is Leucopenia ?

A diminution in the number of white blood-cells in comparison with the normal is known as LEUCOPENIA.

CHAPTER XVII.

EXTERNAL SURFACE.

ALTERATIONS IN SIZE & SHAPE.

1. What is Emaciation?

Emaciation suggests diminution in the size of the body due to inanition and malnutrition.

2. What are the general conditions producing Emaciation?

Emaciation is produced in all pathological processes in which the nutrition is depraved or in which the normal balance between waste and repair is disturbed.

3. What is the average relation between Weight and Height?

The average relation between weight and height, is taken for general guidance only as from 25 to 30 lbs. for each foot in stature.

4. Upon what factors does the Weight of an Individual depend Physiologically?

(i.) The habit of the individual. (ii.) The size of the skeleton. (iii.) The development of muscular tissue. (iv.) The development of adipose tissue and its distribution.

5. What is the clinical significance of pronounced Emaciation in children?

It is to be regarded as indisputable evidence of immproper feeding or of some chronic constitutional disease, such as Rachitis, Tuberculosis or congenital Syphilis.

6. What are the causes of Obesity?

(i.) *Heredity*. (ii.) *Diet*—food and drink. (iii.) *Sedentary habit*. (iv.) *Age*. (v.) *Occupation*. (vi.) *Climate*.

7. In what way does Habit influence Weight of the Individual?

Persons of easy-going, lazy habits are generally fond of the pleasures of the table and do not make sufficient exercise to oxidise even a normal amount of food and as such are inclined to take on an undue amount of adipose to become fatty, which accounts for their more weight, than the persons of active habits and those of worrying restless disposition who exhibit but little sub-cutaneous fat and as such lesser in weight than the former. So habit by helping accumulation or decreases of fat in individual, influences his weight.

8. How does Age influence the Weight?

Certain periods of the life of an individual male or female are prone to add an undue amount of fat in his or her body. As the normal infants are expected to become plumpy, in comparison with their height; the men, at or beyond middle life or the women at or after the climaxis are inclined to become unduly corpulent.

9. How is the Weight influenced by Quantity or Quality of Food or Drink?

Excessive feeding and drinking, especially the taking of starches, sugar, and fat, and the drinking of alcoholic beverages are usually inclined to add more fat to the body, than a normal diet; as such, they influence the weight of the body.

10. How is the Weight influenced by Climate?

The inhabitants of damp, low-lying countries are observed with special frequency to exhibit more corpulence in their bodies than the inhabitants of dry countries who are apt to be spare of build.

11. What are the evil effects of Obesity?

It is apt to lead to illness periodically without apparent cause. It is liable to cause catarrhs and diarrhœa, probably because the self-regulation of temperature is imparied by the thick layer of sub-cutaneous fat and the weakening of the circulation by fatty infiltration of the heart-muscle. It also enfeebles the heart and diminishes heat radiation of the body.

12. What is Dropsy?

Accumulation of serum in the connective tissue-spaces or in one or more of the serous cavities of the body is known by the general name of Dropsy. It is called by special names, according to the differnt position it occupies in the body, e. g., when it is general it is known as *Anasarca*, when involving the serous cavity of the peritonium, as *Ascites*, of the pleura, as *Hydrothorax*, of the cranium as *Hydrocephalus*, of the pericardium as *Hydro-pericardium*; when occurs as effusion into the synovial sac of the joints, as *Hydrarthrosis*; etc.

13. Name some of the causes of Circumscribed Enlargements of the Abdomen.

Circumscribed enlargements of the abdomen may be due to (i.) increase in the size of the abdominal viscera, as the liver, spleen and kidneys, or (ii.) to misplacements of the same, or (iii.) to new formations.

14. Name some of the Tumors which can be traced into the Pelvis.

The tumors that can be traced into the pelvis are—

Cyst of broad ligaments. Hydrometra. Hydrosalpinx. Hæmatosalpinx. Myoma. Pyosalpinx. Hyper-

trophied bladder. Distended bladder. Fibroid
tumor of the uterus. Fibrocystic tumor of the uterus.
Congestion of the uterus. Ovarian cyst. Polypus.
Peritoneal hydatids. Ectopic gestation. Sub-involution.
Tubal cancer or Tubercle.

15. Name some of the Wandering Tumors.

Fatty tumors of intestines. Phantom tumor.
Tumor of the transverse colon. Floating kidney.
Floating spleen. Floating lobe of the liver. Concretions in the intestines. Cancer of the pylorus.
Impacted fæces.

16. Name some of the Lateral Tumors.

Pelvic abscess. Perinephritic abscesses. Pyonephrosis. Sarcoma of the kidney. Parasite of the kidney.
Hydatids of liver or kidney. Encephaloid kidney.
Pelvic Hæmatocele. Hydronephrosis. Enlarged spleen.
Cystic kidney. Appendicitis. Distended gall-bladder.
Fæcal accumulation. Doughy colon (Dysentery). Etc.

17. Name some Fluctuating Tumors.

Abscess of the abdominal walls. Ascites.
Effusion into lesser peritoneal cavity. Distended
bladder. Ectopic gestation. Hydatids. Hydronephrosis. Hydrosalpinx. Lumbar abscess. Ovarian cyst.
Pyosalpinx. Pyonephrosis. Pregnancy.

18. Name some alterations in the Shape of the Back.

Kyphosis. Scoliosis. Lordosis.

19. Describe a Kyphosis.

KYPHOSIS is a posterior curvature of the spinal
cord altering the shape and causing deformity of the
back, which may be even angular. It may be due
to the stooping of the age, Mollities Ossium, Arthritis
Deformans, as part of the changes of the emphysematous chest or caries of the vertebræ. When due to the
latter, the deformity is angular.

20. Give some of its Causes.

See Ans. to the previous Question.

21. Define the term Scoliosis and give some of its causes.

SCOLIOSIS is an alteration in the shape of the back, the curvature being rotary-lateral. It may be due to Rachitis, unequal length of the lower extremities, cerebral and spinal paralyses. Intra-thoracic disease or faulty position among school-girls.

22. What is meant by Lordosis and give some of its causes?

LORDOSIS is an alteration in the shape of the back, in which the normal convex curve of the spine is exaggerated, and may be due to pregnancy, Ascites, abdominal tumors or pseudo-hypertrophic Paralysis.

23. Describe Pseudo-Hypertrophy.

It is a disease of developmental origin, starting in early childhood is observed in a form of muscular dystrophy known as pseudo-hypertrophic Paralysis. It exhibits apparent hypertrophy of certain muscles, e. g., those of the calves and shoulders, associated with the atrophy of others, with exaggeration of the dorso-lumbar concavity. The patient exhibits a waddling gait and when rising from lying on the floor, goes through the process known as "climbing up the thighs." Sensory disturbances are absent. Its course is very chronic and is incurable. Death occurs from inter-current disease.

24. Describe True Hypertrophy.

It is characterized by spasm or rigidity of muscles as soon as they are put into action, relaxation taking place in a few seconds. It is rare as a pathological condition and occurs in Thomsen's disease (Myotonia Congenita).

25. Give the appearance of Inflammatory Swelling of the Muscles.

They lose their normal contour, the outlines of individual muscles being obliterated. They may be associated with cutaneous œdema. The skin may take on an increased color.

26. Give the causes of Muscular Atrophy.

The muscular atrophy may result from (i.) disuse of the parts, (ii.) disease of the upper motor neuron, (iii.) disease of the lower motor neuron, (iv.) disease of the muscles themselves and (v.) disease of the joints.

27. Describe the Atrophy of Disuse.

The atrophy of disuse is due entirely to disturbance of nutrition. It is rarely extreme. It disappears as soon as the affected part is made active. Some of the cases of muscular atrophy attendant upon joint disease belong to this class.

28. Give symptoms and diagnosis of Acute Poliomyelitis Anterior.

The characteristic or diagnostic symptom is *Paralysis* which is abrupt in its onset, and *reaches its maximum in a very short time*, almost at once, attended by flaccidity of the affected muscles. The lege or all four extremities may by involved. The Paralysis of the trunk-muscles occurs often. Nearly always one limb is more severely affected than the others. Unless the case is severe *the Paralysis disappears n part within a few days and some of the affected muscles riecover their functions in part*. The paralyzed muscles *atroplhy* at an early period to an extreme degree. Some muscles are nearly always affeeted permanently. Deformities in the shape of "club-foot" are apt to remain. Among the pre-paralytic symptoms may be mentioned fever, drowsiness or heaviness, irritability, twitchings and jerking, and gastro-intestinal symptoms, which however are not diagnostic.

29. Give symptoms and diagnosis of Muscular Atrophy.

The initial symptoms are muscular atrophy with corresponding loss of power in the affected parts. The hands are usually first affected and there is difficulty in performing delicate manipulations. The muscles of the ball of the thumb waste early. Shoulder-muscles also may be involved first. Beginning at any point it may involve the whole system, converting the patient to a combination of skin and bones or living skeleton only. Deformities and contractures result and lordosis is almost always present. Sensibility is un-impaired. The loss of power is usually proportionate, to the wasting. Irregular pains may precede the onset of wasting.

DIAGNOSIS.— As a rule, it begins in adult life. It begins in the upper extremities and wasting is the first feature and seems to be the immediate cause of the loss of power. The affected muscles do not exhibit, the reaction of degeneration. Fibrillary contractions are common, electric changes occur and the deep reflexes are usually increased. It follows a steady downward course, and is of much slower onset.

30. Give the diseases which may give rise to Joint Lesions.

Acute inflammatory Rheumatism. Chronic articular Rheumatism. Gout. Arthritis Deformans. Gonorrhœai Arthritis. Scarlatinal Synovitis. Simple Synovitis. Hæmophilia. Syphilis. Tuberculosis. Spinal-cord diseases. Rachitis.

31. Diagnose Inflammatory Rheumatism.

Inflammatory Rheumatism or the Rheumatic Fever presents a definite clinical course, which is sufficiently characteristic. Its prodromal phenomena are indefinite and include malaise, headache, general ill-health and slight fever. The stage of invasion is more or less abrupt, and is characterised by a febrile rise of moderate intensity with pains and swellings in the various joint-extremities. The pain is especially prominent. The affected parts exhibit moderate swelling and slight redness. The inflammation does not involve all the joints simultaneously but tends rather to migrate or shift from one joint to the other. Profuse sweat. Temperature—fluctuaing but seldom high. Anæmia, apt to be severe. Leucocytosis moderate, 12000 per c. m. m. Affected joints are more tender.

32. Diagnose Chronic Articular Rheumatism.

It usually occurs in persons passed middle life, who have worked hard and have been exposed to the vicissitudes of weather. It sometimes follows acute inflammatory Rheumatism, *Heredity* also seems to be an important factor, in many cases, in producing these disorders. Though it presents various clinical types the more commonly found ones exhibit pain and stiffness of the various joints, usually without articular swellings. The extent of suffering varies greatly from day to day, the weather having a very important influence. Any number of joints may be involved. With few exceptions the pains are worse in the morning, better from moving about. No impairment of general health.

33. Diagnose Gout.

Repeated attacks of Arthritis, limited to the big toe or to the tarsus, occurring in a member of a gouty family or in a man with dietectic habits of taking excessive quantity of food, particularly of Nitrogenous character and indulgence in alcoholic beverages, leave no doubt as to the existence of Gout. Its clinical features include painful swelling of the metatarso-phalangeal joint of the great toe and a moderate degree of fever and scanty, high-colored urine. The pain is excruciating and especially marked during the night. Exceptionally, other joints such as ankles, insteps, fingers, wrists and knees may be involved. The history of the patient is of paramount importance in the diagnosis of a typical Gout. Age (usually at or beyond middle life), and habits are further diagnostic aids.

34. Give the description of Arthritis Deformans.

It is a diesase of the joints, characterized by inflammatory phenomena and changes in the synovial membranes, cartilage and peri-articular structures, and in some cases by atrophic and hypertrophic changes in the bones. It is due to occult focal infections, particularly from tonsils and teeth. It may be acute or chronic. The acute form occurs especially in children and young adults. Clinically it depicts many types, the main divisions being peri-articular, atrophic and hypertrophic. The causes include heredity, young adult life, the female sex, the neuropathic constitution and defective hygienic surroundings. In the *acute form* the lesions generally commence in one of the smaller joints, especially in the metacarpo-phalangeal articulation and invade rapidly the larger ones. Symmetry of articular involvement is the rule.

In the CHRONIC FORMS, it nearly always begins in the joints of the fingers, and involve all the joints of the body, producing deformities and immobilities in all the invaded parts. Marked and rapid atrophy of the muscles, controlling the movements of the affected parts are almost invariably present. They become contractured later, increasing the deformities.

Constitutional disturbances, such as Anæmia, general debility and emaciation are usually well-marked. The fever is usually moderate and the pulse rate is rapid in proportion to the fever.

Difficulties may be encountered to distinguish it from—

(i.) The *Rheumatic Fever* (Acute Inflammatory Rheumatism) but the presence of thickening in a joint, rapid muscular atrophy, the relatively high pulse rate in relation to the fever speak against rheumatic fever. The affected joints are rarely as tender as in Rheumatic Fever, and the smaller joints are more often involved ;

(ii.) The *Gonorrhœal Arthritis* ; but in the latter the small joints are usually not attacked so often, and after an onset with Polyarthritis the majority of the affected joints usually clear, *leaving one joint particularly involved*, which is rare in the former ; careful search for Gono-cocci decides the issue ;

(iii.) The *Gout*, when the joint-changes are not marked ; marked peri-articular changes speak for the latter.

35. Diagnose Gonorrhœal Arthritis.

In Gonorrhœal Arthritis the larger joints are usually affected particularly the knees. The local symptoms include pain and swelling of the affected joints, which are not hot to the touch, nor markedly red. Its tendency is to remain in the joint or joints which it first attacks and does not shift from one part to another as in inflammatory Rheumatism. The fever is absent. It occurs more frequently in the males than in females. The presence of Gono-cocci is a definite indication.

36. Diagnose Simple Synovitis.

The SIMPLE SYNOVITIS is a local joint affection, which presents no difficulty to diagnosis, unless otherwise complicated.

37. Give the Joint-lesions of Rachitis.

The joint-lesions of Rachitis are usually restricted to the wrists and ankles due to enlargement of the long bones of the localities. They present ring-like appearances without external evidence of inflammation. They appear very early in the course of the disease. Other joints may also be involved.

38. What is the indication afforded by the "Clubbed Fingers"?

They indicate *enfeeblement of the circulation* due to passive congestion of the parts resulting from their peripheral situation.

39. Give a description of the Hand in Paralysis Agitans.

The hand in Paralysis Agitans presents a deformity which is almost pathognomic and has been aptly described as the "writing-hand" i. e., the position which the hand assumes when grasping a pen for writing. There is *no joint-enlargement* and the *deformities are more characteristic* than those of the shaking palsy. The hand deviates towards the ulner border of the forearm and may be associated with a coarse tremor.

40. Describe Dactylitis and give its Relationship with Tuberculosis.

Dactylitis is a fusiform enlargement of the bone, the maximum diameter being about the middle, associated with redness, heat and thickening of the soft parts. It occurs as manifestation of Tuberculosis or Syphilis. Its natural course is to caries and necrosis.

In Tuberculosis it is observed more frequently in children and usually in association with evidences of Tuberculosis elsewhere and is dependent upon an osteo-myelitis of the phalanges and produces a fusiform enlargement of the affected phalanges. There is a strong tendency to spread to adjacent parts.

41. Describe the Syphilitic Dactylitis.

In Syphilis it is due to a gummatous infiltration of the bones or surrounding structures—the ligamentous and sub-cutaneous structures presenting a tense, hard or soft and semi-fluctuating swelling. When the gummatous infiltration breaks down, the pathological process may extend to the joints and bones. It is a manifestation of the *tertiary* and *inherited Syphilis* and runs *a painless course* which is distinctive.

In primary Syphilis, the gummatous process may invade the phalangeal bones and manifest itself clinically by a slowly progressive enlargement of the affected phalanx or phalanges, associated with pain and redness, ending in ulceration and suppuration with extensive disorganisation of the parts.

42. Decribe the Enlargement of the Lymphatic Glands.

Enlargement of the lymphatic glands may be *local* or *general*. The *local enlargements* are due to *infections* within the area drained by the lymphatic vessels, which are received by the enlarged glands. The enlargement of the glands of the neck and sub-maxillary region are frequently due to infectious processes from the mouth and throat, such as carious teeth, stomatitis, tonsillitis and pharyngitis etc., as also acute infections like Measles, Scarlatina, Variola and Diphtheria. There may also be secondary involvement from malignant tumors, such as enlargement of the axillary lymphatics from mammary cancer, and the enlargement of the supra-clavicular glands from malignant disease of the mediastinum.

The principal causes of the *general enlargements* of the lymphatic glands are Tuberculosis, Syphilis and Lymphadenoma (Hodgkin's Disease), though the resulting enlargements may be limited to certain parts of the body.

43. Tell the cause of Localised Swelling of the Lymphatic Glands.

See the *Ans.* to the previous Question.

44. Give in general the distribution of Lymphatic Glands of Head and Neck.

(i.) SUB-OCCIPITAL and (ii.) MASTOID—are distributed in the posterior half of head. (iii.)

PAROTID—anterior half of head, orbits, nose, upper jaw, upper part of the pharynx, (iv.) SUB-MAXILLARY—the lower gums, lower part of the face, and front of the mouth and tongue, (v.) SUPRA-HYOID—anterior part of the tongue, chin and lower lip, (vi.) SUPERFICIAL CERVICAL—external ear, side of the head and neck, and face, (vii.) RETRO-PHARYNGEAL.—nasal fossæ and upper part of the pharynx, and (viii.) DEEP CERVICAL (*upper set*)—mouth, tonsils, palate, lower part of the pharynx, posterior part of tongue, nasal fossæ, interior of the skull, and deep parts of head and neck; (*lower set*)—lower part of neck, and joins the axillary and mediastinal glands.

45. Give in general the distribution of Lymphatic Glands of the Upper Extremity.

(i.) SUPRA-CONDYLOIDS—are distributed in three inner fingers, and (ii.) AXILLARY—upper extremity, dorsal and scapular regions, front and sides of the trunk and breast.

46. Give in general the distribution of Lymphatic Glands of the Lower Extremity.

(i.) ANTERIOR TIBIAL AND POPLITEAL—are distributed in the legs, (ii.) INGUINAL (femoral set) in the perinæum; (horizontal set) in the umbilicus, buttocks and genitals, (iii.) ILIAC—in the pelvic viscera, (iv.) LUMBARS—in the uterus, ovaries, testes, kidneys and (v.) SACRAL— in the rectum.

47. Describe Tubercular Adenitis.

Tubercular Adenitis is met with at all ages, but more common in children than in the adults. In it the submaxillary glands are first involved, which are frequently bilateral but larger on one side than on the other. Not only the submaxillary group, but the glands above the clavicle and in the posterior cervical triangle, may be involved. As they increase in size, individual tumors can be felt—whose surface is smooth and the consistence firm. They may remain isolated, but more commonly they form large knotted masses. They may be painful or tender, especially during the period, they increase in size. Most of the cases sooner or later undergo suppuration. The disease is frequently associated with coryza, eczema of the scalp, ear or lips and with Conjunctivitis and Keratitis. When the glands are large and grow actively there is fever. The subjects are usually anæmic, particularly if suppuration occur. The progress of this form of Adenitis is slow and tedious. Death is rare. In some instances, Tubercular Adenitis acts as a focus for general infection.

48. What classes of Lymphatic Enlargements we have in Syphilis?

IN THE PRIMARY SYPHILIS, closely following the initial sore the inguinal glands become enlarged.

WITH GENERAL INFECTION, numerous lymphatics throughout the body, but especially the supra-condyloid and the posterior cervical exhibit some degree of enlargement. They are rarely of large size and are freely movable beneath the skin.

In the late stages of Syphilis, the lymphatic glands of the affected parts enlarge.

Gummatous tumors of the lymphatic glands are the only form of great syphilitic enlargement of the lymphatic glands.

49. Give a description of Hodgkin's Disease.

HODGKIN'S DISEASE is a disease characterized by the universal or general enlargement of the lymphatic glands, with progressive Anæmia, fever of irregular curve and duration, and the enlargement of the spleen, the fundamental symptom being the enlargement of the lymphatic glands. It is first manifested only in the lymph nodes of the neck, but is soon followed by the involvement of the glandular structures of the axilla, thorax, abdomen and groins; the enlargement grows to a remarkable size, occurring about the internal organs such as, lungs, heart, stomach, intestines, gall-ducts, uterus, etc., produce dangerous symptoms, by interfering with their functions, by reason of the pressure exerted upon them. They are hard like stones, painless and exhibit no tendency to break down or suppurate. *The spleen also is enlarged*, but is usually not great—it occurs early in the course of the disease and is an important diagnostic symptom. Skin changes—distinctive.

THE TYPES OF HODGKIN'S DISEASE are ACUTE LOCAL, GENERAL and SPLENOMEGALIC.

50. What Tumors are found in the Glands?

LYMPHADENOMA. Syphilitic and Tubercular ADENITIS. Infective GRANULOMATA—Tuberculous, Syphilitic and Actino-mycotic. ADENOMATA. GOITRES —of the thyroid. MUMPS and PAROTITIS— of the parotid and sub-maxillary glands. TUMORS— of the pituitary and pineal glands. CANCER and SARCOMA— of the thyroid.

51. What Tumors and Enlargements are found about the Neck?

(i) The enlargement of the thyroid glands, commonly known as GOITRE, which exhibits itself as a tumor situated at the level of the thyroid cartilages and upper end of the trachea. (ii.) Inflammation and (iii.) swelling of the parotid and sub-maxillary glands, resulting in the formation of tumor known as PAROTITIS or MUMPS.

52. Outline the varieties of Enlargements of the Thyroid Gland.

(i.) ADENOMATA—simple or malignant.

(ii.) INFECTIVE GRANULOMATA—from Tuberculosis, Syphilis and Actino-mycosis.

(iii.) CANCER or SARCOMA—of the thyroid.

(iv.) GOITRE—Parenchymatous, cystic and exophthalmic.

53. Diagnose Goitre.

Goitres are readily differentiated from other enlargements of the neck by their upward movement during deglutition. In simple parenchymatous Goitre the enlargement or tumor is smooth and firm involving the whole or part of the thyroid gland. The cystic variety is globular in shape, with smooth surface, well-rounded outline and a sense of fluctuation if the walls are thin. The exophthalmic Goitre is firm and elastic to the touch and pulsations are plainly evident in it. In the last variety exophthalmos and rapid action of the heart (Tachy-cardia) are characteristics; tremor, excessive sweating, diminished electrical resistance of the tissues, œdema, polyuria, amenorrhœa and in the male—impotence constitute other symptoms of note. The pressure phenomena, if the enlargement is large, are present in all the varieties.

54. Give symptoms of Mumps.

The characteristic symptom of Mumps is the swelling of the parotid glands. The initial symptom is fever, which rarely rises above 101°F. with pain just below the ear on one side, where a slight swelling is noticed, which increases gradually, and within 48 hours there is great swelling of the neck and side of the cheek. The swelling is never indurated and boggy in palpation. The other side usually becomes affected within a couple of days and the whole neck is surrounded by a collar of doughy infiltration, and stiffness and pain make movements of the jaws difficult. There is a special liability to Orchitis in male and Mastitis in females. The swelling lasts for 8 to 10 days, from onset to resolution.

Occasionally the disease is very severe and characterized by high fever, delirium and great prostration.

55. Name some of the Physiological Discolorations of the Skin.

The color of the skin becomes *mnddy pale*—bordering on the sallow or ashy, in the old age. Poor constitution also produces changes in the color of the skin, disproportionate to the age. It becomes *"tan"* i. e., of brown or bright red appearance under the influence of an out-of-door life and *sunburnt* under the exposure to the sun's rays. Exposure to constant wind and storm also discolors the skin, not under covering of the clothing.

56. Give indications afforded by the Pallor of the Skin.

Pallor, which comes on suddenly and persists, especially if it is attended by symptoms of collapse, is indicative of internal *hæmorrhage*.

Pallor of gradual onset is certain evidence of bad health. When of a severe grade, it is suggestive of one of the forms of Anæmia or of a diathetic disorder.

57. Give indications afforded by the Increased Redness of the Skin.

Increased redness of the skin in the normal constitution suggests, sudden emotional changes, especially from anger.

In chronic ill-health, it suggests the unstability of the vaso-motor mechanism.

58. Give the Discoloration of Jaundice.

The color of the skin in Jaundice becomes *yellowish,* due to staining of the tissue by the bile. In mild cases, only a yellowish tinge is detected, while in the severe cases, it is intense and may be associated with a greenish hue.

59. Give varieties of Jaundice.

Jaundice is classified into the following varieties :—

(i.) Obstructive Jaundice. (ii.) Non-obstructive or the Toxic and Hæmolytic Jaundice. (iii.) Hereditary Icterus. (iv.) Icterus Neonatorum.

(v.) Icterus Gravis or the Malignant Jaundice or Acute Yellow Atrophy. (vi.) Emotional Jaundice.

60. Give symptoms and diagnosis of Addison's Disease.

SYMPTOMS.—The cardinal symptoms of Addison's Disease are—(i.) *Pigmentation of the skin*, which may be general or in patches, the grade of coloration ranging from a light yellow to a deep brown or even black; (ii.) *muscular and cardio-vascular asthenia*; and (iii.) the gastro-intestinal symptoms such as—nausea, vomiting, diarrhœa, anorexia, etc.

Pain in the back may be an early and important symptom.

DIAGNOSIS.— In the presence of the three cardinal symptoms as described above the diagnosis of Addison's disease is made promptly, but it is scarcely justifiable without the *asthenia*, which is the most characteristic feature of the disease. The occurrence of fainting fits, of gastric irritability are important indications. In doubtful cases, the causes of unusual pigmentation of the skin is sought for and a tuberculin test is made.

61. What changes in the skin are incident to Arsenical Poisoning?

ARSENIC may cause a most intense pigmentation of the skin, which may be local or general. In color, it may vary from a yellowish-brown tint to a deep bronze. As a general rule, wide diffusion of pigmentation usually presents light discoloration.

62. Name some diseases which cause a Pigmentation of the Skin.

Syphilis, Addison's Disease, Vagabonds' Disease, Exophthalmic Goitre, Pellagra, Arthritis Deformans, Cancer, benign tumors of the uterus and ovaries, chronic Interstitial Nephritis and Tuberculosis of the peritoneum.

63. Describe Syphilitic Pigmentation of the Skin.

A persistent pigmentation of the skin over the parts which have been the seat of eruptions or ulcerations is one of the features of Syphilis. In the primary stage, sometimes a slight pigmentation of the surface, persists for some time. In the secondary stage, the cicatrices are at first pigmented; later, assume a clear white tint.

CHAPTER XVIII.

THE NERVOUS SYSTEM.

1. Describe the method of eliciting the Knee-Jerk.

To elicit the KNEE-JERK, the leg to be experimented should be placed over the other and allowed to hang *perfectly limp and lifeless*, so that no involuntary rigidity is permitted to interfere with the reaction. The knees should be *bared*. A slight blow applied smartly on the patellar tendon causes a movement of the foot forwards i. e. the foot is suddenly jerked upwards. It is present in health.

2. Describe the method of eliciting the Ankle-Clonus.

The ANKLE-CLONUS is elicited by pressing the sole of the foot of the patient with the hand of the examiner—the heel resting on his knees and the limb slightly flexed at the knee-joint. A quick succession or clonic series of contractions is obtained if the pressure is kept up. This is a pathological condition.

3. Tell how to obtain a Knee-Jerk with the patient in bed.

The patient should lie on his back and the thigh is flexed at right angle with the body, with the knee nearly at right angle with the thigh, the foot remaining supported loosely in the palm of the examiner's hand, care being taken that the patient exerts no effort to maintain the limb in this position. A blow is then applied in the patellar tendon, as described in Q. 1 above; the knee-jerk then takes place.

4. In what diseases is the Knee-Jerk abolished?

The knee-jerk is abolished in disease or injury to the afferent nerve, efferent nerve or spinal gray matter. They are not obtained in Locomotor Ataxy and Infantile Paralysis.

5. What is the clinical significance of Increased Knee-Jerk?

It is significant of increased true reflex irritability, as in severance of brain from cord and in lateral sclerosis.

6. Describe the method of eliciting the Plantar Reflex.

It is excited by irritation of the sole of the foot, which produces movements of the foot and toe.

7. Describe the method of eliciting the Cremaster Reflex.

It is produced by irritation of the skin on the inside of the thighs; the resulting movement is sudden retraction of the testicle on the corresponding side.

8. Describe the method of eliciting the Gluteal Reflex.

It is produced by irritation af the skin over the buttock, which produces contraction of the glutei.

9. Describe the method of eliciting the Abdominal Reflex.

It is produced by irritation of the skin over the side of the abdomen on a line perpendicular to the nipple. The resulting movement is a contraction of the rectus muscle of the corresponding side.

10. Describe the method of eliciting the Epigastric Reflex.

It is produced by irritation of the side of the thorax on the line of the nipple. The resulting movement is a dimpling of the epigastrium.

11. In what diseases are the Superficial Reflexes abolished?

The superficial reflexes are abolished in—nerve injuries, Neuritic Paralysis, lesions of the spinal nerve-roots and Acute Anterior Poliomyelitis.

12. What is Hemiplegia?

When the one lateral half of the body is paralysed it is known as the Hemiplegia.

13. Describe the method used in determining the Loss in Motor Power.

The method used in determining the loss of motor power includes—an inspection of the affected parts while at rest or during attempts at voluntary motion; the resistance by the patient to passive motion; and the use of dynamometers.

14. What is Paralysis?

A complete loss or great diminution of the power of motion in one or in a number of voluntary muscles by reason of a lesion of the motor nervous apparatus.

15. What is Paraplegia?

Paralysis of the body, usually of the lower extremities, including the bladder and rectum and occasionally of the upper extremities. It may be of traumatic or congenital origin or due to the disease of the cord.

16. What is Monoplegia?

Paralysis of a single limb or a group of muscles is termed as Monoplegia.

17. What is the use of Dynamometer?

Dynamometer is used for measurement of the muscular strength and determining the existence of Paralysis in any part of the body. Its special value is found in enabling one to compare the strength of the paralyzed muscles from time to time.

18. Describe the Gait of Hemiplegia.

The affected leg is dragged after the other one has advanced, or is swung around in a semicircle when advanced.

19. Describe the Gait of Spastic Paraplegia.

In Spastic Paraplegia, i.e., in Paraplegia associated with rigidity of the paralyzed parts the limbs move as in one piece; the toes scrape the ground; owing to the spasm of the abductor muscles, the limbs are drawn in front of each other, or the toe of the advancing foot catches in the heel of the one in front.

20. Describe the Gait of Paraplegia.

When associated with flaccidity of the affected muscles peculiarities varying with the distribution of the Paralysis and the associated deformities will be observed. If there is weakness or loss of power of the anterior tibial group of muscles owing to alcoholic excesses the patient is unable to perform dorsal flexion of the feet; hence when walking, the feet droop, and the patient, lifts them high by making unusual flexion of the knee and hip, i.e., a high-stepping gait with dropped feet.

21. Describe the Ataxic Gait.

In the Ataxic Gait, in-co-ordination is marked and it interferes with walking.

22. Describe the Waddling Gait.

A waddling gait is observed in pseudo-hypertrophic Paralysis. The patient when walking raises his pelvis by the bending of the body towards the side of the affected limb. When standing, the patient tilts the pelvis markedly forwards.

23. Describe the In-co-ordination of Gait in Cerebellar Disease.

The in-co-ordination of Gait in cerebellar disease is of a reeling nature.

24. What is a Babinski's Sign?

Babinski's Sign is a modification of the plantar reflex.

25. Name the Superficial and Deep Reflexes.

Superficial Reflexes—Plantar, Gluteal, Cremaster, Abdominal, Epigastric and Scapular.

Deep Reflexes—Tendon Reflexes as Knee-jerk, Ankle-clonus and Triceps-jerk.

26. Name the different classes of Paralysis as to Location of the Lesion.

1. *Cerebral Paralyses* are of hemiplegic or monoplegic types—the lesion being within the cerebrum, peduncles, pons, or medulla.

2. *Spinal Paralyses* are of paraplegic types—the lesion being in the pyramidal tracts or motor cells of the anterior cornua.

3. *Peripheral Paralyses* are usually monoplegic in type—the lesion being along the course of one or more of the peripheral nerves.

27. Name the Lesions of Sudden Onset, causing Cerebral Paralysis.

i. *Traumatism.*—(a) Lacerations of brain subance or compression by depressed bone. (b) Meningeal or intracerebral hæmorrhages. (c) Inflammations—Cerebritis or Meningitis.

ii. *Hæmorrhages.*—(a) Meningeal—following blows or falls, Bright's disease, arterial degeneration of chronic alcoholism, syphilitic vascular disease, and in children from violent paroxysms of coughing. (b) Intra-cerebral—following miliary Aneurysms and vascular degenerations.

iii. *Vascular occlusions.*—(a) Thrombosis—arterial and venous. (b) Embolism—single or multiple.

28. Name the Lesions of slow Onset causing Cerebral Paralysis.

(i.) Tumors. (ii.) Exostoses. (iii.) Pachymeningitis Chronica. (iv.) Abscess. (v.) Disseminated and other types of Sclerosis. (vi.) Meningo-Encephalitis. (vii.) Syphilitic, Alcoholic and Senile Degenerations.

The last three are of very slow onset.

29. Give in detail the symptomatology of Complete Hemiplegia.

In Complete Hemiplegia the patient is unable to move a single muscle of the arm or leg and is obliged to lie in bed. The face is also involved on the same side as the arms and leg. Associated with the same there may be Paralysis of the tongue. If the patient attempts to take a deep breath, the chest on the affected side does not expand as freely as the healthy side. When Hemiplegia is of sudden onset it is often attended with loss of consciousness.

30. Give in detail the symptomatology of Paralysis from Cerebral Hæmorrhage.

Paralysis of the arm and leg of one side of the body; sometimes one side of the face is also paralysed. It may or may not be associated with unconsciousness. In those cases in which consciousness is not disturbed, the occurrence of Paralysis is easily recognized. The patient is usually restless, but, moves the limbs on one side of the body only. If the facial muscles are involved, there is a relaxation of the cheek in the paralyzed side. Relaxation and want of tonicity in the muscular system of the affected side; by instituting passive motions, the normal muscles always exhibit a certain degree of resistance, while the paralyzed ones not at all.

31. Give in detail symptomatology of Paralyses from Laceration of the Brain.

The symptoms come on immediately after the reception of the injury. Loss of consciousness is most prominent, profound disturbance of cerebral functions.

32. Give in detail the symptomatology of Apoplexy.

The premonitory symptoms, though of an indefinite character are—vertigo, mental and physical weakness, sensory disturbances, etc.

The onset is usually sudden and may or may not be associated with unconsciousness, the patient cannot be roused. The face is injected, sometimes cyanotic or of an ashen-gray hue. The pupils vary; usually they are dilated, sometimes unequal, and always—in deep coma, and inactive. The respirations are slow, noisy and accompanied with stertor—sometimes Cheyne-Stokes rhythm may be present. The cheeks are blown out during expiration, with spluttering of the lips. The pulse is usually full, slow and of increased tension. The temperature may be normal, but is often found sub-normal; in the course of a few hours it rises, ordinarily not higher than 103° F., or more, offering a very unfavorable prognosis. The urine and fæces are usually passed involuntarily. If the arm or leg is lifted it drops 'dead' on the affected side, while on the other it falls more slowly. Relaxation of the muscles of the affected side; rigidity may also be present. The head and eyes may be turned to one side.

In some cases, the onset is not so abrupt, the patient may not lose consciousness, but in course of a few hours there is loss of power (Paralysis), unconsciousness comes on gradually, and deepens into profound coma. The attack may occur during sleep—the patient may be found unconscious or wakes to find that the power is lost on one side.

33. Give in detail the symptomatology of Thrombosis (cerebral).

It is preceded by symptoms of general character resulting from the impoverished condition of the brain or from general malnutrition. Headache (early and very severe), vertigo, dullness of intellect, sensation of numbness and formication, gradually deepening coma, vomiting and convulsions are common. In the majority of cases the onset is gradual, several hours are required for a full development of the symptoms—the first manifestation being a gradually increasing Hemiplegia. Initial fall of the temperature, with subsequent rise.

34. Give in detail the symptomatology of Embolism (cererbal).

It is liable to occur in young subjects who have had Rheumatic Fever or some heart trouble generally a Mitral Stenosis. Its onset is sudden without any premonitory symptoms but sometimes with intense headache. In general, its symptoms are similar to those of cerebral hæmorrhage already described. Unconsciousness, Hemiplegia, or convulsions. Aphasia is especially frequent.

35. Give the causes of Brain Abscess.

The CAUSES of the Brain Abscess are—(i) *Traumatism*. (ii) *Diseases of the middle ear, mastoid cells, nasal passages* and *accessory sinuses*. (iii.)*Septic processes*, such as ulcerative Endocarditis, Localized bone disease, suppuration in the liver, certain inflammation of the lungs,—as metastitic condition and complication of Empyema. (iv.) *Tuberculosis*.

36. Diagnose Abscess of the Brain.

IN ACUTE CASES, the finding of the etiological factors is of highest importance. The history of the injury followed by fever, marked cerebral symptoms, the onset of rigors, delirium and perhaps Paralysis make the diagnosis certain.

The CHRONIC ABSCESSES offer greatest diagnostic difficulties. The symptoms resemble those of cerebral Tumor. If the petient have a history of trauma or localized lung or pleural trouble and suffered for weeks and months with slight headache or dizziness, the onset of a rapid fever, especially if it be intermittent or irregular and associated with rigors, intense headache and vomiting points strongly to the presence of intra-cranial suppuration. The lumbar puncture is important in the differentiation of Meningitis and also the pulse rate. The pulse is rapid in Meningitis, while slow in abscess, irrespective of temperature. The presence of a cause, normal or subnormal temperature point to the abscess rather than Meningitis or Thrombosis. The percussion of the skull may also aid to the diagnosis : the note which is normally dull, becomes much more resonant in the case of abscess.

37. Name the Spinal Paralyses of Slow Onset.

Progressive Muscular Atrophy. Subacute and chronic Poliomyelitis.

38. Name the Spinal Paralyses of Rapid Onset.

Paralyses from—(i.) fractures and dislocations of the vertebræ ; (ii.) punctured or gunshot wound of the spinal cord ; (iii.) meningeal hæmorrhage ; (iv.) intramedullary hæmorrhage ; and (v.) ischemia of the lumbar swelling of the cord.

39. Name the Spinal Paralyses associated with Muscular Atrophy.

Acute—Poliomyelitis Anterior.

Chronic—Chronic Poliomyelitis. Progressive Muscular Atrophy. Amyotrophic Lateral Sclerosis. Acute Descending Paralysis (Landry's Paralysis).

40. Name the Spinal Paralyses associated with Pains in the Extremities.

Locomotor Ataxia. Cervical Hypertrophic Meningitis. Malignant disease of the vertebræ. Tumors of the cord and meninges. Pachy-meningitis with vertebral caries.

41. Name the Spinal Paralyses not associated with early Atrophy or servere Pains.

Ataxic Paraplegia. Spastic Paraplegia. Disseminated Sclerosis. Diffuse Sclerosis. Acute Myelitis. Thrombotic Softening.

42. Give in detail the diagnosis of a case of Acute Poliomyelitis Anterior.

The Paralysis reaches its acme at once and makes no further progress. The paralyzed parts are flaccid. The deep and superficial reflexes are destroyed, some of the affected parts regain their activities, usually within 3 weeks, not infrequently within a few days, while the others remain permanently impaired. The reaction of degeneration is characteristic. The paralyzed muscles atrophy at an early period; the skin becomes cold and clammy and presents a bluish or mottled appearance.

43. Give in detail the diagnosis of a case of Chronic Poliomyelitis Anterior.

The Chronic Poliomyelitis Anterior—is of gradual onset and runs a rapid course; area of the Paralysis tends to increase from the beginning for sometime. The legs are affected first and the Paralysis iecreases gradually often implicating the arms at the same time. The affected muscles are flaccid and undergo atrophy: *reaction of degeneration*. The superficial and deep reflexes are destroyed. Fibrillary twitching almost always present. There is no loss of sensibility. Pains absent or very slight.

44. Give in detail the diagnosis of Spinal Progressive Muscular Atrophy.

Onset very slow. Wasting is the first feature and seems to be the immediate cause of the loss of power. Usually the muscles of the thumb are affected first and gradually the interossei and lumbricales. The affected muscles do not exhibit the reaction of degeneration. The deep and superficial reflexes are diminished only when the atrophy is profound. Fibrillary contractions. Muscles react to Faradism.

45. Give in detail the diagnosis of a case of Amyotrophic Lateral Sclerosis.

A disease of adult life. Paresis of the upper extremities—the first symptoms usually consist of numbness or formication in the fingers; then follow the motor weakness, with more or less rapidly progressive muscular atrophy. Twitchings and rigidities of these muscles precede the atrophy, and may amount to absolute contracture. Similar signs in the lower extremities with exaggeration of deep reflexes, in the second stage. The terminal stage is usually characterised by involvement of the muscles of the lips, tongue, pharynx and larynx and the mind is affected.

46. Diagnose giving symptomatology of Acute Ascending Paralysis.

The first sign is aching and soreness of the parts about to be paralyzed; then weakness in both lower extremities which increases rapidly, until the loss of power of the same is absolute. The area of the Paralysis increases from the first. After the feet, legs and the thighs are attacked and rendered functionless. Afterwards muscles of the trunk are involved followed by those of arms. It finally attacks the muscles of respiration and ends fatally.

The paralyzed muscles are flaccid, but rarely undergo any atrophy. No loss of knee-jerk and normal electrical reactions. Reaction of degeneration may be observed. The bladder and rectum retain their normal functions.

47. Diagnose giving symptomatology of Loco Motor Ataxia.

It runs a prolonged course which may be divided into three stages, viz., *preataxic stage, ataxic stage* and *paralytic stage* ; and exhibit a very large number of varied symptoms during its course. In the pre-ataxic stage the most important symptoms are lightning pains (at first slight but later assume a sharp, darting character, momentary in duration and of great severity), absent knee-jerks (decidedly suggestive), and certain eye-changes but notably pupillary disturbances (pupils react normally to accommodation but fail to respond to the stimulus of light—which is most diagnostic). Later, come the disturbance of gait. unsteadiness when the eyes are closed, the ocular paralyses, bladder and renal disturbances, etc.

In diagnosis the above symptoms are distinctive. In doubtful cases the Wasserman Reaction and a study of the spinal fluid are of great help.

48. Diagnose giving symptomatology of Spinal Meningitis.

The first symptom is a severe chill, associated with *pain iu the back* and sharp pain all over the body and *extremities*. Tenderness of the spine with spasm and *rigidity* of the muscles of the back, resulting in opisthotonos i.e., stiffness of the back and neck. As the disease progresses Paralysis develops, which may become complete. There may be constipation and retention of urine and fæces. In fatal cases, coma and delirium may precede death.

A *causative factor, pains in the back and extremities* and *rigidity* are the distinctive features in the diagnosis of Spinal Meningitis. *Kernig's sign* is very important, Lumbar puncture is also valuable, as it furnishes the nature of the infecting micro-organism.

49. Diagnose giving symptomalotogy of Ataxic Paraplegia.

Its onset is very slow. The trouble begins with tired feeling in the legs; an *unsteadiness of gait gradually develops* with progressive weakness and is a well-characterized feature. The patient finds himself unstable when standing with heels and toes approximated and eyes closed. The rigidity of the legs comes on slowly, but is rarely extreme. The sharp lancinating pains of ataxia are very exceptional, but *pain in the back* is frequent. *The reflexes are exaggerated from the very outset* and the ankle clonus is marked. The in-co-ordination may extend to the arm. All the symptoms gradually increase in intensity over a long period, until complete Paralysis finally develops, when the in-co-ordination becomes less prominent feature, and the rigidity of the paralyzed limbs appears. The sphincters—both vesical and rectal become usually involved. Sometimes mental disorders are observed late in the disease.

50. Diagnose, giving symptomatology of Spastic Paraplegia.

Its clinical feature is a progressive loss of power of the extremities, beginning with as a mere weakness or possibly as *stiffness* in the legs, developing into more or less complete Paralegia *with tonic spasm* and very *marked exaggeration of the deep and superficial reflexes*. Babinski reflex is present. The rigidity is specially prominent in the extensor muscles. Occasionally the patient complains of a dull aching pain in the back or in the calves. The spastic gait is characteristic. the disease is of slow onset always.

51. Diagnose, giving symptomatology of Disseminated Sclerosis.

As the pathological changes are scattered in foci of different sizes throughout the central nervous system, the symptomatology of the disease is quite varied and cannot be said to have a standard. It is characterized clinically by Paralysis, jerky tremor, eye symptoms (mainly Amblyopia, Nystagmus, and Diplopia), scanned speech, vertiginous sensations or other phenomena according to the distribution of the lesions. It runs a prolonged course, often marked by period of improvement. Prognosis highly unfavourable.

52. Give symptoms and diagnosis of Progressive Bulbar Paralysis.

The disease begins with slight defect in the speech and difficulty in pronouncing the dentals and linguals or by vocal fatigue indicating loss of power over the lips and tongue. Finally there is dysphagia. The Paralysis starts in the *tongue* and the superior lingual muscle undergoes atrophy and finally the mucous membrane is thrown into transverse folds. Fibrillary tumors are also seen in the process of wasting. Sometimes the symptoms appear on one side, but they may develop suddenly on both sides. Its Prognosis is absolutely unfavourable.

53. Give symptoms and diagnosis of Pseudo-Hypertrophic Paralysis.

The disease is of very slow onset and progress and is limited to certain ages from 4 to 20. The first sign of the malady is a tendency to fall from trifling causes. A peculiar "waddling gait" is observed next. Certain muscles, particulary those of the calves and shoulders present undue prominence, giving idea of strength, while others exhibit marked atrophy. Paresis, knee-jerk, and electrical reactions —normal in the early stage. No loss of sensibility. Pains absent or very slight.

54. Give symptoms and diagnosis of Juvenile Muscular Atrophy.

A disease of the early life—first manifestation in the muscles about the shoulders. The muscles of the upper arm become involved next (muscles of the forearm usually escape). Finally invades the lower extremities—the muscles of the hips and thighs sffected first. (The legs are affected late—may even escape entirely.) The peculiarities of gait and posture observed in Pseudo-Hepertrophic Paralysis are frequently present.

55. Give symptoms and diagnosis of Syringo-Myelia.

Clinical course and symptoms are varied. Its special symptoms are weakness and muscular wasting in the hands, loss of all forms of sensation, and painless whitlows in the fingers, with recurring deep ulcerations. Painlessness of the lesions and dissociation of the sensory phenomena constitute the characteristic symptoms upon which the diagnosis of Syringomyelia is based.

56. Give symptoms and diagnosis of Multiple Neuritis.

The most important groups of the Multiple or General Neuritis are—The Acute Polyneuritis, Recurring Multiple Neuritis, Alcoholic Neuritis, Multiple Neuritis in infectious diseases, the metallic poisons, and Endemic Neuritis.

Electrical condition—a loss of Faradic irritability and a marked decrease in Galvanic irritability of the muscles and nerves are important symptoms. Muscular *atrophy is present*, but does not take place until the *Paralysis* has become an obtrusive phenomenon and its diagnosis depends upon the grouping of the Paralysis, the presence of *insensibility* when sensory nerves are involved, and the presence of one of the *causes* of Neuritis. The value of anæsthesia as a diagnostic symptom is great. Pain may be present, but it is usually absent.

57. Give symptoms and diagnosis of Arthritic Muscular Atrophy.

It comes about as a result of joint disease, the muscles of the affected limb undergoing atrophy owing to the rest enforced upon them. The nerves also may be affected producing neuritis, manifesting its characteristic muscular atrophy with the typical reaction of degeneration.

58. Differentiate Cerebral and Spinal Palsies.

CEREBRAL PARALYSES—are usually of hemiplegic types i. e., limited to one lateral half of the body ; they may also invade one particular member when they are said to be MONOPLEGIC. They are associated with spasticity to some extent.

SPINAL PARALYSES—assume paraplegic types. Sensory disturbances is more severe on the opposite side to that in which the motor function is most disturbed. Some of them i. e., those dependent upon lesions of the motor-tract within the pyramidal tracts are associated with spasticity, while the others, having their origin in the motor-cells of the anterior cornua are characterized by flaccidity and atrophy of the functionless muscles.

59. Diagnose giving symptomatology of Freidrich's Ataxia.

It is of gradual onset and characterized by the development of an in-co-ordination, first in the lower extremities—the gait resembling more the gait of Alcoholic intoxication than of Loco Motor Ataxia, later extending to other portions of the body, *ulimately affecting the arms*, within a short time. The voluntary movements of the arms become irregular and jerky. Finally disturbances of speech and nystagmus develop.

60. Diagnose giving symptomatology of Acute Myelitis.

The patient first experiences a dragging or heaviness of the limbs, gradually increasing in intensity until it amounts to absolute Paralysis. Shortly after the motor weakness, *sensory disturbances* appear manifesting numbness and formication of the affected muscles which increase more or less rapidly to complete anæsthesia. *Trophic disturbance, Paralysis of the bladder and rectum, rapid wasting, electric changes,* and *fever* are characteristics. There is a girdle sensation at a point corresponding to the upper limit of the inflammation and above the same a band of hyperæsthesia—almost always present and also characteristic. Tendency to bed-sores on all parts exposed to pressure—early.

61. Diagnose giving symtomatology of Softening of the Cord from Thrombosis.

The symptoms of the thrombotic softening of the spinal cord are almost indistinguishable from those of Acute Myelitis. Etiological factors—atheroma and Syphilis play an important part in the diagnosis.

62. Describe the characteristics of a Post-Typhoid Neuritis.

Pain and Paralysis are the characteristics of Post-Typhoid Neuritis. The legs may be affected or the four extrmities. The Paralysis is of atrophic variety, and exhibits the reaction of degeneration.

63. Describe the characteristics of Arsenic Neuritis.

The prominence of the motor symptoms is the characteristic of Arsenical poisoning. The legs are more affected than the arms, particularly the extensors and peroneal group. Paralytic phenomenon most prominent feature.

64. Describe the characteristics of a Post Lead Neuritis.

It involves mainly the musculo-spiral nerves.

65. Describe the characteristics of Erbs' Palsy.

The patient cannot raise his arms at the shoulder, nor can he flex the forearm at the elbow; the movements of the wrists are unimpaired and the arm when flexed at the elbow can be extended by the unaffected triceps.

66. Describe the characteristics of complete Paralysis of the Arms and give the cause.

The plexor is involved in complete Paralysis of the arms. It is always traumatic in origin.

67. What is the Lesion producing "Winged Scapula"?

The Paralysis of the serratus magnus muscle.

68. What are the symptoms resulting from a Paralysis of the Circumflex?

Muscular atrophy; flattening of the shoulder; the patient cannot raise the arm at the shoulder.

69. What are the symptoms resulting from a Paralysis of the Musculo-spiral?

Weakness of grasp of the affected hand—inability to extend the hand and fingers. Slight formication and numbness.

70. What is the clinical significance of a "Double Wrist-Drop"?

Double musculo-spiral Palsy resulting from simultaneous injuries of both the nerves.

71. Name some of the Peripheral Palsies affecting the Lower Extremities.

Paralysis of the quadriceps extensor. Paralysis of the anterior crural nerve. Paralysis of the obturator nerve. Paralysis of the superior gluteal nerve. Paralysis of the gluteus maximus. Sciatic nerve Palsy. Paralysis of the tibius anticus, long extensor of the toes, the peronei, the extensor of the little toe (external popliteal or peroneal nerve). Paralysis of the internal popliteal and posterior tibial nerve. Paralysis of the external plantar nerve.

72. Describe Foot-Drop.

The foot-drop or dropped-foot is a manifestation of the loss of power of extension of the foot upon the leg and extension of the first phalanges of the toes, due to the Paralysis of the external popliteal or peroneal nerve.

73. What is Astrosia Abasia?

Motor in-co-ordination in standing and walking. It is not paralytic in character, but indicative of two separate and distinct conditions, viz., hysterical and and vertiginal. The hysterical one is easily distinguished by its association with the stigmata of hysteria —the patient is unable to walk or stand, and yet she is able to move her limbs perfectly when lying. In the other one, the patient when walking, will suddenly fall to the ground, often forward; it seems to him that his legs give way; when sitting, he will suddenly bend forward, his head dropping on the chest, and his body seems to lose its power of support; in either case, normal strength returns in a minute or two; there is never loss of consciousness.

74. Describe Multiple Neuritis affecting the Lower Extremities.

In Multiple Neuritis of Alcoholic origin, the Paralysis usually begins in the lower extremities; the extensors are affected more than the flexors and there is the characteristic condition known as the foot-drop. The affected muscles undergo atrophy and become flabby. When walking, the patient presents the characteristic "steppage gait."

75. What portions of the Nervops System is diseased in cases of Hemiplegia?

Cerebral portion.

76. What portion of the Nervous System is usually involved in cases of Paraplegia?

Spinal portion.

77. What portion of the Nervous System is usually involved in cases of Monoplegia?

Peripheral portion.

78. What is the clinical significance of a Paralysis arising from Injury in which there is a short interval of Comparative Health between the Time of the Injury and the Onset of Symptoms?

Meningeal hæmorrhage.

79. Describe the characteristics of the Organic Headache.

The main characteristic of organic headache is *the constancy of the pain.* Frequent associations of the organic headache are nausea and vomiting (with clean tongue), fever, delirium, and optic Neuritis.

80. Name some of the Diseases in which the Organic Headache occurs.

Tumor of the brain. Abscess of the brain. Meningitis. Hydrocephalus. Intra-cranial Hæmorrahage. Etc.

81. In which of the Brain Diseases the Headache is most prominent?

Meningitis.

82. What are the rules governing the relation between the Seat of the Pain and the Site of the Lesion in Oganic Headache?

There is no essential relationship between the location of pain and the side of the lesion. When the disease is limited strictly to the meninges, the pain is almost invariably present over the seat of the lesion—further removed from the meninges the given lesions are, the less likely the pain is a guide as to its locality.

83. Name the varieties of Circulatory Headaches.

Congestive headache and Anæmic headache.

84. Differentiate Congestive and Anæmic Headaches.

CONGESTIVE HEADACHE.—It is usually associated with marked throbbing of the blood-vessels of the head and neck, and suffusion of the face. The action of the heart is greatly accelerated. The mental condition is one of irritability. The patients' sufferings are aggravated by the recumbent posture, and by repeated acts of coughing.

ANAEMIC HEADACHE.—The pain is usually symmetrical, and situated in the vertex, sometimes immediately at the back of the orbit. Aggravated after hæmorrhage, greatly releved by lying down. The characteristic anæmic cardiac murmur is present.

85. Name some of the Toxic Causes of Headache.

Syphilis. Diabetes. Malaria. Septicæmia. Uræmia. Rheumatism. Lithæmia. Etc.

86. Name the special features of the Rheumatic Headache.

The rheumatic headaches are especially apt to be associated with soreness of the scalp, and are aggravated during spells of damp or cold weather. They are usually of a dull, heavy, aching character.

87. Name the special features of the Malarial Headache.

The special feature of the Malarial headache is its *periodicity*—comes on at a fixed hour every day or every other day. They are usually situated near one or the other supra-orbital foraman.

88. Name the special features of the Syphilitic Headache.

The special features of the Syphilitic Headache are its *severity* and nocturnal aggravation. The pains are boring and splitting and there is considerable tenderness of the scalp.

89. Name the Organs which may produce Reflex Headaches.

Eyes. Ears. Nose and Throat. Intestinal tract. Sexual organs.

90. What condition of the Eyes is specially liable to lead to Headache?

Errors in refraction.

91. What is the usual situation of the so-called Headache from diseases of the Female Sexual Organs?

Usual situation of the so-called headache from diseases of the female sexual organs is almost invariably situated in the vertex or in the occiput.

92. What do you understand by the term "Neuropathic" Headaches?

Headaches originated from the diseases of the nervous system, such as, Epilepsy, Hysteria, Neurasthenia, etc., are termed neuropathic headaches.

93. Define Tremor.

Tremor is an involuntary trembling or agitation of the body, or some portion of it caused by more or less rhythmical alternate contractions and relaxations of the antagonistic muscles.

94. Describe the Asthenic Tremor.

The tremulous movements occurring during the course of diseases other than those of the nervous system are of the asthenic variety. They are significants of extreme debitily present.

95. Under what circumstances are the Asthenic Tremors observed?

It is observed after prostrating diseases and after hæmorrhages and sexual excesses.

96. Describe the Senile Tremors.

Senile tremors are tremulousness during muscular movements in the old age. Always fine tremors, which begin in the hands and often extend to the muscles of the neck, causing slight movements of the head. The tremulous parts are affected with a peculiar rigidity.

97. Describe the Tremor from Alcohol.

The Alcoholic tremor is usually noticed in the arms, face and tongue and is often associated with local muscular twitchings. It is very prominent owing to the restlessness of the Alcoholic subjects. It is usually worse in the morning and is promptly relieved by a drink of Whiskey. It recurs only on movement.

98. Describe the Tobacco Tremor.

Tobacco tremor is of a very fine character and is due to excessive smoking in the old age.

99. Describe the Tremor of the Paralysis Agitans.

The tremor of the Paralysis Agitans may be noticeable in the four extremities or confined to hands or feet. In the early stage of the disease the tremor is observed only when the affected part is at rest, though it ceases during sleep, any attempt at a voluntary movement may check the tremor, but it returns with increased intensity. Any emotion exaggerates the movement.

100. Describe the Tremor of Disseminated Sclerosis.

The tremor of Disseminated (or Multiple) Sclerosis is *jerky* in character and is one of the important symptoms. It consists of irregular movements or rapid oscillations of a part during any voluntary motion, which ceases when the patient is at rest.

101. Name the Toxic causes of Tremors.

The toxic causes of tremors are—
Tobacco. Tea, Coffee, etc. Lead. Mercury. Chloral. Opium. Alcohol. Uræmia.

102. What is the significance of sudden onset as applied to Paralysis?

It signifies that the lesion must be either traumatic or circulatory in origin.

103. Define Spasm.

Spasm is used to indicate convulsive muscular contractions or movements which involve a limited portion of the body.

104. Define Convulsions.

The convulsion is a nervous disorder characterized by more or less widespread muscular contractions and relaxations in rapid alteration or by prolonged muscular contractions attended with loss of voluntary control of muscles.

105. Define Tonic Spasm.

A tonic spasm is one characterized by prolonged or sustained muscular contractions. It is a spasm characterized by rigidity.

106. Define Clonic Spasm.

A clonic spasm is one characterized by alternate contractions and relaxations.

107. Describe the Epileptiform Convulsions.

Localized convulsions, occurring usually without loss of consciousness are known as Epileptiform convulsions. Their essential features are: the tonic followed by clonic convulsions. The paroxysms may be preceded by a localized sensation known as the *aura*. They may occur in Epilepsy, Hysteria, organic disease of the brain, certain blood states, as uræmia, lithæmia, etc., and from reflex irritation.

108. What diseases are characterized by Epileptiform Convulsions?

See Ans. to the previous Question (Q. 107). Convulsions of this nature suggest the presence of the lesion in the cortical motor areas.

It is always confined to one-half portion of the body and not attended by loss of consciousness. It may be succeeded by Paralysis of the convulsed parts.

109. What is a Hysteroid Convulsion?

Paroxysm of *co-ordinated* convulsive movement with hysterical symptoms is known as a Hysteroid convulsion.

110. What conditions are characterized by Hysteroid Convulsions?

1. Various organic diseases of the brain. 2. Epilepsy. 3. Hydrophobia. 4. Various organic and toxæmic states in individuals of Hysterical temperament.

111. Describe the Jacksonian Epilepsy.

Epileptiform convulsions are known as Jacksonian or cortical Epilepsy. See Ans to Q. 107.

112. What are the usual causes of Epileptiform Spasms in young Children?

Organic diseases of the brain. From reflex irritation. Dentition.

113. What is Habit Spasm?

Half-voluntary spasmodic movements, the results of habit are known as the Habit Spasms. E.g., winking of the eyelids, jerking of the face, etc.

114. Describe Choreic Movements.

Choreic movements are irregular involuntary movements of the voluntary muscles, occurring both during rest and attempts at motion. They interfere with the accuracy of the voluntary movements and may be described in a single word: "Restlessness."

115. What is Hemianæsthesia?

Partial or complete loss of the sense of feeling in a lateral half of the body is known as Hemianæsthesia.

When there is anæsthesia of one-half of the face and of the opposite side of the body it is known as alternate Hemianæsthesia.

116. What is Paranæsthesia?

When the loss of sensation is limited to the lower extremities, it is known as Paranæsthesia.

117. What is Monoanæsthesia?

When the loss of sensation is limited to one part of the body, it is known as Monoanæsthesia.

118. What is Paræsthesia? What is its Clinical Significance?

When the sensation is perverted or altered, it is known as Paræsthesia. It is symptomatic of some organic or functional disorder.

119. Name the conditions which may be accompanied by Convulsions.

Epilepsy. Hysteria. Organic disease of the brain. Reflex irritation. Toxic conditions, such as Uræmia, Lithæmia, etc. Tetanus. Tetany. Strychnia poisoning.

120. Describe the Convulsions of Epilepsy.

The convulsions of Epilepsy are paroxysmal and consist of tonic and clonic spasms and associated with *unconsciousness*. The duration of the convulsive period is short, and spasms *jerky*.

See also Ans. to Qs. 107 and 108.

121. Describe the Convulsions of Hysteria.

The convulsions of Hysteria consist of tonic or clonic spasms and co-ordinated movements, simulating voluntary movements which may be described as "struggling", repeated with utmost irregularity.

See also Ans. to Qs. 109, 110.

122. Describe the Convulsions of Organic Brain Disease.

The typical convulsions of the organic brain disease are of the so-called Jacksonian type. Between the seizures there is a history of headache, vomiting, optic Neuritis, vertigo, and other symptoms of cerebral disease.

See also Ans. to Qs. 107 and 111.

123. Describe the Convulsions of Reflex Irritation.

The convulsions of reflex irritation closely simulate those of Epilepsy, but their onset is not so sudden and unconsciousness not so profound. Their duration are indefinite and are apt to be followed by others in quick succession. Reflex convulsions nearly always give a history which points out the seat of causative irritation.

124. Describe the Convulsions of Toxic Conditions.

The convulsions produced by the various toxic conditions also closely simulate those Epilepsy, with the only difference that their duration are more prolonged.

125. Differentiate Hysteria from Epilepsy.

HYSTERIA.	CONDITION	EPILEPSY.
Emotional disturbance.	— Cause —	Absent.
Palpitation, malaise, choking, bilateral foot aura.	— Premonitory Symptoms —	Unilateral or epigastric aura.

HYSTERIA.	CONDITION	EPILEPSY.
Often gradual.	— Onset —	Sudden.
At the onset.	— Scream —	During seizure.
Active.	— Eyes —	Pupils dilated and fixed.
Partially retained.	—Consciousness—	Immediately lost.
Rigidity or "Struggling"; throws limbs and head about.	—Convulsion—	Rigidity, followed by "Jerking," rarely rigidity alone.
Nil.	— Mouth —	Frothing.
Lips, hands and more often, other people or things.	— Biting —	Tongue.
Never.	—Micturition—	Frequent.
Normal.	—Temperature—	Elevated.
Never.	—Defecation—	Occasional.
Often half an hour or several hours.	— Duration —	A few minutes.
To control violence.	— Restraint —	To prevent accident.
Spontaneous or artificial.	—Termination—	Spontaneous.

126. What are the Tetanic Convulsions and in what conditions are they found?

Tetanic convulsions are consisted of tonic spasms, the only characteristic feature of them being extreme rigidity of the body. They are found in Tetanus, Hysteria, Strychnia poisoning and Tetany.

127. Give some instances of Local Spasms.
Athetosis. Jerkings. Twitchings. Etc.

128. In what conditions the Local Spasms are found?

The local spasms are found in—
1. Organic diseases of the brain. 2. Hysteria.
3. Habit-spasm. 4. Cerebral and Spinal Menin-

gitis. 5. Various occupation neuroses. 6. From reflex irritation.

129. Give the "Stigmata" of Hysteria.

The hysterical stigmata are observed in the inter-paroxysmal period. Prominent among them is the *mental condition*—the characteristic *Hysterical temperament*. Sensory distubances are usually par- and hyperæsthesia, less frequently anæsthesia. Disturbances of taste and smell. More or less headache. Pains which may affect any or all portions of the body. Hysterical Paralysis. Hysterical spasms. Tremor. Etc.

130. Describe the condition known as the "Convulsive Tic."

The condition characterized by sudden arrhythmic and involuntary contractions of muscles is known as the CONVULSIVE TIC. The movements are first noticed in the muscles of the face which may extend to any portion of the body; later speech is involved. Finally the mind is involved and the patient turned insane usually. The patients exhibit a remarkable tendency to imitate.

131. In what conditions may we have Opisthotonos as a Symptom?

Opisthotonos may occur in Tetanus, Strychnia poisoning, spinal Meningitis and Uræmia.

132. In what diseases are Choreic Movements found?

Choreic movements are found in Chorea, Hysteria, organic cerebro spinal diseases and reflex irritation.

133. What is Athetosis?

Athetosis or the mobile spasm is characterized by involuntary movements of the fingers and toes, and inability to keep them still. It is due to some lesion or functional derangement of the brain or spinal cord and especially liable to occur in Spastic Hemiplegias and Diplegias of infancy.

134. Describe Huntingdon's Chorea.

It is a hereditary disease, resembling in character chorea of childhood, occurring in the *adult life*, generally between the ages 30 to 50. The choreic movements begin gradually in the upper half of the body and slowly increase in distribution and intensity. The eye-balls are often affected, and the mental condition is very frequently impaired. It runs a very chronic course and is essentially incurable.

135. Describe Huntingdon's Senile Chorea.

It attacks people of advanced ages. The movements are especially liable to affect the upper part of the body, particularly the face and tongue interfering seriously with articulation. The mind remains unaffected. The presence of strangers and unusual excitement aggravates. The patient is quiet during sleep and the general health is not impaired.

136. Describe Huntingdon's Post-Hemiplegic Chorea.

It follows the attacks of Hemiplegia and the movements are limited to the affected extremities, simulating closely typical chorea. In the vast majority of cases it is associated with Hemianæsthesia, especially in its early stages. Sometimes there is associated an in-co-ordination varying from slight instability to pronounced ataxia.

137. Rigidities may occur in what Diseases?

Rigidities may occur in cerebral affections, spinal affections, diseases and lesions of the peripheral nerves, functional nervous disorders and joint affections.

138. What Spinal Cord Affections are associated with Rigidity?

Acute Myelitis. Acute Meningitis. Chronic Meningitis. Scrofulous Pachy-meningitis from vertebral caries. Meningeal hæmorrhage. Spastic Paraplegia. Amyotrophic Lateral Sclerosis. Bulbar Paralysis. Tumor of the spinal cord. Disseminated Sclerosis.

139. How do you examine the Tactile Sense?

The tactile sense or the sense of touch may be tested by writing on the skin with a hard-pointed instrument, with the patient blind-folded, to preclude his vision from making up for any deficient sensibility. Acuteness of the sensation, is verified by the recognition of the smaller character of the types written. Or, it may be tested by drawing a tuft of cotton or a camel-hair brush over the suspected area: the sensation is intact if the patient perceives the touch, disturbed if he does not.

140. How do you examine the Temperature Sense?

The temperature sense is conducted by applying two test-tubes containing hot and cold water in irregular alternation to the surface of the body.

141. How do you examine the Pain Sense?

The pain sense may be tested by pinching a fold of skin, or by pricking with a needle or by the application of a Faradic brush.

142. How do you examine the Muscular Sense?

The muscular sense is determined by the ability of the patient to recognize weights.

143. What Peripheral Nervous Affections are capable of producing Anæsthesia?

Simple Neuritis. Multiple Neuritis. Herpes Zoster.

144. Peripheral Anæsthesia may be symptomatic of what conditions?

It may occur as a symptom of—

(i.) Exposure to cold. (ii.) Defective circulation. (iii.) Excessive indulgence in tea. (iv.) Leprosy. (v.) Changes in the cutaneous structures. (vi.) The various acroparæsthesiæ.

145. Diagnose a Simple Neuritis.

To diagnose a Simple Neuritis main reliance is placed on its characteristic symptoms, *pain*, with tenderness, *weakness*, *anæsthesia* and *paræsthesia* of the area supplied by the affected nerve. Etiology also is taken in account. The character of the pain is steady, and is of a boring or stabbing character.

146. Diagnose a Multiple Neuritis.

See Ans. to Q. 56 of this Chapter.

147. Diagnose a Post-Typhoid Neuritis.

See Ans. to Q. 62 of this Chapter.

148. Diagnose a Post-Alcoholic Neuritis.

In a post-Alcocolic Neuritis the combination of "*wrist-drop*" and "*foot-drop*" with congestion of the hands and feet is quite characteristic. Among the most striking features are most peculiar and almost characteristic *mental disorder* and *delirium*—the patient loses all appreciation of time and place, and describes with circumstantial details long journeys which he says, he has recently undertaken, or tells of persons whom he has just seen. The previous history of the patient is important.

149. Diagnose an Arsenical Neuritis.

See Ans. to Q. 64 of this Chapter.

150. Diagnose a Beri-Beri.

To diagnose a Beri Beri, its special phase a Neuritis, should be kept in mind. The types of the disease give the idea as to symptomatology. It often sets in with catarrhal symptoms, followed by pains and weakness in the limbs and lowering of the sensibility in the legs, with the occurrence of paræsthesia. The *atrophic* types display the features of an Acute Multiple Neuritis with severe pains and muscular weakness succeeded by atrophic Paralysis. In the *hydrophic* types in addition to Neuritis, the œdema soon becomes the most marked feature with cardiac Dropsy. The *pernicious* types are characterized by the symptoms of the foregoing, pursuing a rapidly fatal course with cardiac break-down.

151. Diagnose an Influenzial Neuritis.

Influenzial Neuritis involves various cranial and spinal nerves and is more likely to appear as a sequel than during the illness. All forms are not uncommon and in some cases are characterized by marked disturbance of motion and sensation. There may be severe pain or more or less widely distributed Paralysis.

152. Anæsthesia of the Throat may be due to What?

Anæsthesia of the throat may be due to functional or hysterical origin and occurs in—(i.) Hysteria. (ii.) Post-diphtheritic Paralysis. (iii.) Bulbar Paralysis. (iv.) As part of Hemianæsthesia.

153. Anæsthesia of the Rectum may be due to What?

Rectal anæsthesia also may be due to functional or hysterical origin and may occur in—

(i.) Hysteria. (ii.) Loco Motor Ataxia and other affections of the spinal cord. (iii.) Widespread cerebral degeneration.

154. General Hyperæsthesia occurs in What Conditions?

It may occur in—

(i.) Hysteria. (ii.) Hydrophobia. (iii.) Cerebrospinal fever.

155. Hemi-hyperæsthesia occurs in What Conditions?

It may occur in—
(i.) Hysteria. (ii.) Disease of the Pons Varolii.

156. Name some of the causes of the "Bearing Down" Sensation.

Some of the causes of the "bearing down" sensations are—
(i.) Diseases or conditions affecting the uterus, especially membranous Dysmenorrhœa. (ii.) Hæmorrhoids. (iii.) Undue fullness of the bladder. (iv.) Prolonged standing.

157. Name some of the causes of "Cold and Chilly" Sensation, in the Normal or Sub-Normal Temperature.

COLDNESS may be due to Hysteria, Lateral Sclerosis, Myxœdema, Neurasthenia or Syringo-myelia.

CHILLINESS may be a prodromal symptom of an attack of migraine.

158. Name some of the causes of the Sensation of Faintness.

It may be present as an accompaniment of—
The various forms of Anæmia, Angina Pectoris, Fatty Degeneration of the heart, Thrombosis of the pulmonary artery, Pneumothorax, thoracic Aneurysm, Ascites, cardiac neuroses, flatulent distension of the stomach and intestines; it may be present as the result of emotion, fatigue, excessive heat, painful affections, depressing poisons, and as evidence of shock after injuries; some women experience faintness from the fœtal movements during pregnancy.

159. Describe the Girdle Sensation.

The GIRDLE SENSATION is a sensation as though a band had been tied around the pelvis or one of the limbs. It is a symptom of affections of the spinal cord and may be found in Loco Motor Ataxia, Chronic Myelitis, injury or tumor of the spinal cord, and inflammation or tumor of the spinal meninges, and in some cases of spinal Sclerosis.

After prolonged vomiting or repeated paroxysms of violent cough a similar sensation may be felt, corresponding to the insertion of the diaphragm, and due to a strain of that muscle.

160. Give some of the causes of Numbness and Tingling.

(i.) NUMBNESS AND TINGLING IN THE FEET—

Loco Motor Ataxia, Myelitis, and Chronic Spinal Meningitis.

(ii.) IN THE FINGERS AND TOES—

Arthritis Deformans and Tetany.

(iii.) In the fingers and occasionally in scalp and feet—Acro-paresthesia.

(iv.) Certain poisons may also cause numbness.

161. Name some of the causes of Pain.

Neuralgia. Neuritis. Diseases of the spinal cord. Reflex pains. Pains from various toxæmiæ. Rheumatism. Gout. Hysteria. Anæmia.

162. Describe the Pain of Neuralgia.

The pain of Neuralgia is not constant, but paroxysmal, and may be described as stabbing, burning or darting in character. The skin may be exquisitely tender in the affected parts. Before the onset of the pain there may be uneasy sensations, sometimes tingling in the part which will be affected.

163. Describe the Pain of Neuritis

The *pain* is the most important symptom of *Neuritis*. It is of a boring and stabbing character and is usually felt along the course of the nerve and in the parts in which the nerve is distributed. The nerve itself is sensitive to pressure. It is often intensified at night and by changes in weather to cold or damp.

164. Describe the Pain of Spinal Cord Disease.

Pains originated from spinal cord disease manifest themselves either as *backache* or *spinal irritation* or *peripheral* or *eccentric pains*. The first two may occur from a great variety of other affections. Organic spinal pains are especially liable to occur in conjunction with Meningitis and disease of the vertebræ; in the former as sensitiveness over the bones themselves and in the latter between the vertebræ which become more severe when arising from malignant disease of the bones or meninges.

The *eccentric* or *peripheral pains* may arise (i.) from irritation of the sensory nerve-roots and (ii.) from irritation of the sensory conducting tracts in the cord itself They are almost always bilateral and symmetrical. The pains arising from the former are often of a severe darting character, while those from the latter are generally dull in character and are apt to be confounded with the pains of rheumatism.

The *girdle sensations* around the waist or trunk are also manifestations of a very eharacteristic pain accompanying spinal diseases. (See Ans. to Q. 159 of this Chapter.)

165. Describe the Pains of Spinal Cord from Reflex Conditions.

The pains of spinal cord from reflex conditions are—

(i.) Pain over the fourth and fifth dorsal vertebræ—from disease of the stomach, especially however from gastric ulcer. (ii,) Pain over the 7th to 9th dorsal vertebræ—from diseases of the colon. (iii.) Pain over the last dorsal and all the lumbnr vertebræ—from uterine diseases.

166. Describe the Pains of Spinal Cord from Toxic Causes.

The toxic causes of spinal pains are some acute infectious diseases as Typhoid Fever, Small-pox, etc.

Follicular Tonsillitis. Malaria, Syphilis, Diabetes. Uræmia and Lithæmia.

167. Describe the Pains of Spinal Cord from Hysteria.

Pain in the spinal cord is practically present in every hysterical subject, with great sensitiveness to touch, limited to particular regions of the spine. The pain is sometimes spontaneous, while in others occurs only when evoked by pressure; it may be limited to the spinal processes, or it may be diffused laterally into the muscles.

The so-called sensitive spine is generally associated with hysterical Neuralgia which occurs in neurotic subjects.

168. Describe the Pains of Rheumatism and Gout.

The pains of Rheumatism and Gout are for the most part fixed.

See also Ans. to Qs. 31, 32 and 33, of Chap. XVII.

169. Name some of the causes of Sharp Pains.

Angina Pectoris. Appendicitis. Dissecting Aneurysm. Ectopic gestation. Gout. Pleurisy. Pneumothorax. Spinal Hæmorrhage. Acute inflammations of serous membranes.

170. Name some of the causes of Dull Pains.

Chronic inflammation of serous membranes. Inflammations of mucous membranes and visceral parenchyma.

171. Name some Causes of Paroxysmal Pains.

Angina Pectoris, Aneurysm, Appendicitis, Colic, cerebral tumors, distended bladder, Dysentery, Dysmenorrhœa, Floating Kidney, Lead Colic, Lumbricci, Loco Motor Ataxia, Neuralgia, parturition, renal calculus, Cholera, strangulated Hernia, etc.

172. Name some causes of Radiating Pains.

Acute Aortitis. Angina Pectoris. Aneurysm. Atony of the Stomach. Caries or contraction of the spine. Gastritis. Hepatic Colic. Hip-joint disease. Neuralgia. Renal Calculus. Spinal hæmorrhage. Spinal Meningitis. Uterine Fibroids. Vesical Calculus. Etc.

173. Name some causes of Shifting Pains.

Flatulence, Hysteria, Loco Motor Ataxia, Spinal cord tumor. Tape-worm. Trichinosis.

174. Name some causes of Gnawing Pains.

Abdominal aneurysm. Caries of the spine. Cancer of the stomach. Descending thoracic Aneurysm. Gout. Lithæmia. Periostitis. Spinal Meningitis.

175. Name some causes of Pain increased by Motion.

Acute inflammatory diseases. Abscess. Caries of the spine. Fractures. Gout. Glandular Fever. Lumbago. Neuritis. Oophoritis. External and internal Pachy-meningitis. Peri-Nephritis. Acute Pleurisy. Pneumonia. Pleurodynia. Acute Rheumatism. Sciatic Neuritis. Spinal Meningitis. Spinal cord tumor. Salpingitis. Weil's disease.

176. Name some of the causes of Pain increased at Night.

Loco Motor Ataxia. Neuritis. Osteitis. Periosteitis. Renal Calculus. Rheumatism. Syphilis.

177. Name all the causes of Pain in the Face.

Disorders of the teeth. Facial Neuritis. Tic Douloureux. Diseases of the ears. Disease of the accessory nasal sinuses.

178. Describe the Pain of Facial Neuralgia.

The pain of facial neuralgia is of sudden onset, usually of a sharp, darting character, and is paroxysmal, which may recur, usually not lasting more than

2 minutes. These attacks may recur every few minutes or they may be long in their return. They may be caused from inflammation of one or more branches of the trigeminus and brought about by exposure to cold, especially to direct draughts of cold winds on the face. If of the fifth nerve, it is called Tic Douloureux or Prosopalgia.

179. Describe the Pain of Disease of the Middle Ear.

The diseases which cause pain in the middle ear are acute catarrhal and acute purulent Otitis Media. In acute catarrhal cases, though the pains sometimes may be of darting character usually are not severe, neither they are always present; they are aggravated during coughing, sneezing and eructations. In the acute purulent cases the pains are severe and are usually continuous, and may be attended with secondary fever and brain symptoms.

180. Describe the Pain of Tic Douloureux.

See Ans. to Q. 178 above.

181. Describe the Pain of Angina Pectoris.

See Ans. to Q. 57 of Chap. XII.

182. Describe the Pain of Brachial Neuritis.

The *pain in the arm* is the prominent symptomatic feature of Brachial Neuritis and follows the course of the nerves. When the attack is mild, the pain instead of being continuous, is diffused. Motor symptoms are usually absent.

183. Describe the Pain of Erythromelalgia.

The pain of Erythromelalgia may be of dull, heavy or it may be of a atrocious nature, affecting the extremities more often of the feet than the hands and is associated with *great redness* of the parts. In extreme cases, the pain may be constant. It is usually relieved by cool weather. It is worse in summer or when the parts are made to hang down. May be associated with flushing and local fever.

184. Describe the Pain of Phlegmasia Alba Dolens.

The pain is situated in one or both legs and is associated with swelling and white discoloration of the parts. More or less diffuse soreness is always present.

185. What do the so-called "Growing Pains" of Children indicate?

They are regarded as muscular expressions of rheumatism.

186. Name some of the causes of Pain in the Feet.

Rheumatism. Corns and Bunions. Badly-fitting shoes and stockings. Morton's Disease. Tarsalgia. Reflex pains from diseases of the genito-urinary tract. Neurasthenia.

187. What is Morton's Disease

It is a form of Neuralgia affecting the foot, the pain of which starts at the base of the fourth toe, and is aggravated by lateral pressure in the foot.

188. Name the causes of Backache, Intra-spinal.

The causes of the intra-spinal backache are—

Cerebro-spinal Meningitis. Spinal Pachymeningitis. Internal spinal Meningitis. Myelitis. Syringo-myelia. Tumor of the spinal cord. Hæmorrhage into the cord or meninges.

189. Name the causes of Backache, Vertebral.

Caries of the vertebræ. Cancer of the vertebræ. Arthritis Deformans. Sacro-iliac disease.

190. Name the causes of Backache, Intrathoracic.

Aneurysm of the Aorta. Mediastinal tumors. Œsophageal disease.

191. Name the causes of Backache, Local.

Muscular (Myalgia or Lumbago). Arterial. Lumbar Abscess.

192. What Constitutional Diseases may produce Backache?

Hysteria. Neurasthenia. Acute Infectious diseases. Anæmia of all kinds. Sexual excesses or bad sexual hygiene.

193. Name some of the causes of Backache, Intra-abdominal.

Renal (as in Acute Nephritis, Calculus, etc.). Hepatic (as in Cancer of liver, Lithæmia, Floating Liver). Gastric (as in ulcer, atonic Dyspepsia, Gastritis, gastric neuroses, flatulence). Pelvic (as in Cystitis, diseases of the female genital organs, prostate, rectum and anus). Intestinal (as in indigestion, Tympanites, constipation). Miscellaneous (as in Aneurysm of the abdominal aorta, Appendicitis, and abdominal tumors).

194. What is the meaning of the word Coma?

Abnormally deep or prolonged sleep or a state of unconsciousness from which the patient can be but partially, if at all, aroused.

195. What is the meaning of the word Stupor?

The word stupor means—suspension of sense, either complete or partial.

196. What is the meaning of the words Coma Vigil?

The words COMA VIGIL means a comatose condition in which the patient lies with open eyes, but unconscious and delirious.

Chap. XVIII.]   THE NERVOUS SYSTEM   299

197. Coma is symptomatic of What Conditions?

Coma is symptomatic of—

Cerebral traumatism Apoplexy. Cerebral Embolism and Thrombosis. Cerebral tumor. Cerebral abscess. Cerebral Meningitis. General Paralysis of the Insane. Epilepsy. Narcotic poisonings. Sunstroke. Uræmia. Diabetes Mellitus. Syphilis. Malaria. Cholæmia. Acute Yellow Atrophy of the Liver. Acute infectious diseases of the foudroyant type. Exhaustion in the course of acute diseases. Dyspepsia. Obesity. Narcolepsy. Hysteria. Syncope. In the initial stages of some cases of Insanity. Cerebral malnutrition from weakened heart and degenerated arteries in the old age.

198. Describe the Coma incident to Cerebral Traumatism.

The coma incident cerebral traumatism occurs in compression of the brain from fractured skull, meningeal hæmorrhage, intra-cerebral hæmorrhage, laceration of brain substance, and intra-cranial inflammations. To determine the traumatic origin of the coma, the objective signs of injury as contusions or lacerated wounds of the scalp, bleeding from the ear, etc., and the absence of a history of other possible causes are usually taken into account.

199. Describe the Coma incident to Idiopathic Cerebral Hæmorrhage (Apoplexy).

The coma incident to Apoplexy is attended by stertorous breathing and other allied symptoms described in Ans. to Q. 32 of this Chapter.

200. Describe the Coma incident to Cerebral Tumor.

The coma incident to cerebral tumor may occur as a paroxysmal symptom (usually in association with or as a sequence of a convulsive seizure), or a terminal phenomena.

201. Describe the Coma incident to Cerebral Abscess.

To determine the origin of the coma incident to cerebral abscess, the presence of signs of conditions liable to produce suppuration is taken into account and the diagnosis is entirely based upon such signs.

See also Ans. to Q. 36 of this Chapter.

202. Describe the Coma incident to Epilepsy.

The coma incident to Epilepsy is in the majority of cases, of short duration. To diagnose its Epileptic origin, See Ans. to Q. 120 of the Chapter.

203. Describe the Coma incident to General Paralysis of the Insane.

The coma incident to the General Paralysis of the Insane simulates the coma of Apoplexy and occurs during the course of the disease. Some of them are exact clinical counter-parts of true apoplectic seizures coming on suddenly like Apoplexy while others come on gradually in the course of 24 hours.

204. Describe the Coma incident to Alcohol.

The coma incident to Alcohol or drunkenness is rarely profound. Odor of Alcohol in the breath is a positive sign. It may be profound owing to personal susceptibility or the taking of abnormally large quantities.

205. Describe the Coma incident to Opium.

The coma incident to Opium appears within an hour of taking the drug. After a brief period of excitement the patient becomes drowsy and quickly passes into a condition of absolute stupor, with complete muscular relaxation all over the body. The pupils are contracted to the minimum and do not react to light.

206. Describe the Coma incident to Illuminating Gas.

The coma incident to illuminating gas, leads the sufferer to complete unconsciousess, the cause of which is detected by the odor of the gas permeating the room.

207. Describe the Coma incident to Sunstroke.

The coma incident to sunstroke is rarely profound. Weather condition with high fever makes the diagnosis easy. It is attended with restlessness with cold, clammy surface, weak pulse and even delirium.

208. Give in detail the features of Uræmic Coma.

The uræmic coma may develop gradually without any convulsion. Frequently it is preceded by headache, and the patient gradually becomes dull and apathetic, with or without any indication of renal disease. Twitchings of the muscles may occur, particularly in the face and hands. In some cases torpor persists for weeks or months. The tongue is usually furred and the breath very foul and heavy.

209. Give in detail the features of Diabetic Coma.

The diabetic coma displays three different features. (i.) Without any previous dyspnœa or distress the patient may be attacked with headache, a feeling of intoxication, thick speech, and a staggering gait and gradually falls into deep coma. Or, (ii.) particularly after exertion, the patient is attacked suddenly with weakness, giddiness and fainting; the hands and feet become cold and livid, the pulse small, and respiration rapid; the patient becomes drowsy and death occurs within a few hours. Or, (iii.) typical dyspnœic coma, in which with loud and deep breathing, the pulse grows weak, and the patient gradually sinks and dies.

210. Give in detail the features of the Coma in Hysteria.

The hysterical coma is never profound, but is disturbed by laughing, crying, hysteroid spasms and talking. The facial expression is different from that observed in cases of unconsciousness due to all other causes. The paroxysm is usually preceded by emotional disturbances.

211. Define the term Delirium.

Delirium is a disturbance of cerebral functions manifested in the imparied action of the nerve-centres, characterized by hallucinations, incoherent thought, speech and action.

212. Give in detail the Delirium in Hysteria.

The delirium in Hysteria occurs in a condition which may be spoken of as *status hystericus*. The patient may be confined to bed for weeks and months, entirely oblivious to their surroundings, with deliriums, which may simulate those of delirium tremens, particularly associated with loathsome and unpleasant animals. Deliriums and hallucinations may alternate with emotional outburst of an aggravated nature.

213. Give some of the causes of Delirium.

The exciting causes of delirium are—
Toxæmiæ. Asthenia. Nervous disorders. Certain poisons.

214. Describe the Delirium found in some Fevers.

Of the fevers in which delirium usually occurs the most important are—Typhoid Fever, Scarlatina, Intermittent and other Malarial fevers, Yellow Fever, Influenza, and Septic fevers.

In TYPHOID FEVER the delirium occurs usually in the second and third week and in most instances it is of a low, muttering type.

In SCARLATINA, the delirium is a prominent and early symptom.

In INFLUENZA, the delirium may be of the active, wild variety.

In SEPTIC FEVERS, the delirium is low and muttering.

215. Describe the Delirium found in Acute Mania.

In delirium of Acute Mania the utterings of the patient when taken singly are apparently bright and witty; when taken as a whole, they are the veriest nonsense. The patient is mentally and physically active. Vulgarity of the language is present in many instances.

216. Describe the Delirium found in Delirium Tremens.

The patient talks constantly and incoherently; he is incessantly in motion and desires to go out and attend to some imaginary business. He exhibits an expression of terror or horror and endeavors to escape from his imaginary enemies, even resorting to violence. It is worse at night. The delirium usually continues for five or six days, after which it subsides and the patient slowly regains his strength.

217. What constitutes an Electrical Examination?

An investigation into the reactions of the affected parts, to both Galvanic and Faradic currents constitutes an Electrical examination.

218. What forms of Batteries are used?

For electro-diagnostic purposes, two forms of batteries are used, viz., the Faradic Battery and the Galvanic Battery.

219. What is the usual Strength of the Galvanic Machine?

The usual strength of the Galvanic machine should be not less than 50 volts.

220. What is the meaning of the Sign CaCLC?

In a galvanic battery the muscular contractions are more readily obtained by applying the negative pole and closing the current, which is called CATHODAL CLOSING CONTRACTION or briefly CaCLC.

221. Give the meaning of the Terms CaOC, AnOC and AnCLC.

CaOC.—or CATHODAL OPENING CONTRACTION indicates muscular contractions which take place on breaking the circuit with the negative poles applied.

Note :—A greater strength of current is necessary to affect this result.

AnOC.—or ANODAL OPENING CONTRACTION indicates muscular contractions at the positive pole on breaking the circuit of the Galvanic current.

AnCLC—or ANODAL CLOSING CONTRACTION indicates muscular contractions at the positive pole when the current completes the circuit.

222. What is the order of Irritability of Muscles as to Contraction in response to Galvanism?

(i.) CaClC. (ii.) AnOC. (iii.) AnClC. (iv.) CaOC.

223. What precautions are necessary in the Application of a Battery?

In the application of a battery every attention must be paid to details. The electrodes must be properly covered and moistened with warm or salt water, and the battery must be in perfect order.

224. What is meant by the Motor Point?

It indicates the point where a nerve enters into a muscle or a point where the nerve comes nearest the cutaneous surface.

225. What will you note in a Faradic Examination?

In a Faradic examination the diminished, absent or increased muscular contractions are noted.

226. What will you note in a Galvanic Examination?

Besides the nature of the muscular contractions, both "quantitative" and "qualitative" alterations should be noted.

227. What is the Alteration Theory?

It is a theory to explain the Galvanic phenomena of living tissues, which may be summed up as follows:—

Protoplasm when injured or excited in its continuity becomes negative to the uninjured part; when heated becomes positive; and the surface-polarisation diminishes with excitement and in the process of dying.

228. Define and give the significance of the Reaction of Degeneration.

The change in Reaction to electric stimulation of the degenerated nerves and muscles is known as the "Reaction of Degeneration". The degenerated nerve fails to excite in both Faradic and Galvanic currents, but the muscle though fails in Faradic, *responds in a slow and lazy* manner, instead of being sharp, quick, lightninglike as in a normal muscle; the contraction is often produced by a weaker current and the AnClC may be greater than CaClC. It is of diagnostic value, as it indicates a lesion affecting a motor nerve or its nuclear cells. It is present in Acute

Poliomyelitis, nerve injuries and inflammations and in degenerations of the nuclei of the cranial nerves. It is of especial value in prognosis ; if partial (slight diminution of both Faradic and Galvanic excitability), the disease will probably last one or two months ; if complete will last much longer.

229. What does Simple Diminished Irritability mean and where it is found?

It means slight changes in the muscular irritability while the nerve reacts normally, or nearly so. It may be found in cerebral palsies after the Paralysis has lasted 3 or 4 months, in certain spinal cord diseases, as Amyotrophic Lateral Sclerosis, and after slight injuries and inflammations and in certain muscular conditions, as Arthritic Muscular Atrophy, atrophy from disease and myopathic atrophy.

CHAPTER XIX.

CEREBRAL LOCALIZATION.

1. Give the general Anatomy of the Brain.

The brain is said to consist of (i.) the CORTEX or srface—subdivided into LOBES, LOBULES, CONVOLUTIONS, FISSURES and SULCI, (ii.) the CENTRUM OVALE or central white substance (conducting tracts)—subdivided into PROJECTIONS FIBRES, COMMISSURAL FIBRES and ASSOCIATION FIBRES ; and (iii.) the BASAL GANGLIA —subdivided into the OPTIC THALAMI, the CORPORA STRIATA, CORPORA QUADRIGEMINA and the CORPORA GENICULATA

2. What Landmarks are used in Cerebral Localisation ?

Anatomical, Physiological and Pathological knowledge, and clinical experience.

3. What is the Fissure of Sylvius ?

The FISSURE OF SYLVIUS is the cleft between the anterior and middle lobes of the brain. It begins at the base of the brain at the anterior perforates pace, and, passing outward to the external surface of the hemisphere, divides into 2 branches—one vertical ; the other, horizontal (the longer one).

4. Where is the Fissure of Rolando ?

It is situated about the middle of the outer surface of the hemisphere. It commences at or near the great longitudinal fissure, half an inch behind the midpoint between the glabella and the external occipital protuberance, and runs downward and forward to terminate a little above the horizontal limb of the fissure of Sylvius.

5. Where is the Parieto-Occipital Fissure?

It commences about midway between the posterior extremity of the brain and the fissure of Rolando, and runs downward and forward for a variable distance becoming indistinct below.

6. Where is the Motor Area of the Cortex?

It occupies the convolutions around the fissure of Rolando, and turns over the edge of the hemisphere into the marginal convolutions of the mesial surface.

7. What portion of the Motor Area controls the Movements of the Feet and Legs?

The motor area of the feet and legs occupies the convolutions bordering on the longitudinal fissure, both on the median and outer surface of the brain. It is the backward portion of the motor area of the Cortex.

8. What portion of the Motor Area controls the Movement of the Head and Eyes?

The very lowest portion.

9. What portion of the Motor Area controls the Movements of the Arm?

The upper portion on either side of the fissure of Rolando.

10. What portion of the Motor Area controls the Movements of the Trunk?

The marginal between the LEG and ARM areas.

11. What is the most important Function of the Occipital Lobes?

The function of vision.

12. Where is the Auditory Centre?

It is situated in the hinder part of the first and possibly the second temporal convolutions.

13. In Cerebral Localization what Two Essential Points should be taken into consideration?

(i.) The *nature*, and (ii.) the *location* of the lesion.

14. What do you understand by a Destructive Lesion of the Brain?

The lesion of the brain produces two classes of symptoms, viz., DIRECT and INDIRECT. The direct symptoms may be DESTRUCTIVE or IRRITATIVE. The lesions which produce destructive symptoms are known as the destructive lesions, while those producing irritative symptoms are known as the irritative lesions of the brain.

15. What is an Irritative Lesion of the Brain?

See Ans. to the previous Question.

16. What Muscles have Bilateral Representation?

The muscles of the *trunk*, *larynx* and *pharynx*.

17. Lesions of the Frontal Lobes give rise to What Symptoms?

Symptoms indicating mental impairment.

18. Lesions of the Motor Area give rise to What Symptoms?

The lesions of the motor area produce *paralytic* or *convulsive* symptoms according as the lesions are destructive or irritative.

19. Lesions of the Temporo-Sphenoidal Lobes give rise to what Symptoms?

They produce disturbances of the auditory functions. The *destructive lesions* cause deafness; the *irritative lesions*—auditory hallucinations, and even convulsions produced by auditory auræ.

20. What is Aphasia?

This is a complex condition in which the will to speak exists and also the ability to speak, but the connection between the two is broken down. When the patient speaks, the words which he utters may be well-pronounced, but are not those which he wishes to utter. It is associated with disorganisation of Broca's convolution.

21. Define "Motor" and "Sensory" Aphasia.

The motor Aphasia is characterized by inability to express ideas in speech, symbols or gestures, or inability to write. It is almost invariably associated with right-sided Hemiplegia.

The sensory Aphasia is characterized by inability to understand spoken words (*word-deafness*) o written or printed words (*word-blindness*).

22. Where is the Centre for Visual Memories?

It is situated in the angular gyrus. Lesions in this centre produce *word-blindness*.

23. Lesions of the Corpora Quadrigemina produce What Symptoms?

They produce at first, an in-co-ordination of movement, very closely simulating that arising from cerebellar disease; it is aggravated on voluntary movement. Next the eye muscles are paralysed—the superior and inferior recti bearing the brunt.

24. What symptoms may we have from Lesions in the Pons Varolii?

They produce paralyses of the hemiplegic type with symptoms of motor disturbances. Irritative phenomena, such as convulsions involving both arms or both legs, semi-convulsive paroxysms of coughing, trismus, marked pupillary contractions are liable to occur. Temperature disturbances are common.

25. Lesions in the Crura Cerebri produce What Symptoms?

Symptoms vary with the situation and size of the lesion. If the lesion is intra-crural, it produces Weber's syndrome (alternate Hemiplegia of the oculo-motor type) associated with hemianæsthesia. If the lesion is sub-crural and sufficiently large in size, it produces Hemiplegia with bilateral motor culi palsy.

26. Lesions in the Cerebellum produce What Symptoms?

Lesions of the lateral lobes produce no symptom.

Lesions of the middle lobe produce, in-co-ordination of gait, simulating that of intoxication. Knee-jerks may be either present or absent. Loss of vision—frequently observed.

The tumor of the cerebellum is apt to be associated with optic Neuritis, vomiting, and deafness, or loss of vision.

27. Lesions in the Optic Chiasm prodce What Symptoms?

The lesions of the central portion produce bilateral Hem anopsia.

The lesions attacking the outer portion produce nasal Hemianopsia.

28. What is Hemianopsia; what are the Varieties?

Hemianopsia is blindness of one-half of the visual field in one or both eyes—*unilateral* when affects the one, *bilateral* when affects the both.

Other varieties are—

LATERAL or VERTICAL Hemianopsia, when the affected half-field is separated from the normal half by a vertical dividing line; HORIZONTAL Hemianopsia when the dividing line is horizontal.

TEMPORAL Hemianopsia, when the affected half-field lies towards the temporal side; BI-TEMPORAL

Hemianopsia if both the temporal half-fields are involved.

NASAL Hemianopsia, if the nasal half-field is affected.

HOMONYMUS Hemianopsia, if the nasal half-field of one eye and the temporal half-field of the other are involved.

29. What is the usual Status of Functional Hemianopsia?

Migraneous seizures.

30. Give in general the Functions of the Brain.

The BRAIN is the seat of conscious as well as instinctive intelligence and mental activities. It controls and directs the voluntary movements, and regulates in a measure the vaso-motor, trophic and secretory mechanisms of the body.

31. Give the Motor Tracts of the Brain and Spinal Cord with their respective Functions.

The cerebro-spinal MOTOR TRACTS or paths are of *two* classes; the DIRECT or VOLUNTARY and the INDIRECT motor tracts.

(i.) THE DIRECT MOTOR TRACT.—It is a long continuous strand of fibres, composed of single neurons originating from cells in the CENRTAL CONVOLUTIONS, puts the CORTEX directly in contact with motor cells of the PONS VAROLII, MEDULIA OBLONGATA and SPINAL CORD of the opposite side. It is concerned with *all voluntary movements of the body*.

(ii.) THE INDIRECT MOTOR TRACT.—The root of this tract is in the ANTERIOR CENTRAL CONVOLUTION, and to some extent in the FRONTAL LOBE. Fibres from the nerve-cells of these regions pass down into the PONS VAROLII, surround the nerve-cells known as the PONS NUCLEI and terminate there. From the pons nuclei NEURAXONS cross through the median lines into the CORTEX and end there. From here the nerve-cells send fibres through the PEDUNCLES into the SPINAL CORD, where they pass along mainly in the LATERAL FUNDAMENTAL COLUMNS, to conduct finally with the ANTERIOR HORN CELLS. This tract is concerned in the *co-ordination of bodily movement* and in *the higher reflex* and *automatic acts. Playing musical instruments and the involuntary use of the hands and limbs in work or games of skill are under the control of this mechanism.*

32. Give the Sensory Tracts with their respective Functions.

The SENSORY TRACTS are more tortuous and broken than the motor tracts. They are also classified as DIRECT and INDIRECT, and are concerned in bringing tactile, muscular and general sensations from the remoter parts of the body to the cortex of the brain.

The DIRECT SENSORY TRACT is made up of—

(a) A PERIPHERAL SENSORY NEURON— nerve-fibre from the *periphery* to the *spinal ganglia*, and through the same by way of *the posterior root of the spinal cord* to a group of cells lying in the *posterior horns*, where it meets and surrounds with its end brush a second sensory cell.

(b) A SPINAL-THALAMIC NEURON— nerve-fibre from the second sensory cell described above, crosses to the *lateral column* of the other side of the spinal cord, through the *anterior commissure* and runs up to the *optic thalamus*, passing through the *lateral ascending tract*, the *medulla oblongata* and the *pons Varolii*, where it sends its terminal to a third cell.

(c) A THALAMIC-CORTICAL NEURAXON— nerve-fibre from third cell at the optic thalamus to the *cortex* of the *central convolutions*.

Note:—Some direct sensory tracts go from the posterior roots to the columns of Goll and Burdach and thence to the optic thalami and central convolutions.

The direct sensory tracts, carry for the most part, the *sense fo touch, pain* and *temperature*.

THE INDIRECT SENSORY TRACT is made up of—

(a) A PERIPHERAL SENSORY NEURON —nerve-fibre from the periphery to the posterior root, *as above described*.

(b) A SPINAL-CEREBELLAR NEURON— nerve-fibre from the second sensory cell passes directly into the posterior column of the cord of the same side and ascends till it reaches the upper end, and crossing there over to the other side in the sensory decussation reaches the cortex of the cerebellum, where it terminates.

(c) A CEREBELLAR-THALAMIC NEURON—nerve-fibre from the cerebellar cell which *takes up the impulse carried on by (b) neuron passes through the superior cerebellar peduncle to the red nuclei and optic thalamus, where it terminates*.

(d) A THALAMIC-CORTEX NEURON— nerve-fibre from the optic thalamus to the cortex of the central convolutions.

Note :—Other indirect sensory tracts go from the sensory roots to the cells of the column of Clark, thence by the direct cerebellar tracts to the cerebellum, thence to the red nuclei and thalamus. and finally to the brain cortex.

The indirect sensory tracts are concerned with *the sensation from the muscles and joints* which have to do with co-ordination, and with *visceral sensations*. The *automatic* and *psycho-reflex acts* are performed through the indirect sensory and indirect motor tracts.

33. Give the Functions of the Pre-frontal Lobes of the Brain.

The pre-frontal lobes or that part of the brain in front of the pre-central convolution, are one of the higher or ASSOCIATION centres. THEIR FRONTAL PARTS are concerned with *volition* and *the power of self-control*, *concentration of thought aud attention,* while the posterior parts contains *centres for the movements of the head and eyes.*

Lesions in this part of the brain cause *changes of character* as is evidenced by peevishness and irritability of temper, mental enfeeblement, lack of power to concentrate the mind or to control the acts or emotions.

34. Give the Functions of the Central Convolutions of the Brain.

This part of the brain is also called the SENSORI-MOTOR AREA. It is concerned in the production of nervous impulses which cause *voluntary motions of the body,* and also *the centre for the cutaneous sensations of the parts corresponding to the muscular groups which it supplies.* Its lower part, known as the CENTRAL OPERCULUM, is a *centre for the movements of the larynx, mouth, tongue and face.* Above this and about the middle third of the central convolutions is the *centre for the movements of the shoulder, arm, hand and fingers.* Further up near the longitudinal fissure, and extending over into the mesial surface and back into the superior parietal lobule, is the area for *the trunk hips, feet and toes.* The base of the first and second frontal convolutions is *the centre for movement of the eyes.*

35. Where are the Centres of Special Senses?

The special senses have two centres—the *primary* and the *secondary.* The primary centres are connected with the ganglia at the base of the brain; the secondary centres are stituated in the cortex, at the occipital, parietal and temporal lobes.

36. Where are the Centres for Vision?

The PRIMARY CENTRE FOR VISION is in the posterior part of the optic thalamus, the external geniculate body, and anterior corpora quadrigemina.

The SECONDARY CENTRE is situated in the *occipital lobe,* and particularly upon its mesial surface, and in that of the cuneus, known as the calcarine fissure.

> Note :—Each occipital lobe is the centre for visual impulses from the corresponding half of the retina of each eye. The total destruction of both occipital lobes, or even of a considerable portion of them involving the median surface causes blindness. Destruction of one lobe causes half-blindness or Hemianopsia.

37. Where are the Centres for Hearing?

The PRIMARY CENTRE FOR HEARING is in the posterior tubercle of the corpora quadrigemina and the internal geniculate body.

The SECONDARY CENTRE is in the cortex of the first and second convolutions of the TEMPORAL LOBE.

> Note :—Destruction of one temporal lobe causes deafness in the opposite ear.

38. Where are the Centres for Smell?

The PRIMARY CENTRE FOR SMELL is in the olfactory lobes.

The SECONDARY CENTRE is probably in the anterior part of the limbic lobe, the uncus and in part of of the hippocampal convolution.

39. Where are the Centres for Taste?

The PRIMARY CENTRE for taste is not known.

The SECONDARY CENTRE is in the hippocampal convolution.

40. Give the Centres for Memories.

The CENTRE FOR THE MEMORIES OF THE ARTICULAR MOVEMENTS OF SPEECH is in the posterior part of the third left frontal convolution.

The CENTRE FOR THE MEMORIES OF THE MOVEMENTS OF WRITING is thought to be at the posterior part of the second left frontal convolution.

The CENTRE FOR THE MEMORIES OF ORDINARY CO-ORDINATE MOVEMENTS is probably in the interior parietal lobule.

The CENTRE FOR THE VISUAL MEMORIES OF WRITTEN LANGUAGE is in the angular gyrus, extending backward from there into the occipital lobe.

The CENTRE FOR THE AUDITORY MEMORIES OF SPOKEN LANGUAGE is in the posterior part of the first and the corresponding upper part of the second temporal convolution.

> Note :—In the right-handed people all the memory centres are in the left cerebral hemisphere; in the left-handed people all the memory centres are in the right hemisphere.

41. Give the Functions of the Thalamus Opticus.

It is connected by its projecting fibres, with the frontal, parietal, occipital and temporal lobes of the cortex.

The fibres that go to the occipital cortex are connected with the optic tract, and as such with the *function of vision*. It seems to have some relation to the *expression of emotions*.

The fibres that go to the temporal lobe are connected with the auditory tract, and as such with the *function of hearing*.

It is probably also the *primary centres for sensations of touch, muscular sense*, and perhaps for *smell* and *taste*.

CHAPTER XX.

SPINAL LOCALIZATION.

1. Give a description of the General Anatomy of the Spinal Cord.

The SPINAL CORD or the MEDULLA SPINALIS is a slender, cylindriform neural structure occupying the upper two-third of the vertebral canal, connected above with the brain, through the medium of the bulb, and passing through the cervical and dorsal vertebræ to the lower border of the first lumbar vertebra, terminates in the FILUM TERMINALE (a slender filament of gray substance), which lies in the midst of the nerve-roots forming the CAUDA EQUINA.

It is divided into CERVICAL, DORSAL or, THORACIC, LUMBAR and SACRAL portions, corresponding with the nerves it gives off. They are respectively 4″, 10½″, 2″, and 1½″ long. Its average diameter is 1 C.M. and has two SWELLING or ENLARGEMENTS, the cervical and lumbar. It is surrounded by THREE MEMBRANES, one after another, externally by DURA MATTER (having protective function), centrally by ARACHNOID (having serous function), and internally by PIA MATER (having vascular function), all of which are continuous with the corresponding envelopes of the brain.

It is composed of WHITE MATTER or nervous substance *externally* (its chief portion), and GRAY MATER or nerve-fibres *internally* in its axial or central portion ; the latter is so arranged, that it looks like two crescentic masses on the surface of a transverse section of the cord, connected together by a narrower portion or ISTHMUS ; a MINUTE CANAL, lined by a layer of columnar ciliated epithelium containing a fluid called CEREBRO-SPINAL-FLUID, runs through the centre of this isthmus, in a longitudinal direction through the whole length of the cord and opens above at the 4th Ventricle, at the back of the Medulla Oblongata and pons Varolii. The WHITE MATTER increases in quantity from below upward; the GRAY MATTER is greatest in the cervical and lumbar and least in the dorsal region—it acts as a centre for and a distributor of nerve-impulses.

The spinal nerves arise from the spinal cord by two roots, anterior and posterior; there are 30 pairs of such spinal nerves—8 in the cervical, 12 in the dorsal, 5 in the lumbar and 5 in the sacral portion of the cord.

> Note :—The spinal cord does not extend throughout the entire length of the vertebral column. Its lowermost extremity is on a level with the interspace between the first and second lumbar vertebræ.

2. Describe the Upper and the Lower Motor Neurons.

The UPPER MOTOR NEURON or the upper motor path extends from the ganglion cells in the cerebral cortex, the axis-cylinder process of which passes through the pyramidal tracts, terminating at, but not in immediate connection with the ganglion cells of the anterior gray horns. Any lesion of them is associated with spastic Paralysis, which is attended by excessive action of the tendon and cutaneous reflexes proceeding from all spinal segments below the uppermost level of the lesion.

The LOWER MOTOR NEURON commences in the ganglion cells of the anterior gray horn above-named, and the nerve-fibres emanating therefrom, and terminates in the muscles. Lesions limited to them produce symptoms referred to the disturbed function of the affected segment and to no others.

3. What portion of the Cord governs Sensations?

The *postero-external* column of the cord, which is known as the column of Burdach governs all sensations.

4. What portion of the Cord governs Motion?

The motor neurons.

5. Where does the Sensibility to Pain lie?

The sensibility to pain lies apparently in the *Gray Matter* near the gray (posterior) commissure.

6. Where is the Centre for Heat Sense?

It seems to lie near the gray commissure.

7. Where is the Centre for Muscles Sense?

This centre is probably in the postero-median column of the spinal cord.

8. What portion of the Cord controls the Bladder and Rectum?

The lumbar enlargement.

9. What Centres lie in the Medulla?

The MEDULLA OBLONGATA or the upper enlarged portion of the spinal cord contains the *centres of cranial nerves* and in it also are various *reflex* and *automatic centres controlling* and *regulating the vaso-motor system, respiratory* and *cardiac rhythm, visceral movements* and *secretions*.

10. What are the Functions of the Cervical Section of the Cord?

The CERVICAL SECTION of the spinal cord is the root of 8 pairs of the spinal nerves :—

THE UPPER OR THE 1st FOUR CERVICAL PAIRS are distributed in the occipital region and the neck, and *supply motion to the muscles which rotate the head and draw it back and sideways* ; one branch the PHRENIC, supplies the diaphragm and *assists in fixing the thorax in forced inspiration*.

THE LOWER 4 CERVICAL PAIRS (and the 1st dorsal) are distributed—the short nerves to the shoulders and trunk and the long nerves to the upper extremities (arm) and *supply motion to muscles toro tate the posterior edge of scapula when the arm is raised, to elevate the shoulders, to raise the arm, to rotate the humerus* (inward, forward and outward), *to rotate the arm, to depress the shoulder, to pull the arm backward, forward, downward and the side, to flex the forearm, to extend the forearm, to turn the head upward and to extend and to flex the wrist, phalanges, thumb and fingers.* THE 8th CERVICAL WITH THE 1st DORSAL—*flex the wrist and the 1st phalange, the 2nd and 3rd phalanges of the third and fourth fingers and extend the scond and third phalanges.*

> Note:—The diseases of the upper cervical group are spasms, Paralyses, and Neuralgias. Of the lower cervical group—spasms (occupation neuroses), Neuralgias, numb hands, and neurotic œdema.

11. What are the Functions of the Dorsal Section of the Cord?

THE DORSAL SECTION OF THE SPINAL CORD is the root of another 12 pairs of the spinal nerves, of which the 1st is the largest and belongs functionally to the arm nerves; they carry motor and sensory fibres te the voluntary muscles, skin and other tissues of tho trunk-wall, and splanchnic fibres to the lungs and abdominal viscera.

THE UPPER SIX DORSAL NERVES are mainly *inspiratory in function*; they also *extend and rotate the dorsal and cervical vertebræ.*

THE LOWER SIX are *expiratory* nerves. They also assist in *compressing the abdominal viscera* and in *flexing, extending and rotating the spine.*

12. What are the Functions of the Lumbar Section of the Cord?

The LUMBAR SECTION OF THE SPINAL CORD is the root of the next 5 pairs of spinal nerves, whose POSTERIOR BRANCHES supply the erector spinæ, interossei, multifidus spinæ, and inter-spinales muscles and also the skin of the back. THE ANTERIOR BRANCHES

OF THE UPPER FOUR unite to form the LUMBAR PLEXUS and THE FIFTH sends most of its fibres to the SACRAL PLEXUS. The LUMBAR PLEXUS have 6 BRANCHES, the FIRST FOUR of which are comparatively short and *supply sensation to the abdominal wall and external genitals*, the LAST TWO are longer and mixed nerves and supply *the hip and knee-joints, the muscles of the anterior, inner and outer part of the thigh, the skin over this region and inner side of the leg and dorsum of the foot.*

13. What are the Functions of Cauda Equina?

The CAUDA EQUINA is made up of five lumbar, five sacral and coccygeal nerve-roots. *The sacral nerves are the main agents in station and locomotion ; they control the legs entirely and also the posterior muscles of the thigh and buttocks ; they give sensation to these parts.* They carry also fibres that *regulate the sexual function* (the second sacral—*erection centre* and third sacral—*ejaculation centre*), *bladder* (fourth sacral), and *rectum* (fifth sacral).

14. Differentiate (i.) Lesions of the Lower End of the Spinal Cord, (ii.) Cauda Lesions, and (iii.) Lesions of the Peripheral Nerves.

(i) The LESIONS OF THE LOWER END OF THE CORD—

There is little pain or sensory irritation at first, but later, dissociation of sensations. Fibrillary contractions and involuntary twitchings of the leg muscles. Paralysis, involving the lower limbs ; it is flaccid, and is followed by atrophy. The visceral centres are involved. The symptoms usually come on rapidly (in a few days), and the motor *disturbances are more conspicuous and troublesome than the sensory disturbances.*

> Note :—If the Conus is not implicated, the Paralysis does not seriously involve these centres or the muscles of the pelvic girdle.

(ii) The CAUDA LESIONS.—

(a) Due to *tumor*
(b) Due to *injury*
— There is often severe pain felt in the bladder and along the course of the sciatic nerves, usually bilaterally, followed after a time by anæsthesia in the course of the sciatic nerves. There is little motor irritation and Paralysis follows slowly, accompained with pain. The sensory symptoms are all along prominent. The sexual, bladder and rectal centres are later paralyzed. The course is progressive.

> Note :—The symptoms of the lesions due to Tumor come on slowly, but sudden when due to injury.

(c) Due to *compression*—The symptoms are much the same as above, but there is less motor disturbance and there may be no involvement of the visceral centres.

(iii) The LESIONS OF THE PERIPHERAL NERVES—
Sciatic pains, tender points ; the pains are not so severe, and there is no marked anæsthesia. There may or may not be Paralysis and sensory and motor symptoms go together, the former slightly predominating. Symptoms come on rather rapidly.

> Note :—The lesion may be unilateral.

15. Describe in detail the Circulation of the Cord.

The branches from the vertebral, ascending cervical and superior intercostal arteries supply blood to the spinal cord from THE ABOVE, and branches from the dorsal intercostal, lumbar and sacral arteries FROM BELOW. They send off small branches which enter the spinal canal through the foramen magnum above and intervertebral foramina at the sides ; they pierce the dura mater and are distributed on the pia mater and in the cord. The veins enter the pia mater and the cord by passing along the nerve roots. The arteries predominate in total capacity in the anterior plexus and central arteries, the veins predominate in the posterior plexuses and peripheral vessels. The central arteries are larger and longer than the peripheral. Hence the blood circulates more quickly and under greater pressure in the central gray of the cord.

16. What are the Functions of the Multipolar Cells?

The associative or column nerve-cells, which have their origin in group of nerve-cells lying in the central parts of the GRAY MATTER of the cord, and produce numerous short and COMMISSURAL FIBRES are known as the MULTIPOLAR CELLS. The SHORT FIBRES unite different levels of the cord and the COMMISSURAL FIBRES unite the different halves of the cord.

17. Give the General Function of the Spinal and also of the Special Centres in the Cord.

The spinal cord is a conductor and centre of nervous action. It represents the lowest evolutionary level of the development of the nervous system. Its general function falls into two categories : (i.) FUNCTIONS OF THE WHITE MATTER—*conduction*; and (ii.) FUNCTIONS OF GRAY MATTER—the reflection of afferent impulses, and their conversion into efferent impulses (*reflex action*), the gray matter being *the centre and distributor of nerve impulses*.

(i.) FUNCTIONS OF THE DIFFERENT PARTS OF THE WHITE MATTER—

(a) THE COLUMNS OF GOLL—conduct special sensations from the muscles, articulations and tendonous sheaths *via* the roots on the same side. Lesions in this region cause loss of the sense of position of the limbs, of the power of estimating weights, and of co-ordination of muscular effort (ataxia).

(b) THE COLUMNS OF BURDACH— pathway for all kinds of afferent impulses, conduct to a certain extent the tactile sensations. Lesions

in this region may cause pain, anæsthesia, ataxia and loss of reflexes.
- (c) THE ANTERO-LATERAL ASCENDING TRACT—conducts sensations of pain and temperature.

    > Note : The direct and crossed pyramidal tracts carry motor impulses from the brain to the anterior horns. The cross pyramidal tract crosses in the medulla to the opposite side to that where it originates, and passes down the lateral column to connect the motor cells of the anterior horn. The direct pyramidal tract runs down in the anterior column, and at different levels sends fibres across through the anterior commissure to the motor-cells of of the anterior horns.

(ii.) FUNCTIONS OF THE DIFFERENT PARTS OF THE GRAY MATTER—
- (a) CLARK'S COLUMN—conduct impulses from the viscera relating to equilibrium and sense of position.
- (b) AUTOMATIC CENTRES—
    - (1) CILIO-SPINAL CENTRE—controls *the contraction and dilatation of the puds.*
    - (2) GENITAL CENTRES—control *erection, ejaculation* and *parturition.*
    - (3) RECTAL CENTRE—controls *defæcation.*
    - (4) BLADDER CENTRE—controls *micturition.*
    - (5) VASO-MOTOR CENTRES (certain subsidiaries)—send out *rhythmical impulses* and control *blood-pressure,* and *constriction* and *dilatation of the vessels.*
- (c) CELLS OF THE POSTERIOR HORNS— Sensory in function and are connected with *tactile, pain* and *temperature* sensations.
- (d) TROPHIC CENTRES— regulate the *nutrition of joints, bones* and *skin.*

18. What are the principal Irritative Symptoms in Spinal Cord Disease?

Pains and paræsthesias of the back and limbs. Hyperæsthesia and feelings of constriction around the waist. Rigidity. Spasms. Exaggerated reflexes. Irritability of the visceral and vascular functions.

> Note: The more superficial and meningeal the disease the more are the symptoms irritative.

19. What are the principal Depressive and Destructive Symptoms of Spinal Cord Disease?

Anæsthesia. Ataxia. Paralysis. Wasting. Loss of power over visceral centres.

> Note—The more central and myclonic the disease, the less the irritation and the more the Paralysis and visceral disturbance.

20. What is the Common Form of Paralysis in Spinal Cord Disease?

Paraplegia.

21. What is Common Form of Paralysis in Brain Disease?

Hemiplegia.

22. What is the Common Form of Paralysis in Multiple Neuritis?

Quadruplegia.

CHAPTER XXI.

THE EYE.

1. What constitute a complete Eye Examination?

A *complete* examination of the eye should include the examination of the eye-lid, conjunctiva, cornea, sclerotica, iris, fundus oculi, the motor apparatus of the eyes, the state of the refraction and the state of vision.

2. What are the generally accepted causes of Swelling of the Eyelids?

The swelling of the eyelids results from *general* or *local* causes.

GENERAL CAUSES—Dropsy. Chronic and acute Nephritis. Anæmia. Arsenical Poisoning. Iodism.

LOCAL CAUSES— Inflammatory affections of the eyes. Hay Fever. Angeio-neurotic œdema. Urticaria. Conjunctivitis. Etc.

3. Name some Toxic causes for Swelling of the Eyelids.

Arsenical Poisoning. Iodism. Etc.

4. Describe a Chancre of the Lids.

A Chancere of the eyelid presents ulceration which is small and indurated. The discharge is *slight*, may amount to nothing more than a mere moisture.

5. What is von Græfe's Sign?

In Exophthalmic Goitre, the upper lid fails to move in complete harmony with the eyeball when the latter is directed downwards, but remains in a state of spasmodic elevation. This is known as *Græfe's Sign*.

6. What is Stellwag's Sign?

In Exophthalmic Goitre there may be slight retraction of the upper lid. This is known as Stellwag's Sign. The palpebral aperture is disproportionately great in comparison with the exophthalmos. This may be complicated with Græfe's Sign.

7. Describe the Motor Disturbance of the Eyelids.

The motor disturbances of the eyelids manifest themselves as *Paralysis* and *spasm*.

The PARALYSIS may be either *Lagophthalmos* i.e., the inability to close the eye, or *Ptosis* i.e., partial or complete inability to raise the upper lid.

The SPASMS are manifested as *Blepharospasm, nictitating spasm*, and *fibrillary twitchings of the lids,*

8. Outline the varieties of Conjunctivitis.

(i.) Simple Catarrhal Conjunctivitis. Chronic Catarrhal Conjunctivitis. Exanthematous Conjunctivitis. Phlyctenular Conjunctivitis or Scrofulous Ophthalmia. Purulent Conjunctivitis—Gonorrhœal Ophthalmia and Ophthalmia Neonatorum. Croupous Conjunctivitis. Diphtheritic Conjunctivitis. Follicular Conjunctivitis. Granular Conjunctivitis.

9. Name symptoms suggestive of Corneal Disease.

The symptoms of corneal disease are *Objective* and *Subjective*.

The OBJECTIVE symptoms are—
Pericorneal injection. Loss of transparency. Ulcerations. Deformities. Vesicles and Tumors.

The SUBJECTIVE symptoms are—
Pain. Photophobia. Blepharospasm.

10. Give the varieties of Diplopia.

The simple Homonymous Diplopia. Th rossed Diplopia.

The SIMPLE or HOMONYMOUS is produced by *convergent squint*. In it the right-hand image is seen by the right eye and the left-hand image is seen by the left eye.

The CROSSED DIPLOPIA is produced by *divergent squint*. In it the right eye sees the left-hand image and the left eye the right-hand one.

> Note :—A red glass placed before one eye will color the corresponding image.

11. What Error in Refraction is mostly responsible for Headaches ?

Astigmatism.

12. What is Lagophthalmus, and what are its Causes ?

Lagophthalmus indicates an inability to close the eyes.

Its CAUSES— may be *paralytic* or *mechanical*.

The *paralytic causes* may be due to disease of the seventh cranial nerve or peripheral facial palsy.

The *mechanical causes* may be due to cicatrical contraction of the skin overlying the lids or unusual protruberance of the eyeballs as from Exophthalmic Goitre and retro-ocular tumors.

13. What is the essential cause of Morning Ptosis ?

Exhaustion—occurs mostly in weak women.

14. Name the Condition of the Eye associated with Blepharospasm.

Tonic spasm of the orbicularis palpebrarum.

15. What is the "Habit Spasm" as referred to the Eye ?

Winking movements of the eyelids are known as "habit spasms". Nictitating spasm constitutes one of the varieties of "habit spasms".

16. In examining a conjunctival disease what points should be taken into consideration?

Both *objective* and *subjective* symptoms should be considered. See Ans. to Q. 9 of this Chapter.

17. Describe the Discharges of the Eye met with in Conjunctivitis.

In Conjunctivitis the discharges may be *mucous, muco-purulent* or *purulent*.

The MUCOUS DISCHARGE is clear and more or less watery. It is characteristic of simple Catarrhal Conjunctivitis.

The MUCO-PURULENT DISCHARGE is consisted of mucus infested with thick yellowish flocculi. It is found in Acute and Chronic Catarrhal Conjunctivitis and Granular Ophthalmia.

The PURULENT DISCHARGE presents a thick creamy consistence and is of a yellowish-green color. It is found in Purulent (Gonorrhœal) Ophthalmia and Catarrhal Conjunctivitis.

> Note :—The associated symptoms in Gonorrhœal Ophthalmia are much more virulent.

18. In what conditions do we find Dryness of the Conjunctiva?

In *collapsic states* and in *facial Paralysis*.

19. Describe the Diphtheritic form of Conjunctivitis.

The Diphtheritic Conjunctivitis is due to infection of the conjunctiva with *Klebs-Laffler* bacili, which in the majority of cases are secondary to faucial or nasal Diphtheria. The *pseudo-membrane*, which is comparatively *thick* and covers the conjunctiva of the globe and lids, presents a *gray color* and is *closely adherent* to the surface beneath and *can only be removed with force*.

leaving a raw, bleeding surface. The onset of the disease is sudden and progress rapid. Swelling of the lids, with marked induration, is an early symptom. The discharges are serous and blood-streaked. Constitutional symptoms are well-marked. It is a serious affection and the sloughing of the cornea, with total destruction of the affected eye is a common sequel.

20. Describe the Croupous form of Conjunctivitis.

It presents the picture of a simple Conjunctivitis plus the appearance of the *false-membrane*, which is seen mainly upon the palpebral conjunctiva. Though soon renewed and leaves a raw, bleeding surface, *the flase membrane can be removed with comparative ease.* It runs a prolonged course, which may be greatly shortened by proper treatment. The diagnosis cannot be made positively without a bacteriological examination of the exudate.

21. What are Phlyctenules and of what are they Diagnostic?

The phlyctenules are little vesicles or blisters on the epidermis, cornea or conjunctiva, which tend to break down aud form small ulcerations at their apices. They are reddish in color and are generally multiple and surrounded by a network of blood-vessels, the unaffected portion being fairly clear.

They constitute, *the diagnostic symptom* of phlyctenular Conjunctivitis and Phlyctenular Keratitis.

22. Give symptoms and appearance of Trachoma.

The APPEARANCE.—It is at first characterized by sago-like elevations of the palpebral conjunctiva, and later by fibrous and cicatrical tissue that by friction produces pannus.

The SYMPTOMS.— In the beginning discrete elevations with some little thickening of the lids. Moderately severe conjunctival inflammations are associated in more advanced and acute cases. Conjunctival thickening. Corneal opacities.

It is also known as Granular Conjunctivities or Granular Lids or Granular Ophthalmia and is exceedingly chronic and very resistant to treatment. It is due to a specific *diplococcus*.

23. Give the appearance of Ecchymoses affecting the Conjunctiva.

The ecchymoses affecting the conjunctiva appear as solid red patches, at first bright, later becoming dark.

24. Name all the diseases of the Conjunctiva.

The diseases of the conjunctiva include the following :—

(i.) *Conjunctivitis*—for its *varieties* see Ans. to Q. 8 above.

(ii.) *Pterygium*.

(iii.) *Symblepharon*.

25. Give the symptoms and appearance of Catarrhal Conjunctivitis.

SYMPTOMS.—Sensations of heat and burning in the eye, obscuration of vision by the increased production of mucus and a mild degree of photophobia. Mucous discharge.

APPEARANCE.—Conjunctival injection, i.e., formation of a more or less marked, coarse scarlet network of tortuous blood-vessels in the conjunctiva. In severe cases it is associated with œdema of the sub-conjunctival tissue (chemosis).

> Note :—The intensity of the injection is an index of the severity of the affection.

26. Give the symptoms and appearance of Chronic Catarrhal Conjunctivitis.

SYMPTOMS.— Besides the symptoms of Acute Conjunctivitis, there is a slight muco-purulent discharge from the eyes.

APPEARANCE.—A mild grade of conjunctival injection. The edges of the lids are red.

27. Give the symptoms and appearance of Phlyctenular Conjunctivitis.

SYMPTOMS.—Phlyctenulæ upon the conjunctiva. Lachrymation.

APPEARANCE.—See Ans. to Q. 22 above.

28. Give the symptoms and appearance of Purulent Conjunctivitis.

SYMPTOMS.— A high degree of conjunctival injection, with more or less Chemosis and sensitiveness of the parts to manipulation. The discharge is at first serous and may contain some blood; it soon becomes mixed with pus, finally entirely purulent.

APPEARANCE.—A high degree of conjunctival injection with more or less œdema of the sub-conjunctival tissue. Swelling and redness of the lids.

29. Give symptoms and appearance of Follicular Conjunctivitis.

SYMPTOMS.—Lachrymation, mucous discharge and conjunctival injection.

APPEARANCE.—Formation of small elevations, especially in the fornix conjunctivæ, with slight thickening of the lids and conjunctival injection.

30. Give symptoms and appearance of Pterygium.

SYMPTOMS.—Conjunctival irritation.

APPEARANCE.—A triangular patch of thickened conjunctiva, the apex pointing towards the pupil, the fan-shaped base extending towards the outer part of the eyeball. In its earlier stage, it is coursed by numerous blood-vessels, which converge at the apex.

31. Give symptoms and appearance of Pingueculæ.

SYMPTOMS.—They cause no inconvenience other than their appearance.

APPEARANCE.—Small yellowish white elevations or spots situated between the cornea (not upon it) and the canthus of the eye.

32. What is Symblepharon?

Symblepharon is an abnormal adhesion of the eyelids to the eyeball due to burn, wounds, etc. It usually follows Granular Ophthalmia and Diphtheritic Conjunctivitis.

33. Give the objective symptoms of Corneal Disease.

The objective symptoms are:—
(i.) Pericorneal injection. (ii.) Opacities. (iii.) Ulcerations. (iv.) Deformities. (v.) Vesicles. (vi.) Tumors.

34. Give the subjective symptoms of Corneal Disease.

The subjective symptoms are:—
Pain, photophobia and blepharospasm.

35. Describe in detail Pericorneal Injection.

The pericorneal or ciliary injection appears as a diffuse *rose-colored band* about the edge of the cornea, which in reality consists of very fine and closely-placed small, straight vessels radiating from the edge of the cornea. It is suggestive of disease of the cornea, iris, or ciliary body.

36. How does it differ from Conjunctival Injection?

The PERICORNEAL INJECTION remains stationary during the manipulation of the conjunctiva, while CONJUNCTIVAL INJECTION moves with the manipulation.

37. What are the causes of Loss of the Transparency of the Cornea?

The causes are :—

(i.) Inflammatory infiltration of the cornea. (ii.) Formation of cicatrices in the cornea. (iii.) Accumulation of pus within its substance. (iv.) The Arcus Senilis.

38. Describe the Arcus Senilis.

The Arcus Senilis is a ring or narrow band of fatty degeneration of the corneal tissue along the corneal edge. It usually occurs in the aged, hence it derives its name as such. It may also occur in younger subjects due to degenerative changes.

39. Describe a Simple Ulcer of the Cornea.

A simple ulcer of the cornea is small in size and superficial and exhibits no tendency to perforation. It is usually cured without causing any permanent structural defects.

40. Describe a Serpiginous Ulcer of the Cornea.

A serpiginous ulcer of the cornea is caused by breaking down of an infiltration of the central corneal tissue. It tends to spread in both surface and depth and its margins exhibit a disposition to slough. The rest of the cornea is inflamed and irritated. It pursues a malignant course and is liable to be associated with ritis and Hypopyon.

41. Describe a Marginal Ulcer of the Cornea.

The marginal ulcer involves the cornea near its circumference. It runs a slow course.

42. Name some Deformities of the Cornea.

The deformities of the cornea are :—

(i.) KERATO-CLONUS or KERATO-GLOBUS— Distension or protrusion of the cornea. The distension is transparent, regular and cone-shaped, the apex of the cone being the centre of the cornea.

(ii.) BUPHTHALMUS—Extensive distension of the cornea, preventing closure of the lids.

(iii.) STAPHYLOMA— Bulging of the cornea in the form of a tumor.

43. Describe Herpes as it affects the Cornea.

Herpes corneæ is characterized by the appearance of groups of small vesicles confined to the cornea alone. It may occur as an idiopathic affection and exhibits a remarkable tendency to recurrence. It may also occur as a manifestation of Herpes Zoster when it is associated with intense pain and local anæsthesia. When the vesicle ruptures, ulcer follows the same.

44. Give symptoms and appearance of Retinitis.

SYMPTOMS—The characteristic symptom is the *loss of transparency of the retina*. Hæmorrhages may be present.

APPEARANCE.— Diffused haziness or circumscribed opacities and swellings. In advanced cases— areas of exudation are exhibited as *white spots*, which may be confluent or discrete.

45. Give symptoms and appearance of Retinitis Albuminuria.

SYMPTOMS.— Hyperæmia of the disc, which may even be swollen and its outline indistinct. Hæmorrhages. Small spots, usually withish, though some times yellow or gray, in the retina around the disc, which usually form a broad, white belt around the disc, separated from the latter by a space of grayish infiltration.

APPEARANCE.—*Small white spots in stellate form about the macula*, together with a whitish belt which surrounds the disc.

46. What is the Prognostic Value of Retinitis Albuminuria in Interstitial Nephritis?

In the majority of cases it is to be accepted as evidence of advanced renal changes, and death occurs within six months or a year after the appearance of Retinitis.

47. Describe the appearance of Diabetic Retinitis.

Numerous white spots, grouped irregularly, appear about the macula.

48. Describe the appearance of Leukæmic Retinitis.

The retina is much swollen and the blood-vessels are greatly dilated. The entire retina assumes a pale or yellowish hue. Hæmorrhagic extravasations and whitish or yellowish spots of exudation are also observed.

49. Give the Functional Disturbances of the Retina.

The functional disturbances of the retina are :—
(i.) Toxic Amaurosis. (ii.) Hysterical Amblyopia.
(iii.) Hyperæsthesia of the retina. (iv.) Hemeralopia.
(v.) Nyctalopia.

50. What are the Toxic Amauroses, and in what conditions are they found?

The *Toxic Amauroses* occur either as manifestations of Uræmia or from lead, Quinine, and Salicylic Acid poisonings or from tobacco-poisoning in Alcoholic subjects.

51. Describe the Tobacco Amaurosis.

The *Tobacco Amaurosis* is characterized clinically by the obscuration of central vision, especially for colors, notably red and green. It occurs especially in subjects who indulge to excess in Alcohol. Chewing tobacco is more injurious than smoking.

Note :—If not properly treated, organic changes in the optic nerve may develop.

52. Describe the Hysterical Amblyopia.

The hysterical Amblyopia is characterized by limitation of the visual fields, which may occur either as an isolated symptom or in association with other hysterical symptoms.

53. What is Hemeralopia?

Night-blindness. The vision is good in day. It is a symptom of several diseases of the eye, of failure of general nutrition, etc.

54. What is Nyctalopia?

It is the reverse of Hemeralopia. In this condition the subject sees better by night or in semi-darkness than by daylight.

55. What is Optic Neuritis?

Optic Neuritis is inflammation of the optic nerve. It may occur as a *papillitis* or inflammation of the head of the nerve, a *Neuro-Retinitis* or descending neuritis, a *Peri-Neuritis*, or a *Retro-bulbar Neuritis*.

56. Give all the causes of the Optic Neuritis.

The causes of Optic Neuritis are:—

Brain tumors. Abscess of the brain. Meningitis. Thrombosis. Multiple Neuritis. Nephritis. Diabetes. Infectious fevers, such at Scarlatina, Typhoid Fever, Variola, etc. Syphilis. Lead-poisoning. Severe-hæmorrhages. Exposure to cold. Local lesions, as orbital diseases, e. g., tumors, caries, Periostitis, etc.

In women—Anæmia. Chlorosis. Menstrual disturbances.

57. Describe the appearance of an Optic Neuritis.

The disc exhibits an increased redness and its borders are obscured. Swelling—the form of the disc lost entirely and its location is recognized only by the point of convergence of the vessels.

58. What is the clinical significance of an Optic Neuritis?

Usually the acuity of vision, the color-sense and the normal fields are more or less affected.

59. What is its Prognostic significance as to Sight?

The sight is not necessarily disturbed, usually however it is affected and the prognosis depends entirely upon the causative factors. Some cases may subside, leaving no disturbance of vision, while severe cases may go on to absolute blindness.

60. What are the causes of the Optic Atrophy?

(i.) PRIMARY CAUSES.— Brain tumor. Locomotor Ataxia. Disseminated Sclerosis. General Paresis. Orbital lesions. Hydrocephalus.

(ii.) SECONDARY— After Neuritis.

61. Give symptoms, appearance, and course of Scrofulous Keratitis.

SYMPTOMS.— *Glandular enlargments. Anæmia.* Persistent coryza, with excoriation of the nostrils. Post-nasal Adenoids. Well-marked photophobia. Profuse lachrymation.

APPEARANCE.—One or more phlyctenulæ on the surface of the cornea, associated with more or less ocular injection.

COURSE.—Chronic; while treatment brings great relief, the causes at work tend to its frequent recurrence.

62. Give symptoms, and appearance of Interstitial Keratitis.

SYMPTOMS.— The characteristic symptom is *gradually increasing opacity*—in the initial stage. More or less pain and lachrymation and the phenomena of sasociated dyscrasiæ.

APPEARANCE.—At first the cornea becomes opaque and the epithelial surface presents a dull aspect. It is soon invaded by very delicate and closely-situated blood-vessels, which give a reddish blush to the cornea.

63. Give symptoms, appearance and course of Episcleritis.

SYMPTOMS.— Slight pain. Conjunctival and peri-corneal injection. Lachrymation. Slight photophobia.

APPEARANCE.—A purplish and somewhat raised patch in the sclerotica, at a short distance—from the limbus corneæ.

COURSE.— The disease runs a course from three to four weeks, with remarkable tendency to recurrence.

64. How do you determine Intra-Ocular Tension?

If the intra-ocular tension is increased, the purple-patches referred to in the previous question, are more extensive and better defined than in Episcleritis.

65. What symptoms point to Diseases in the Iris?

They include alteration in the appearance of the iris and severe pain with peri-corneal injection.

66. Give symptoms, appearance and course of Iritis.

SYMPTOMS.— Severe pain. Peri-corneal injection. *Diminution in the size of the pupil and its inactivity.* Adhesion of the iris to the lens.

APPEARANCE.— The iris presents a dull or lustreless appearance. The size of the pupil is diminished.

COURSE.—It runs an acute course and is amenable to early and proper treatment. If improperly treated there is occlusion of the pupil, with dense adhesions between the iris and crystalline lens.

67. Give causes of Iritis.

The causes of Iritis are—
Syphilis.   Rheumatism.   Gout.   Diabetes.   Tuberculosis.

68. How do you examine the Pupillary Reaction?

To examine the pupillary reaction as to light, the patient should be placed, so that a good light falls upon his eyes, which *must be carefully covered*. Then the covering is to be removed suddenly from one and the effect noticed. The result having been determined, the observation should be repeated upon the other eye.

> Note :—Normally the admission of light should be followed by pupillary contraction.

69. How do you determine the Pupillary Movements during Accommodation?

To determine this the patient is required to fix his gaze upon an object held close to the eyes, say 8 or 10 inches. Then he is directed to look at some distant object.

> Note :—Normally, in the former case the pupils should contract, while in the latter, the pupils dilate.

70. Describe Argyll-Robertson Pupils.

The pupils which respond to accommodation but not to light are known as Argyll-Robertson pupils. It is an early symptom of Loco Motor Ataxia and General Paralysis of the Insane and possesses a high diagnostic value.

71. What is Hippus?

Spasmodic pupillary movement, independent of the action of light is known as Hippus. Contractions and dilatations occur in rapid succession. This is observed in Acute Meningitis, disseminated Sclerosis, Hysteria, Epilepsy and in some cases of tuberculous mediastinal glands.

72. What is Mydriasis?

Abnormal dilatation of the pupil of the eye is known as Mydriasis.

73. What is Myosis?

Abnormal contraction or smallness of the pupil of the eye is known as Myosis.

74. What do you understand by the Consensual Reaction of the Pupils?

Consensual reaction means unanimous action. When light is thrown into one eye, causing the pupil of that eye to contract, it would be seen that the pupil of the other eye also behaves in like manner, though the latter received none of the light stimulus. If in a case of blindness due to, say, optic nerve atrophy the affected eye be stimulated by light, there will be no pupillary movement of the either eye; if the companion eye be stimulated, both the pupils will exhibit the consensual reaction as in health.

75. Refusal of the Pupils to contract in a Case of Blindness is suggestive of what?

It is suggestive of the lesion being in the lower portion of the visual tract.

76. Under what conditions may Mydriasis be present?

Mydriasis may be present under the following conditions :—

(i.) In the forced movement discharged from the

medulla ; vomiting, swallowing, chewing, forced respiration. (ii.) Destruction of the optic nerves; Amaurosis. (iii.) Irritation of the sympathetic nerves. (iv.) In irritation of the cilio-spinal region of the cord. (v.) In encephalic Anæmia. (vi.) In cerebral softening ; in acute Dementia. (vii.) In Hydrophobia. (viii.) In Glaucoma. Etc.

77. Under what conditions may Myosis be present?

(i.) In local irritation or painful affections of the eyeball. (ii.) In irritation of the oculo-motor nerve. (iii.) In Paralysis of the cilio-spinal region of the spinal cord. (iv.) In encephalic congestion. (v.) In the early stages of cerebral tumor. (vi.) In small hæmorrhages into the cerebellum. (vii.) In convulsions arising from menigo-encephalitis. (viii.) In uræmic coma. Etc.

78. What are some of the causes of Paralysis of the Accommodation?

Some of the causes of Paralysis of the accommodation or loss of power of accommodation for near vision are :—

Paralysis of the ciliary muscle. Paralysis of the iris. Diphtheria. Syphilis. Tuberculosis. Etc.

79. Give symptoms of Atrophy of the Optic Nerve.

SYMPTOMS.—Gradual decrease of acuity of vision. Concentric limitation of the visual field. Loss of color sense. Dilatation and immobility of the pupil. The sense of sight may remain good for a long time.

Ophthalmoscopically, the disc presents an opaque, bluish or grayish white appearance and often has a cup-shaped appearance The vessels are few in number and more or less reduced in size and the lamina cribrosa may become plainly visible.

> Note :—The diagnosis is based upon the ophthalmoscopic findings.

80. What is Exophthalmos?

Abnormal prominence or protrusion of the eyeballs is known as EXOPHTHALMOS. It occurs as a symptom of orbital growths or retro-ocular œdema, and is one of the characteristic symptoms of Exophthalmic Goitre.

81. What is Enophthalmos?

Retraction or recession of eyeballs in the orbit is known as ENOPHTHALMOS. It is observed in collapsic conditions and in wasting diseases.

82. Give the Nerve-supply of the Muscles of the Eye.

The muscles of the eye are supplied by the *third fourth* and *sixth cranial nerves*. The *fourth* or *patheticus* supplies the *superior oblique* muscle; the *sixth* or *abducens* supplies the *external rectus*; and the *third* or *motor oculi* supplies the remaining muscles, both external and internal.

83. What are some of the causes of Ocular Palsies in (a) Adults: (b) Children?

(a.) The causes of ocular palsies in ADULTS are—
Syphilis. Rheumatism. Infectious diseases. Organic brain diseases of a sarcomatous or tuberculous nature. Disseminated Sclerosis. General Paralysis of the Insane. Etc.

(b.) The causes in CHILDREN are :—
Congenital. Tuberculosis. Some infectious diseases, especially Diphtheria.

84. What symptoms are complained of in Ocular Palsies.

The cardinal symptom is *Strabismus*—marked by defective movement of the eyeball in the direction of action of the affected muscle or muscles. Diplopia. False projection of the visual field i. e., the ability of the patient to judge correctly the position of objects becomes impaired. Greater secondary deviation of the sound eye.

85. What is Primary Deviation?

By deviation is meant a turning aside from the normal. In strabismus or paralytic squint, the deviation of the visual axis of the squinting eye is known as PRIMARY DEVIATION.

86. What is Secondary Deviation?

Deviation of the covered healthy eye when the squinting eye fixes is known as SECONDARY DEVIATION. This deviation is greater than that observed in the affected eye.

87. Describe Homonymous Diplopia.

See Ans. to Q. 10 of this Chapter.

88. Describe Crossed Diplopia.

See Ans. to Q. 10 of this Chapter.

89. What is Concomitant Squint?

When the squinting eye has full range of movement it is known as the concomitant squint. It is due to refractive errors.

90. What is Convergent Squint?

When the squinting eye is turned to the nasal side the squint is known as convergent squint. It is due to the spasmodic affections of the ocular muscles, and Paralysis of the superior oblique muscle and external recuts.

91. Give symptoms of Paralysis of the Third Nerve?

The symptoms include—

Abolition of all movements of the eye, with the exception of abduction and rotation downwards and outwards. The power of accommodation is lost, and the pupil is moderately dilated and does not react to light.

When the Paralysis is complete, there is drooping of the upper eyelid (ptosis), and deviation of the eyeball *outwards* and *downwards*.

When all the eye-muscles are paralysed, there is a slight protrusion of the eyeball.

92. Give symptoms of Paralysis of Superior Rectus.

The symptoms of Paralysis of the superior rectus are :—

Deviation of the eye *downwards*, with slight divergence; *crossed diplopia*—aggravated when the patient tries to look upwards. The false image is seen above the true, and is tilted, in the case of the affection of the left eye, to the patient's right.

93. Give symptoms of Paralysis of Internal Rectus.

The symptoms of Paralysis of the internal rectus are :—

Crossed diplopia. Divergent strabismus.

94. Give symptoms of Paralysis of Inferior Rectus.

The symptoms of Paralysis of the inferior rectus are :—

The eye deviates upwards and slightly outwards. The relative position of the images is converse to that of Paralysis of the superior rectus, as described above.

95. Give symptoms of Paralysis of the Fourth Nerve.

The symptoms of Paralysis of the fourth nerve are :—

Loss of movement of the eye *downwards and inwards*. Convergent strabismus. *Simple diplopia*.

96. Give symptoms of Paralysis of the Sixth Nerve.

The symptoms of Paralysis of the sixth nerve are :—

Loss of power in the external rectus. Convergent strabismus. Homonymous diplopia.

97. What symptoms may result from Muscular Insufficiency?

Insufficiency of ocular muscles may produce:—

Strabismus. Asthenopia. Diplopia. Irregular movements of the eyeball. Etc.

98. What is Nystagmus, and what is its Diagnostic Value?

Nystagmus is a rhythmical oscillatory movement of the eyeballs, generally *lateral* (may also be vertical or rotary). It is associated with some *local changes* such as opacities of the cornea and lens and degenerative diseases of the choroid and retina; it occurs in some *diseases of the nervous system* such as Disseminated Sclerosis, Freidrich's Ataxia, Meningitis, meningeal hæmorrhage, Thrombosis of the cerebral sinuses, tumor, and local softening. Lesions in the Pons, Optic Thalamus and Corpora Quadrigemina have also caused it.

Its diagnostic value is that it is a *positive proof of organic disease*.

99. Give the conditions associated with Irregular Movements of the Eyeballs.

The irregular movements of the eyeballs are associated with:—

Ocular palsies, muscular insufficiencies, refractive errors, labyrinthine disease, chronic Hydrocephalus, Meningitis and Hysteria.

100. What is the clinical significance of Conjugated Deviation of the Head and Eyes?

The clinical significance of conjugated deviation of the head and eyes is: the paralytic or spasmodic involvement of the external rectus of one eye and the internal rectus of the other and the sterno-mastoid muscle on the side opposite to the direction of the movement. It is frequently observed in cerebral hæmorrhage, brain tumor and Meningitis.

101. How do you test the Acuity of Vision?

The ACUITY OF VISION is determined by certain *test-types* standardized for *normal vision* at different distances, e. g., TWENTY type legible at 20 feet, TEN type at 10 feet, etc. The distance from which the patient is able to read them is measured, and the *record of vision* is that distance divided by the distance at which the same is legible by the normal eye. Thus, if the TWENTY type can be read at 10 feet, the record of vision is $\frac{10}{20}$.

> Note:—Each eye should be tested separately, care being taken that the one not in use is well-covered.

102. How do you test for Astigmatism?

The test for ASTIGMATISM is ordinarily conducted over a diagram consisting of a number of *lines* of uniform width, drawn in different directions; the lines are clear, sharply defined, and not too narrow. The patient is directed to look at the diagram, and if the eye is astigmatic, some of the lines will appear clear, and others more or less indistinct.

103. How do you test Visual Field?

The test for VISUAL FIELD is conducted by an instrument called the PERIMETER.

104. How do you test Muscular Equilibrium?

The test for MUSCULAR EQUILIBRIUM is conducted by an instrument called the MADDOX PRISM. The prism is held before one eye, and the patient is directed to look with both the eyes at a lighted candle. If the muscular balance is normal, there will appear *a long red band running at right angles to the axis* at which the prism is held, and *intersecting* the light, which will present the usual appearance as observed with the naked eye. If there is muscular insufficiency, *the red band will not intersect the light,* but *will pass to one or the other side of it,* according to the particular muscles affected.

165. How do you make an Opthalmoscopic Examination?

There are two methods of ophthalmoscopic examination, viz., the *direct* or that with an upright image and the *indirect* or that with an inverted image, both conducted in a dark room, where artificial light such as an Argand gas-burner or a student's lamp is commonly used.

For employing the *direct method* the mirror is held as close as possible to the optic disc of the patient to be examined. The patient is asked to look straight, forward, while the examiner looks in from the temporal side at an angle of about 15°. For the examination of the left eye, the observer's left is used, and for the right eye, the right; the place of the lamp being shifted and the instrument put into the corresponding hand. If the eyes of both be normal in refraction, and in both accommodation be entirely at rest, the details of the eye-ground will be easily seen.

For employing the *indirect method*, the observer holds the mirror 12″ or 14″ from the patient, and brings before the latter's eye, within 2″ of it, a bi-convex lens of two and a half inches focus. This lens condenses the light from the mirror and also collects the emergent light into an inverted image which lies at about $2\frac{1}{2}″$ from the lens, between it and the mirror. The observer examines this aerial image, and not the eye. It is bright, small, and covers a larger surface and shows better the relation of the parts.

CHAPTER XXII.

THE EAR.

1. How do you conduct the Examination of an Ear?

To get a complete knowledge of the Pathological conditions of the ear a systematic method must be followed minutely.

The *history* and the *subjective symptoms* as given by the patient and gathered by the physician by enquiry should be recorded. The temperament, conditions of general health and the presence of any dyscrasia should be noted. Enquiries about sore-throat, coryzas and chronic catarrhs, the use of tobacco and deafness (if hereditary) should be made and noted.

The *objective symptoms* are next gathered by a systematic examination of the ear from all sides. The hearing of both the ears, is tested by the VOICE, watch and TUNING-FORK and is carefully recorded. The internal condition is examined first by direct light, and then by reflected light from a mirror (OTOSCOPE).

2. Give the Anatomy of the Ear.

The human ear is divided into three component parts, viz., the EXTERNAL EAR, the MIDDLE EAR or the TYMPANUM, and the INTERNAL EAR or the LABYRINTH. The *first* comprises the AURICLE or the PINNA, and the EXTERNAL AUDITORY MEATUS: the *second*, the TYMPANUM with two diverticulas, the MASTOID CELLS and PROCESS behind, and the EUSTACHIAN TUBE in front; and the *third* the VESTIBULE, SEMI-CIRCULAR CANALS and COCHLEA. The SURFACE of the external ear is a *dermoid* one, its features are like those of the integument generally; the middle ear or the tympanum is lined by a mucous membrane which is at the same time periosteum to the bone which it overlies, and is continuous with the pharynx *via* the Eustachian Tube. The internal ear or the labyrinth is lined by a serous membrane in immediate relation to and supporting the terminal fibres of a nerve of special sense.

3. Give the Physiology of the Ear.

The external and middle ears are *conducting*, and the internal ear is both *conducting and receptive*. The sounds are caused by vibrations. They are transmitted as waves through the air and concentrate in the funnel-shaped external ear, which conducts them to a vibratory membrane, which in turn transmits them by delicately adjusted osseous levers to another membrane, attached to the inner end of the chain of ossicles ; those corresponding vibrations, like the echoes of the first, set in motion the fluid contained in a bony cavity and through the same pass to the basilar membrane and membrane of Reissner and set the endo-lymph of the canal of the cochlea in motion and ultimately impress the hair-cells at the extremities of the auditory nerve in the cochlea.

4. Give the Method of Diagnosis of an Aural Disease.

The diagnosis of an aural disease must be based upon an accurate knowledge of the normal appearances and Physiological action of the auditory apparatus. Every opportunity should be taken to examine the membrana tympani, its color and movements during inflation and phonation, the appearance of the ossicles if visible, and the hue of the middle ear. The naso-pharyngeal space, the mouth of the Eustachian tube, and the movements of the palato-pharyngeal muscles should be studied closely by methods and instruments as enumerated in Ans. to Q. 1 of this Chapter.

When a patient complains of some functional disturbance of the ear, the determination of the *cause*, *consequence* and *lesion* is indispensible.

5. Name some Symptoms of Ear Disease.

The symptoms of ear disease may be *common* or *uncommon*.

THE COMMON SYMPTOMS.— Deafness or impairment of hearing. Pain. Abnormal discharge. Tinnitus Aurium. Vertigo.

THE UNCOMMON or OCCASIONAL SYMPTOMS.— Sensation as of something moving in the ears. Fullness and pressure in the ears. Resonance of the voice. Itching and soreness in the ears. Double hearing. Inability to tell from what direction sounds come (*Paracusis loci*). Sensation of breathing sounds in the ears. Etc.

6. What is suggested by Sudden Impairment of Hearing?

It is suggestive of plugging of the external auditory meatus, as by cerumen.

7. What is suggested by Sudden Loss of Hearing following (i.) Mumps; (ii.) Scarlet Fever; and (iii.) Influenza?

(i.) Suggestive of auditory nerve lesion.

(ii.) and (iii.) Suggestives of middle ear involvement.

8. What symptom suggests Syphilis of the Auditory Nerve?

Very rapidly increasing deafness, with no other symptoms suggests Syphilis of the Auditory Nerve.

9. What is suggested by Slowly Progressive Deafness of Tinnitus Aurium?

Suggestive of changes in the tympanitic cavity; in the case of old people, auditory nerve Sclerosis.

10. What is suggested by Impairment of Hearing—recent and moderate and not associated with Pain?

Suggestive of catarrh of the Eustachian Tube, mild catarrh of the tympanum or impacted cerumen.

11. What is suggested by very Sudden Deafness following extreme Vertigo and Nausea?

Suggestive of labyrinthine lesion, probably hæmorrhagic.

12. What is suggested by Sudden Deafness following Head Injury, (i.) with the appearance of Blood in the Canal, and (ii.) when a Flow of Serum appears in association with or after the Bleeding?

(i.) Suggestive of rupture of the membrana tympani.
(ii.) Suggestive of fracture of the base of the skull or auditory nerve lesion.

13. What is meant by Tinnitus Aurium? What are its Causes?

The subjective ringing or hissing sound heard in the ears, due to various affections of the tympanum and internal ear. It may also result from alterations in the general vascular pressure, in a variety of diseases, such as, chronic Interstitial Nephritis; heart diseases, Anæmia and overdosing with Quinine, Salycilate of Soda and Alcohol.

14. What is the most common cause of Pain in the Ear?

The most common cause of pain in the ear is inflammation of the middle ear.

15. How do you differentiate Pain from Disease in the Canal?

The pain from disease in the auditory canal is aggravated by pressure within the canal or on the tragus, or by traction upon the auricle or by a chewing motion.

16. How do you differentiate Pain from Disease in the Middle Ear?

The pain of inflammation of the middle ear is aggravated by sneezing and blowing the nose and by pressure below the lobule of the external ear.

17. How do you differentiate Pain from Disease in the Eustachian Tube?

It disappears very promptly on inflation. It is sometimes severe.

18. How do you differentiate Pain from Inflammation of the Mastoid Process?

It is usually aggravated by pressure over the base or apex of that prominence.

19. What is suggested by Pain occurring during the Course of Chronic Suppurative Disease of the Tympanum?

It suggests either the damning up of discharge of the supervention of or increase in already existing caries of the bones.

20. Describe the Vertigo of Ear Disease.

The vertigo of ear disease is due to increased labyrinthine tension or to changes in the labyrinth itself as exudation and hæmorrhage. It is a prominent symptom of Meniere's Disease.

21. What is Meniere's Disease?

It is a disorder characterized by intense *vertigo, deafness, tinnitus aurium*, etc. The lesion is probably in the semi-circular canals, and may be attended with nausea, vomiting and syncope. From a diminution of hearing, the hearing is at last suddenly and totally lost.

22. Describe the Vertigo from Organic Disease of the Brain.

The vertigo may occur from any kind of disease situated in any portion of the brain, and is especially liable to occur in *tumors* in or near the cerebellum. It frequently accompaines Loco Motor Ataxia and Disseminated Sclerosis of the brain and spinal cord.

23. Describe the Vertigo from Cardiac Disease.

The vertigo resulting from cardiac disease is usually due to *failing circulation*, and is aggravated by exertion, strong emotions and causes generally calling upon the heart for extra work.

24. Describe the Vertigo from Epilepsy.

The vertigo of Epilepsy appears without any previous warning and is invariably associated with some *loss of consciousness*. It may be associated with deafness and tinnitus aurium.

25. Differentiate Epileptic Vertigo from Meniere's Disease.

Very quick recovery of the patient from the attack, the absence of any aural disturbance during the inter-paroxysmal period and the invariable association of some *loss of consciousness*, differentiate the Epileptic vertigo from Meniere's Disease.

26. Describe the Vertigo from Hysteria.

The vertigo from Hysteria is recognized by the characteristic temperament of the patient and its association with the usual stigmata of the disease.

27. Describe the Vertigo from Neurasthenia.

The vertigo from Neurasthenia is usually associated with general weakness and sensation of pressure in various portions of the head.

28. Name an Instance where Disturbance in a Special Sense can cause Vertigo.

The *refrative errors* can cause vertigo in association with blurring of sight, frontal and occipital headache, conjunctival irritation and lachrymation.

29. What is Peripheral Vertigo?

The peripheral vertigo may occur from causes, of which the laryngeal and the gastric are of special prominence. The laryngeal vertigo begins with a sensation in the larynx which leads to a severe spasmodic *cough*, at once followed by vertigo and unconsciousness. The attack lasts for a few minutes.

The gastric vertigo is especially liable to be associated with acute and chronic Gastritis and Hyperchlorhydria.

30. Name the Toxic Conditions causing Vertigo.

The TOXIC CONDITIONS which may cause vertigo are—

(i.) POISONOUS DRUGS, such as Belladonna, Cannabis Indica, Alcohol, tea, etc.
(ii.) LITHAEMIA.
(iii.) Bright's Disease.

31. What is the significance of a thin Watery Discharge from the Ear?

It indicates rupture of the membrana tympani and lesion of the labyrinth, caused by a fracture at the base of the skull.

32. What is the significance of a Mucoid Discharge from the Ear?

It indicates the inflammation of the drum cavity.

33. What is the significance of a Purulent Discharge from the Ear?

It indicates inflammation of either the auditory canal or the drum cavity.

If from the CANAL, it is generally attended with diminution of pain.

If from the DRUM CAVITY, its appearance is succeeded by relief of pain.

If *without preceding pain*, it is strongly suggestive of tubercular complication,

34. What is the significance of a Bloody Discharge from the Ear?

It indicates the rupture of the membrana tympani. It may also result from granular tissue.

35. What is the significance of a Brownish, Blackish or Bluish Discharge from the Ear?

It indicates bone disease.

36. What is the significance of a Foul Odor to a Discharge from the Ear?

It indicates decomposition from defective drainage.

37. What is to be suspected, if the Discharge is of Short Duration, and recurs repeatedly?

The disease of the attic. Examination will discover perforations in the membrana flaccida.

38. Give the Tests for Auditory Function.

The AUDITORY FUNCTION is tested by—

(i.) VOICE—Using the tone of ordinary conversation, stage-whisper or the reserve-air whisper.

The examiner stands a few feet away from the patient upon the side of the ear to be tested. The patient is directed to close his eyes, so that he cannot see the lips move. The examiner then utters a variety of words in a conversational tone or wishper and gradually approaches the patient; the distance from which the sound is audible is noted and compared with the distance from which the sound is audible *normally*.

(ii.) INSTRUMENT.—Using *watch* and similar apparatus or the *tuning fork*.

    (a) BY WATCH or similar apparatus : say a stop-watch.—The watch should be standardized by testing a number of normal cases. The examiner holds the watch in the palm with its face towards the hearer's ear which is to be tested, the other ear being closed by the finger, at the normal distance and then approach gradually towards the patient until he can catch the sound ; the distance from which the sound is audible is then measured by a tape-measure and compared with the distance from which the sound is audible normally. *The result is a fraction*, the *denominator* of which is the distance at which the sound is heard normally and the *numerator* is the distance from which the sound is audible to the examining ear.

    (b) BY TUNING-FORK.—For this, two tests are commonly used, those of WEBER and of RINNE.

    WEBER'S TEST.— The vibrating tuning-fork is placed with its base on the vertex, forehead, or against the teeth of the patient. It is heard more distinctly in the affected ear, if the canal or tympanum is involved ; if the labyrinth is involved, it is heard better in the normal ear.

    RINNE'S TEST.— The vibrating tuning-fork is held with its base against the mastoid process, and when the perception of sound ceases and the lines of the fork are held in front of the auditory meatus, *normally* the sound is once more perceived.

If the labyrinth is involved, the hearing is defective and we note the result: "Rinne's test, *positive.*"

If the conducting apparatus i. e., the canal aud tympanum are involved, the vibrations are heard longer over the mastoid than with the fork in front of the ear, and we note the result: "Rinne's test, *negative.*"

39. Describe the Use of Eustachian Catheter.

An Eustachian Catheter is an instrument used for objective examination of the Eustachian Tube for distending or making applications to it. It should be held loosely and moved in gently, so that no injury may be caused, to the mucous membrane and the instrument may follow a crooked passage if such be present. It is introduced through the nose to reach the pharyngeal wall and thence to the mouth of the Eustachian Tube. It helps the diagnosis of naso-pharyngeal, tubal and tympanitic disorders.

40. Name some of the Abnormal Conditions of the Eustachian Canal.

Catarrhal inflammation. Chronic Nasal Catarrh. Adenoid tumors. Chronic inflammation.

41. Describe the Appearance of the Normal Tympanic Membrane.

The color of a normal tympanic membrane is from a bluish to a yellowish-gray, differing at different ages and by Anatomical variations in and around it. It is *lighter* in infants because the dermic layer is thicker, and generally shaded with pink. It has an amber-gray, translucent appearance near the centre, in front, and behind the malleus.

42. What points are to be noted about Tympanic Membrane?

About its polish, translucency, color, hyperæmia, retraction, flattening or bulging, surface, perforation and abnormal growth.

43. How may the Eustachian Tube be examined?

It may be examined by posterior rhinoscopy. Its patency may be determined, by passing air to the tube by means of a catheter or other method and also by the character of the sound, whether the tube is freely open or artresic, and the presence of fluid in the tube and the tympanic cavity.

44. Name some Abnormalities of the Tympanum.

(i.) Loss of its POLISH—due to deposits of foreign matters or presence of desquamating epithelium or wax.

(ii.) Loss of its TRANSLUCENCY—due to inflammatory thickening.

(iii.) Loss of its COLOR—due to inflammation of the middle ear. The membrane may present a bright red surface, later gray and sodden.

(iv.) HYPERAEMIA.

(v.) EXAGGERATED RETRACTION.

(vi.) FLATTENING or BULGING—due to the presence of free fluid in the tympanum.

(vii.) IRREGULARITIES of its SURFACE—due to scars, vesicles, polypi, and granulations.

(viii.) PERFORATION—due to inflammation of the tympanic cavity or traumatism.

45. What does a Bulging or Flattening Membrane mean?

It usually indicates the presence of free fluid in the tympanic cavity.

46. What does a Retracted Membrane mean?

It indicates imperfect ventilation of the tympanum.

47. How are Perforations to be diagnosed?

The perforations are to be diagnosed by inspection or by inflation of the tympanum.

48. Give symptoms of Inspissated Cerumen.

SUBJECTIVE SYMPTOMS.—Ringing in the ears, sudden impairment of hearing, sense of fulness, accompanied, at times with pain and vertigo. There may be an irritating, tickling cough. In the severe forms there may be reeling and staggering.

OBJECTIVE SYMPTOMS.—A blackish or brownish mass obscures the membrana tympani.

49. Diagnose Eustachian Catarrh.

The subjective symptoms of the Eustachian catarrh are sense of fulness, itching, pains in the throat and cough. Associated ear symptoms are tingling and stuffy feelings in the ears, deafness, vertigo, and pain which is sometimes extremely sharp. They are produced by the engorgement of tubes, and the ensuing defective ventilation of the tympanum; the drum-head shows marked retraction. To avoid errors, either in diagnosis or treatment, the ears of all patients should be examined.

50. What is the usual Location of the Furuncles?

The usual location of the *furuncles* is within the auditory canal. The objective appearance of the lesion is that of a circumscribed swelling within the meatus.

51. Give symptoms and diagnosis of Chronic Catarrhal Otitis Media.

SYMPTOMS.—

(i.) SUBJECTIVE.—*Gradually-increasing deafness,* usually associated with and sometimes preceded by tinnitus, and occasionally vertigo. Rarely, the patient complains of some pain and itching.

> Note :—The deafness is marked by impairment of the lower tone, the tones of higher picth being better heard. Weber's test shows hearing better in the affected ear : Rinne's test ; negative.

(ii.) OBJECTIVE.—The canal may be dry, or there may be present an unusual quantity of cerumen. The membrana tympani is opaque and presents a dull surface, or it may be dull and atrophic. The anterior and posterior folds, exaggerated. The drum-head is impaired in its mobility. The Eustachian Tube is commonly less permeable than in health. The light reflex is shortened or absent.

The DIAGNOSIS is based upon the presence of the above subjective and objective symptoms.

52. Give the symptoms and diagnosis of Acute Catarrhal Otitis Media.

SUBJECTIVE SYMPTOMS.—Sense of fulness in the ears, deafness, tinnitus and *pain*. The pain is the most prominent symptom, which increases gradualiy till it perforates the membrane (from 1 to 3 days), when it ceases. After perforation there is a mucoid discharge in the canal. It is aggravated at night or when the patient is lying down. The symptoms are of rapid onset.

In children, it may be complicated with high temperature (103° to 104° F.), vomiting, delirium, convulsions, simulating Meningitis.

OBJECTIVE SYMPTOMS.—Diffuse hyperæmia of the drum-head, particularly of the lower portion. With the stage of exudation, there is a flattening or bulging, and the lusture of the surface is lost.

DIAGNOSIS.— After ascertaining *the cause*, and investigation of the symptoms, the ear should be examined to find out the objective symptoms. Where there are symptoms of cerebral irritation, particularly in children, the eye also is to be examined.

53. Give the symptoms and diagnosis of Acute Suppurative Otitis Media.

SUBJECTIVE SYMTOMPS.—Great pain, and high temperature accompained by deafness, *prostration*, and often delirium. The pain is not relieved until perforation of the membrana tympani takes place. The symptoms are of *sudden* onset and *severe*.

OBJECTIVE SYMPTOMS.—Hyperæmia of the drumhead greatest in its upper part and yellow-colored. Sometimes the upper wall of the lower end of the canal is involved in the hyperæmia and swelling and it may be difficult to find out where the canal ends and membrane begins. The perforation is found to occur frequently in the upper portion of the membrane.

DIAGNOSIS.— Besides the rapidity of the onset, the severity of the symptoms and prostration, a maximum degree of swelling in Sharpnell's membrane, with involvement of the lower end of the canal, is indicative of Acute Suppurative Otitis Media. It is almost never insidious in its attacks, but bold and pronounced.

It is imperatively necessary to recognize the disease early and to treat it actively.

54. Give symptoms and diagonosis of Chronic Suppurative Otitis Media.

SUBJECTIVE SYMPTOMS.—The local symptoms vary with the pathological condition of the ear ; ordinarily *Otorrhœa* or *a purulent discharge* from the ear and *hardness of hearing* are the only symptoms. When the upper portion of the tympanum is involved, it displays most serious consequences, such as, fever, nausea, vertigo, lateral headaches, delirium, increased sensitiveness of the external auditory canal, occasional darts of pain through the aural region and even extension of the inflammation to the mastoid, meninges, and the venous sinuses of the brain. The discharge is very offensive.

OBJECTIVE SYMPTOMS.—Perforation of the drum-head, of any size. Exuberant granulation tissue and polypi are common. The external meatus and the outer surface of the drum-head have a bright-red appearance due to constant passing of the pus and the pharynx is frequently found in a catarrhal stage.

DIAGNOSIS.—Exudation of offensive pus from the ear and the discovery of its cause are the chief diagnostic points of the disease. If the pus is of ordinary color, it shows tympanic granulations; if it is dark and comes from above or behind, it indicates the presence of caries. The prognosis depends upon the constitution of the patient and the eondition of the ear, as revealed by a careful inspection of the tympanum after it had been thoroughly cleansed. The natural course of the disease is towards deeper parts.

55. What are some of the Complications of Purulent Ear Disease?

(i.) Polypi within the tympanum. (ii.) Paralysis of the facial nerve. (iii.) Caries and Necrosis of the temporal bone. (iv.) Mastoiditis. (v.) Cerebral abscess. (vi.) Pyæmia. (vii.) Meningitis. (viii.) Phlebitis and (ix.) Thrombosis of the lateral sinus.

56. Give symptoms of the Internal Ear Disease.

SYMPTOMS.—
(i.) In the auditory-nerve diseases—deafness, vertigo and nausea. There are seldom fever and unconsciousness. The tuning fork is heard better on the good side. The high register of sounds impaired. Very sudden attacks are probably hæmorrhagic.

(ii.) In other cases—sudden invasions of paroxysms of tinnitus associated with vertigo and followed by deafness.

57. How will you diagnose a Polypus in the Ear?

The ear should be syringed and wiped clean, a speculum introduced, and the parts illuminated and examined. A fine probe or a paltinum wire loop pushed between the polypus and the canal walls will inform one about the consistence, mobility, size and attachment of the growth. The spot from which the growth springs should be determined, so that a snare for removal may be applied properly.

58. Give the varieties of Polypi in the Ears.

(i.) ANGIOMAS.—Soft, red, irregular-shaped growths. They are composed of newly-formed network or mesh of blood-vessels held together by connective tissues. When these growths are punctured or torn, copious and alarming hæmorrhage sometimes occurs. They are *very rare*.

(ii.) MYXOMAS.—Structureless *mucin jelly*, held together by anastomosing network of spindle and irregular stellate cells, with a liberal intermixture of fine fibres, and are covered by pavement epithelium, and feel soft and smooth. They are *very rare* and may be readily *mistaken* for a mucous polypus, with which they are to be distinguished with the help of a microscope before a certain diagnosis can be made.

(iii.) FIBROMAS.—Bluish-gray in color and smooth and tough like *callous skin*. They originate in the periosteum of the tympanum and push the mucous membrane as they develop. Though its frequency is next to *mucous polypus* which occurs more frequently, it is easily recognized after cleaning the ear, by the *color, consistency* and *dry-looking surface*. It grows very slowly.

(iv.) MUCOUS.—Purple, pale pink, bluish-red, raspberry red or crimson in color. Their surface is smooth and glistening, a little papillary or lobulated. There is frequently a copious hæmorrhage upon its removal. They grow very fast and spring up rapidly after their removal. They are more frequently seen than the three previous varieties all together.

59. Give the symptoms and diagnosis of the Mastoid Disease.

SYMPTOMS.— A heavy aching pain begins deep in the ear and mastoid, and extends to the occiput, becoming very severe at night; sharp intermitting pains shoot through the side of the head; the skin over the mastoid becomes red, slightly swollen, and sensitive to the touch, and the patient feels chilly uncomfortable and sick. Sometimes there is vertigo, nausea and vomiting. Thrombosis, Pyæmia, Meningitis or cerebral abscess may complicate in severe cases, with convulsions and coma ending fatally.

DIAGNOSIS.—The *pain is deep, severe and radiating*. The discharge from the ear frequently ceases almost entirely. The tissues over the mastoid may not be much affected, but generally are boggy and sensitive. The constitutional disturbance is marked. The subjective symptoms are often more severe, than what the objective symptoms suggest. It may be confounded with acute inflammation of the tympanum, but when relief of pain does not follow a warm douche and a proper paracentesis of the drumhead, one is justified to diagnose the disease as of mastoid origin.

60. What is the relation of a Pharyngeal Disease with an Aural Disease?

The pharyngeal disease is so closely allied to an aural disease, that the former must be suspected as the cause of much trouble in the ear.

CHAPTER XXIII.

X-RAY DIAGNOSIS.

1. Who discovered the X-ray, and in what Year?

The X-ray was discovered by Roentgen, in the year 1895 A. D.

2. Why does the Medical Diagnostician find the X-ray valuable?

The medical practitioner found it to be of considerable value in outlining certain organs of the body, whose borders, by blending more or less with contiguous viscera are uncertain of determination, by the ordinary methods of diagnosis.

3. What property relative to the Fluoroscopic Screen in examining the Tissues of the Body is possessed by the X-ray?

The X-ray possesses the property of making on the fluoroscopic screen *shadows* whose densities are practically in proportion to the densities of the tissues to be examined.

4. What two forms of X-ray Apparatus are chiefly used?

FLUOROSCOPE and RADIOGRAPH.

5. In the use of the X-ray, why is a Dark Room advisable?

In Radiography darkness is not so necessary, but in Fluoroscopy relative, and at times, absolute darkness or exclusion of light is essential.

6. With the Outfit ready for use, describe in general terms the Position of the Patient under Examination.

The patient may stand before the apparatus, or seated in a chair having either a movable or a straight back. Where the organ affected is not affected by position, it is better to have the patient lie prone or supine upon some convenient bed, such as a canvas stretcher or trestles.

7. Describe in general terms the Principles underlying ordinary Radiography.

Ordinary Radiography has as its principle the action of the ray upon a sensitized film, the impression or picture thus made varying in degree with, in general terms, the density of the parts examined.

It is this property of the X-ray, that enables a radiographer to take not only a shaded view of the organs he is examining, but, to some extent a perspective view of them also.

8. Describe the Fluoroscope and Fluoroscopy.

The FLUOROSCOPE.—It is essentially a box made to fit over the eyes so as to exclude all ordinary light, while the end opposite the face portion is covered by a screen coated with *Barium-Platinum Cyanide*. It is held up before the patient, who is interposed between the energized X-ray tube and the instrument, and the screen is made fluorescent by the rays which pass through him. The part to be examined must be in a direct line with the screen end of the instrument as well as the X-ray tube. With the details of position and relation of tube to the patient attended to, the observer looks through the Fluoroscope, and if fluorescence has been well-established, shadows are observed in the Fluoroscope, which varies according to the same rule that obtains in Radiography. Thin patients are readily examined by the Fluoroscope, but in the obese fluoroscopy is sometimes difficult.

FLUOROSCOPY is the viewing of the parts under examination by means of the Fluoroscopic Screen or Fluoroscope.

9. How would you adjust the Spark-Gap in an Adjustable Tube to secure "Low" or "High" Vaccuum?

Adjustment is almost instantly secured by a change made in the length of the spark-gap—*lessened* to secure a low vacuum and *lengthened* to secure a high vacuum.

> *Note* :—Usually, a low vacuum gives a better fluoroscopic view.

10. How the patient should be attired during an X-ray Examination?

The patient should be attired with a thin garment and stripped of all clothing likely to interfere with the finer details of the examination, such as corsets, buttons, buckles, etc. Nothing should be allowed to compress or in any way distort the part under examination.

11. Why it is necessary that the patient should be given an Idea of the Nature of the Examination in advance, and an Explanation be made of the steps of the process?

Otherwise, he may be startled or frightened, or, at an important stage in the examination, indulge in a movement of the body that will depreciate the value of the investigation.

12. Describe Radiography.

The Radiography consists in the substitution of a photographer's plate for the Fluoroscope or screen. The rays act upon the silver-salts in the sensitized plate as do the rays of ordinary light, and produce *shadows showing the various changes in the homogeneity of the part*. The process differs very little from that employed in ordinary photography, except that a camera is not used.

In making a radiogram, the part should be divested of as much clothing as possible, especially of all metal parts. If a limb is bound in splints, the latter need not be removed, if they do not contain pins, etc. Even plaster-of-Paris casts are no bar to the penetration of the X-ray.

The sensitized plates generally used are especially made for the purpose, and are known as X-ray plates.

13. What is the Value of X-ray Examination in Diagnosis?

The X-ray simply deals with shadows made by opaque objects, and determines nothing more than their existence, size, form and situation. This limits X-ray, for purposes of diagnosis, within somewhat narrow conceptions; but, in spite of that its value is inestimable, because it enables the diagnostician to have the proper estimate of internal disease-conditions. Moreover it is not only confirmative, but is often suggestive and conclusive.

14. Give the Fundamental Principles of the X-ray in its Application to Medical and Surgical Diagnosis.

(i.) It simply outlines the contours of the body.

(ii.) It outlines certain organs and tissues of the body.

(iii.) It outlines and locates foreign bodies, which may be within the tissues.

Note:—The decision is to be arrived at by comparing the shadow of the part under examination with the shadow of the part in its normal condition.

15. Compare the Observations mdae by Fluoroscopy with those of Radiography.

Flouroscopy may be said to be a view in gross: Radiography a view in detail. The latter is usually a finer demonstration, and shows effects not possible to obtain by the former.

16. What Evidence is required in Interpreting an X-ray Picture?

A knowledge of all the facts bearing on the case is required in interpreting an X-ray picture.

17. What Disease of the Brain will the X-ray materially assist in diagnosing?

The tumor of the brain.

18. Why is the X-ray of no service in diagnosing Intra-spinal Disease?

The shadows formed by the spine, in the X-ray plate are too indefinite, hence it is of no help to the medical clinician in his diagnosis of intra-spinal disease.

19. Name some of the Affections of the Thorax in which the X-ray is employed to outline.

Pulmonary consolidations, cavities, Emphysema and Tuberculosis. Mediastinal Tumors. Aortic Aneurysm. Enlarged or displaced heart. Pericardial effusions. Pleural effusions. Empyema. Tumors of various kinds. Foreign bodies. Etc.

20. Describe the Influence of Diaphragm on the Fluoroscopic Picture in the Examination of the Thorax in the Living Subject.

The shadow cast by the diaphragm, is restricted on the affected side or sides and usually in the lower part of its excursion.

21. What Diseases of the Thorax will increase the Normal X-ray Fluoroscopic Shadow?

It may be due to Pneumonia or congestion of the lungs or to pulmonary cavities filled with exudate.

22. What Diseases of the Thorax will decrease the Normal X-ray Fluoroscopic Shadow?

Emphysema of the lungs or Pneumothorax.

23. What will suggest a Cavity in the Lung, filled with Air?

The usual lung-fluorescence will be interrupted at the point by an oasis of intenser light.

> Note :—It needs to be confirmed by other tests to make such a diagnosis positive.

24. If a Consolidation Shadow is found under a portion of the Chest-wall which responds normally to Auscultation and Percussion, what would it suggest?

Pheumonic or Tubercular lung affections.

25. If the Congestion and Consolidation of Lungs increase or decrease, what will be their effect on the Shadows?

The density of the shadow will be proportionately greater or less.

26. What is the usual position of the Shadows in Pneumoina?

The shadow will be in the middle portion of the lungs, with the apex and base, very slightly, if at all, shadowed.

27. If during the Convalescence of Pneumonia, the Shadow grows darker at the Base, what would you suspect?

Empyema of the pleura.

28. What would you suspect, if on Examination of the Chest, you find the Fluorescence to be unusually Bright and extended in Area further at the Apex and downward at the Base than is normal, with Diminished Diaphragm Excursion?

Emphysema of the lung.

29. What would lead you to differentiate, in the living subject, between a supposed Fluoroscopic Image of the Spine and that of the Heart?

The shadow of the spine unites with that of the heart at both its upper and lower portions, so requires differentiation. Usually the pulsations of the heart will enable differentiation between them. During a deep inspiration more lung and heart surface is brought into fluoroscopic view, hence the heart is more easily seen.

30. What other Shadows may blend with that of the Heart?

Other shadows are those of the diaphragm, liver and the large blood-vessels. Shadows seen in the region of the heart may be due to tumors or enlarged glands, and to atheromatous arteries,

31. What is the Indication of a Pulsating Shadow in the Right Chest, in Pleural Effusions, in addition to the shadow cast by the Liquid in the Left Chest?

It is the evidence of the displacement of the heart.

32. If, in the Examination of the Chest, the left side is lighted up brightly without the usual Heart-shadow, and on search the Heart-shadow is found on the Right Side, what would that indicate?

It indicates that the heart has been transposed.

33. Give the Nature of the Shadows of Thoracic Aneurysms.

Their shadows are pulsating ones, unless the tumors are filled with clots, in which case pulsations are impeded or absent.

> Note:—In a shadow supposed to be that of an aneurysm, vertebral, sternal and other shadows must be carefully excluded.

34. Why the Shadow of the Heart, in the X-Ray Examination, is greater than the Area of Dullness?

It is due to the fact that some of the shelving borders of the heart do not present themselves against the chest-wall during ordinary physical examination.

35. In examining the Œsophagus and Stomach by the X-Ray, what Mechanical Aids are often used?

Distension by flexible sounds for the ŒSOPHAGUS and by *water* for the STOMACH.

36. If Abnormal Shadows show in the Renal, Urinary, Bladder and Urethral Regions under X-Ray Examination, what may they indicate?

Strongly suggestive of calculus (stone).

37. What are the Drawbacks of a Surgical or Medical Clinician who relies upon someone else to the X-Ray Work for him ?

He must always run the risk of two things : *first*, the radiographer may not supply all the necessary details in his radiogram, and, *second* that he himself may not be able to properly interpret the shadows placed before him in the radiogram.

38. What is the Contribution of the X-Ray to the Medicine and Surgery, in general ?

It has assisted in a most wonderful manner in establishing a new standard of normal conditions and relationship in the living human body ; and has helped in the determination of the existence, character and location of diseased tissues and disturbed relations, in parts, which, for effectiveness, no other means has ever been able to approach.

INDEX

A

Abdomen, enlargement of
    the, 97, 241.
  palpation of the, 97, 98.
  retraction of the, 97.
Abdominal pains, 89, 100, 101, 102, 103, 105.
  causes of the, 100.
  in acute Enteritis, 101.
  in Appendicitis, 101.
  in Cholera Morbus, 102.
  in constipation, 98.
  in Dysentery, 102.
  in duodenal ulcers, 101.
  in epigastrium, 89.
  in gastric affections, 89.
    Cancer, 89.
    ulcer, 89.
  in Hernia, 101.
  in intestinal colic, 103.
    indigestion, 100.
    obstruction, 99.
  in lead-poisoning, 101.
  in nervous disorders, 105.
  in Rheumatism, 105.
Abscess, antero-pharyngeal, 72.
  cerebral, (See Brain, abscess of the).
  latero-pharyngeal, 72.
  œsophageal, 80.
  of the brain, causes of the, 265.
    diagnosis of the, 265, 266.
  of the kidneys, 219.
  of the lingual tonsil, 65.
  of the nasal septum, 129.
  of the rectum, 113.
  peri-pharyngeal, 72.
  peri-nephritic, the cardinal symptoms of, 222.
  retro-pharyngeal, 72.
Accommodation, the Paralysis of, 343.
  pupillary movements during, 341.
Acetonuria, the significance of, in Diabetes, 213.
Acuity of vision, 348.
Addison's disease, 256.
Adenitis, post-nasal, alteration in the mouth in, 51.
  Tubercular, 251.
Æstivo-autumnal parasites, 232.
Age, as cause of obesity, 240.
  effect of, on temperature, 6.
    on pulse rate, 27.
  importance of, in diagnosis, an example, 3.
  influence of, on frequency of respiration, 27.
    on thermometer, 4.
    on weight of the body, 240.
Air, cold, effect of, on respiration, 41.
  rarefied, effect of, on respiration, 41.
Air-passages, obstruction of the, interfering respiration, 43.
Albuminuria, 209, 210.
  conditions which may produce, 210.
  false, 210.
  febrile, probable factors of the, 260.
  in renal diseases, 210.
  Physiological, 210.
  tests for, 209.
Allorhythmia, 30.
Amaurosis, tobacco, 337.
  toxic, 337.
Amblyopia, Hysterical, 338.
Amphoric breathing, 136.
Amyloid degeneration of the kndneys, 221.
Amyotrophic lateral Sclerosis, 268.
Anæmia, appearance of the tongue, in, 59.
  fever associated with, 16.
  secondary, 228.
  splenic, 228.
  symptomatic, forms of leucocytes in, 236.
  with low red blood count, 236.

INDEX

Anaesthesia, of the rectum, 290.
of the pharynx, 76
of the throat, 290.
peripheral, 288, 289.
Anarthria, 154.
Anatomy of the brain, 307.
of the ear, 350.
of the oesophagus, 79.
of the pancreas, 121.
of the pile bearing inch, 112.
of the spinal cord, 318.
of the spleen, 120.
of the stomach, 90.
Aneurysm of the aorta, 197.
obstruction to oesophagus by, 81.
pain in, 195.
Angina pectoris, 198.
pain of, 192.
Anidrosis, 25.
the diagnostic features of, 25.
Ankle-clonus, the method of eliciting, 258.
Anorexia, 88.
the significance of, 88.
Anosmia, 128.
Antero-lateral ascending tract of the spinal cord, functions of the, 325.
Antrum of Highmore, disease of, 127.
Aorta, aneurysms of the, pain in, 195.
symptoms and diagnosis of the, 197.
Aortic area, 187.
diastolic murmur, 190.
insufficiency the pulse of, 33.
murmurs, 190.
notch and its variations, 37
regurgitation, murmurs of, 184.
sphygmographic evidence of, 38.

Aortic second sound, accentuation of, the significance of, 186
stenosis, murmurs associated with, 190
sphygmographic evidence of, 37.
the pulse of, 33.
systolic murmur, the causes of, 194.
Aortitis, the pain of, 195.
Apex-beat, displacement of the, 192.
Aphasia, 154, 310.
differention between Aphonia and Anarthria, 154.
motor and sensory, 310.
Aphonia, 154.
some causes of, 154.
Aphthae, Bednar's, 54, 55.
Aphthous stomatitis, 54.
Apolexy, 264.
Appendicitis, 108..
fever of, 17.
pain of, 101.
Appetite, excessive, 88.
loss of, 88.
perverted, example of, 88.
occurs in, 88.
Arcus senilis, 335.
Argyll-Robertson pupils, 341.
Arms, paralysis of the, 275.
the motor area controlling the movement of the, 308.
Arrhythmia, 28.
causes of, 30.
during convalescence, 31.
reflex causes of, 31.
subjective symptoms of, 31.
the toxic causes of, 30, 31.
vavular lesions, suggesting, 31.

Arsenical poisoning,
  pigmentation of the skin,
    from, 256.
Arterial Tension, high, evil effects
    of, 32.
effect on, from withdrawing
  certain quantities of fluid
    suddenly, 34.
  personal habit leading to, 32.
  sphymographic evidence of 37.
  increased, the causes of, 32.
  low, sphygmographic evidence
    of, 37.
  the causes of, 33.
Arteries, radial, examination of, 33.
Arterio-capillary resistance, conditions producing high tension
    from, 32.
  the general causes of, 32.
Arterio-sclerosis, conditions associated with, 33.
  dependent upon Syphilis, the
  vessels usually attacked in, 34.
  the causes of, 34.
  the great predisposing causes
    of, 38.
  **the influence of nervous
    activity on, 38.**
  the symptoms of, 38, 39.
  **when associated with
    interstitial nephritis, 34.**
Arthritis deformans, 247.
gonorroeal, 248
Astasia Abasia, 276
Asthma, 173.
Astigmatism tests for, 348.
Atelectasis, the symptoms and
    physical signs of, 171,
Athetosis, 286.
Atrophy of disuse, 244..
  muscular, causes of, 244.

Atrophy, muscular, symptoms
    and diagnosis of, 245.
Atrophy of the optic nerve, 348
optic, causes of, 339.
Auditory centre, 308.
Auscultation, 131.
how performed, 131
of the heart, 189.
of the oesophagus, 81.
of the stomach, 82.

B

Babinski's sign, 262.
Back, alteration in the shape of
    the, 242.
**Backache, constitutional diseases
    producing, 298.**
intra-abdominal, the cause
    of, 298.
intra-spinal, the causes of, 297
intra-thoracic, the causes of, 298.
local, the causes of, 298.
vertibral, the causes of, 297.
Bearing-down sensation, the
    causes of, 291.
Bednar's Aphthae, 54, 55.
Beri-beri, diagnosis of, 289.
Bile-duct, 117.
Bladder, conditions of the,
  producing Haematuria 207.
diseases of the, which may
    produce Pyuria, 206.
increased irritability of the,
    the causes of, 216.
**portion of the spinal cord
    controlling the, 320.**
Blepharospasm, condition of the
    eye associated with, 329.
Blood, 225.
**changes, in Anaemia,
    secondary, 228.**

Blood changes, splenic, 228.
in Haemophilia, 229.
in Leukaemia, 227.
pseudo, 229.
in Purpura, 230
in Scurvy, 230.
color-index of the, 235.
cells, 226.
-cells, red, method of
counting, 226.
preparation for counting, 226.
white, differential count of, 227.
method of counting the, 227,
preparations for counting
the, 227
disease of the, with low percentage of haemoglobin, 236
disorders of the, which may
interfered with respiration, 42.
examination, constituents of, 225.
-films, preparations for
staining, 235.
method for preparing, for
Widal reaction, 233.
method of preparation of the
skin surface for taking the, 225.
parasites of the, Malarial, 230.
smear, the process of making
the, 225.
specific gravity of the, 234.
vomiting of, 87.
Blood-vessels, changes in the, how
to recognize, 34.
diseases of the, associated
with pain, 177.
Bradycardia, 28.
brain diseases associated with, 29.
conditions associated with, 28.
Brain, Abcess of the, 265, 266.
Anatomy of the, 407.

Brain, central convolutions of
the, their functions, 315.
destructive lesions of the, 309.
disease, common forms of
Paralysis in the 326.
general functions of the, 312.
irritative lesions of the, 309.
laceration of the, Paralysis
from, 264.
motor areas of the, 308.
motor tracts of the, their
functions, 312.
Paralysis of the, 262, 263.
prefrontal lobe of the, their
functions, 314.
sensory tracts of the, 313.
substance, lacerations of, 264.
vertigo from disease of the, 355.
Breath odor of the, in
Diabetes, 67.
in uraemic coma, 67.
Breath, offensive, affections of the
brain causing, 67.
affections of the stomach
causing, 67.
causes of, 666.
drugs causing, 67.
respiratory diseases
causing, 67.
the most common cause
of, 67.
Breathing, bronchial or tubular,
sound qualities of the, 138.
broncho-vesicular, sound
qualities of the, 138.
ineffectual, diseases and conditions accompanied by, 45.
metamorphosing, 140.
restrained, diseases and conditions accompanied by, 45.

Breathing, shallow or feeble diseases and conditions accompanied by, 45.
slow, diseases and conditions accompanied by, 45.
vesiculo-cavernous, 139.
Bright's Disease, (see Nephritis.)
Bromidrosis, 25.
Bronchiectasis, 173.
Bronchitis, acute catarrhal, 167.
the subjective symptoms of, 176.
Chronic, 172.
Bronchophony, 139, 140.
whispering, 136, 140.
Broncho-Pneumonia, (See Pneumonia Broncho).
Bulimia, 88.
occurs in, 88.

C

Calculi, pancreatic, 122.
renal, 224.
Cancer, of the bile-passages, 118.
of the gall-bladder, 112.
of the intestines, 108.
of the oesophagus, the symptoms of, 80.
of the panceras, 123.
of the rectum, 112.
of the pylorus, 82.
of the stomach, 96.
Canker-Sores, 53.
Cardiac areas, 188.
valvular, 186, 187.
murmurs, 190.
sounds, as heard in the apex, 189.
sounds, decreased intensity of the, 189.
increased intensity of the, 189.
thrills, 193.
diastolic, 194.

Cardiac thrills, pericardial, 193.
presystolic,, 194.
systolic, 193.
Casts, epithelial, 214.
fatty, 214.
hyaline, 214.
granular, 214
pseudo, 215.
tube, 214.
waxy, 204.
Catheter, Eustachian, the use of, 359.
Cauda Equinia, functions of the, 322.
lesions of the, differentiation with lesions of the lower end of the cord and peripheral nerves, 322.
Cells of the posterior horns, function of the, 325.
Centre, auditory, 308.
for hearing, 316.
for heat sense, 320.
for memories, 316.
for musle sense, 320.
for Pain, 320.
for smell, 316.
for taste, 316.
for vision, 315.
Centres, automatic, 325.
for visual memories, 310.
in the medulla, 320.
of special senses, 315.
special, of the cord, 324.
trophic, of the cord, 325.
Cerebellum, lesions of the, symptoms from 311.
Cerebral embolism, 265.
haemorrhage, the paralysis from, 263.
localization, 307.

Cerebral localization, landmarks
    used in, 307.
  what two essential points taken
    into consideration, in 309.
  palsies and spinal, differen-
    tiated, 273,
  thrombosis, 265.
  vomiting, characteristics of, 87.
Cerumen, inspissated, symptoms
    of, 316.
Chancre, of the eyelids, 326.
  of the lips, 49.
Chemical reaction
    of gastric contents, 93.
  of urine, 208, 209.
Chercot-Leyden Crystals, 182.
Chest, 132.
  alar, 135.
  alteration in the shape of, 145.
  bilateral diminution in the
    size of the, 146.
  enlargement of the, 146.
  diseases of the, associated with
    pain, 176.
  decreasing the normal
    fluoroscopic shadow, 372.
  increasing the normal
    fluoroscopic shadow, 372.
  in which, X-ray, is employed,
    371.
  X-ray examination of the, the
    influence of diaphragm on
    the fluoroscopic screen, 371.
  examination of the, condition of
    voice used in, 138.
  flat, 146.
  fluoroscopic image of the,
    differentiaed with that of
    spinal cord, 372.
  inspection of the normal, 134.

Chest, pain in the, frequently
    observed, causes of, 176.
  lines forming the division of
    the normal, 132.
  Palpation of the, qualities of
    sounds to be used in, 135.
  changes in the vocal
    fremitus, 134.
  Vocal fremitus intense in, 135.
  Percussion of the, 135.
  position of the patient, in, 135.
  intensity, pitch and duration
    of the sound, in, 135.
  pterygoid, 145.
  rachitic, 146.
  regions of the, with
    boundaries, 133.
  organs lying in each
    respective, 133.
Cheyne-Stokes Respiration, 43.
  diseases and conditions
    accompanied by, 46.
Chicken Pox, (See Varicella.)
Chief ascending wave, its use
    and alterations, 36.
  determination of the height
    of the upstroke of, 36.
Children, diseases peculiar to, 2.
Chilliness, causes of, 291.
Chole-cystitis, acute infectious, 117.
Chole-lithiasis, 119.
Cholera Asiatica, symptoms and
    diagnosis of, 107, 108.
  Infantum, fever of, 17.
  Morbus, symptoms and
    diagnosis of, 107, 108.
Chorditis Tuberosa, 158.
Chorea, Huntingdon's, 287.
  post-haemiplegic, 287.
  senile, 287.

Chorea, what is, 282.
Choreic movements diseases in
    which they are found, 286.
Chromidrosis, 25.
Circulation, revolution of the, the
        phenomenon of, 192.
    of the cord, 323.
Circulatory System, the, 184.
Cirrhosis of the liver,
        haematefesis of, 87.
Climate, in the etiology of
        obesity, 240.
Clubbed fingers, 249.
Coldness, causes of. 291.
Colon, dilatation of the, 109.
    test-lavage of the, 98.
Columns of Burdach, functions
        of the, 324.
    of Clarke, the functions of, 325.
    of Goll, the functions of, 324.
Coma, Alcoholic, 300.
    definition of, 298.
    Diabetic, 301.
    Hysterical, 302.
    in Apoplexy, 299.
    in Cerebral Abscess, 300.
    in Cerebral Haemorrhage, 299.
    in Cerebral Traumatism, 299.
    in Cerebral Tumor, 299.
    in Epilepsy, 300.
    in Gas-poisoning, 301.
    in general Paralysis of the
            Insane, 300.
    in Opium-poisoinng, 300.
    in Sunstroke, 301.
    symptomatic of, 299.
    Uraemic, 301.
Coma Vigil, 298.
Complications of purulent ear
        disease, 364.

Congenital defect, some
        examples, 2.
Conjunctiva, diseases of the, 332.
Conjunctiva, dryness of the, 330.
    ecchymoses affecting the, 332.
Conjunctival diseases, points to
        be considered in, 330.
Conjunctival injection, compared
    with pericorneal injection, 334.
Conjunctivitis, catarrhal, 332.
    chronic, 332.
    croupous, 300.
    discharges from the eye in, 330.
    follicular, 333.
    phlyctenular, 333.
    purulent, 333.
    the varieties of, 328.
Consolidation, signs of
        beginning, 145.
    signs of complete, 145.
    slight, percussion, respiratory
        and vocal signs of, 144.
Constancy of cough, 179.
Constipation, character of the
        diet causing, 102.
    constitutional causes of, 98.
    definition of, 110.
    frequent use of purgatives
        as a cause of. 110.
    local cause of, 98.
    symptoms that may result
            from, 102.
Continued fever, simple, meaning
        of the term, 12.
    varieties of, 9.
    what is, 9.
**Convolutions, central, of the
        brain, 315.**
Convulsions, conditions that
    may be accompanied by, 283.
    definition of, 281.

Convulsions, Epileptiform, 281, 283, 285.
diseases characterized by, 282.
Hysteroid, 282, 284, 285.
Hysteroid, conditions characterized by, 282.
of organic brain disease, 284.
of reflex irritation, 284.
of toxic conditions, 284.
tetanic, 285.
Convulsive tic, 286.
Cornea, deformities of the 335, 336.
Herpes as it affects the, 336.
marginal ulcers of the, 335.
serpiginous ulcers of the, 335.
simple ulcers of the, 335.
the loss of transparency of the, 335.
Corneal disease, objective symptoms of, 328.
peri injection, the description of, 334.
compared with conjunctival injection, 334.
subjective symptoms of the, 334.
symptoms suggestive of, 328.
tissue, fatty degeneration of the, 335.
Corpora Quadrigemina, lesions of the, symptoms of, 310.
Cortex, motor area of the, 308.
Cough, circumstances in which absent in Pneumonia, 180.
constancy of, what is suggested by, 179.
dry, 179.
diseases and conditions in which they may occur, 179.
factors essential for the production of, 178.

Cough, moist, diseases and conditions in which they may occur, 179.
moist, 179.
night or evening, what is suggested by, 180.
production of, in heart diseases, 180.
reflex, 179.
sensations exciting the, 178.
the mechanism of, 178.
what vtrieties of, should be suppressed, 179.
winter, what is suggested by, 180.
Coughing for a long period, its pernicious effects, 180.
Cranial nerves, affections of the due to interference in respiration, 42.
Crisis, 8.
Crura cerebri, lesions of the, symptoms from, 311.
Curvature, of the spinal cord, exaggerated, 243.
posterior, 242.
rotary-lateral, 243.
Cylindroids, 215.
Cysts, pancreatic, 123.

D

Dactylitis, 249.
its relationship with Tuberculosis, 249.
syphilitic, 249.
Deafness, slowly progressive, of Tinnitus Aurium, 352.
suddden, following head injury, 353.
Influenza, 352.
Mumps, 352.
Scarlet Fever, 352.
vertigo and nausea, 353.

Defervescence, 8.
  by crisis, 8.
  by lysis, 8.
Degeneration, the reaction of, the significance of, 305.
Deglutition sounds, 92, 93.
Degrees, Centigrade converted into Fahrenheit, the process of, 6.
Delirium, definition of, 302.
  causes of, 302.
  in Acute Mania, 303.
  in Delirium Tremens, 303.
  in fevers, 302, 303.
  in Hysteria, 302.
Delirium Tremens, delirium in, 303.
Dentition, appearance of the gums in, 57.
  as it appears in the first set, 57.
  causes of delayed, 57.
  reflex disturbances from 57.
Dengue, fever of, 14.
Deviation, conjugated of head and eyes, 347.
  primary, 345.
  secondary, 345.
Diabetes, mellitus, the cardinal symptoms of, 222.
  odor of the breath in, 67.
  the condition of sweat in, 25.
  the significance of acetonuria and diaceturia in, 213.
Diaphragm, paralysis of the, how recognized, 42.
  the influence of, on fluoroscopic screen, in the X-ray examination of the thorax, 371.
Diarrhoea, causes of, 99.
  definition of, 193.
  diseases in which, may be symptomatic 99, 100.

Diarrhoea, symptoms, of 103.
Digestive Tract, the, 47.
Digital examination of the rectum, 111.
Dilatation of the stomach, 95.
Diptheria, buccal, 54, 75.
  differentiation with follicular tonsillitis, 69.
  the appearance of, 79.
  the prognostic value of a slow pulse, in, 29.
Diplopia, crossed, 345.
  homonymous, 345.
  varieties of, 344.
Disseminated Sclerosis, 270.
  tremors of the, 280.
Drink, influence of, in weight 240.
Dropsy, 241.
Ducts, bile, 117.
  common, obstruction of the 119.
  cystic, obstruction of the, 119.
Dullness, cardiac, increase in area of, 194.
  comparative or relative or deep cardiac, the area of, 188.
  splenic percussion, the normal limits of, 120.
  superficial or absolute, the area of, 188.
  superficial, percussion note in the area of, 188.
Duodenal ulcer, the pain of, 101.
Duodenum, dilatation of the, 109.
Dynamometer, the use of, 260.
Dysentery, symptoms and diagnosis of, 109.
  the pain of, 102.
Dysphagia, 76.
  laryngeal, 158.
Dyspnoea, diseases and conditions accompanied by, 46.

INDEX

Dyspnoea, expiratory, 44.
diseases and conditions accompanied by, 46.
inspiratory, 44.
diseases and conditions accompanied, by, 46.
laryngeal, the causes of, 155.
varieties of, 43.

E

Ear, 350.
Anatomy of the, 350, 351.
cerumen in the, inspissated, symptoms of, 361.
disease, internal, symptoms of, 364.
method of diagnosis, of the, 351.
purulent, complications of the, 364.
relationship with pharyngeal disease, 366.
symptoms of the, 352.
vertigo of the, 354.
discharge from the, 356, 357.
bloody, 357.
brownish, blackish or bluish, the significance of, 357.
foul odor, significance of, 357.
mucoid, the significance of, 356.
of short duration but recurs repeatedly, 357.
purulent, the significance of, 356.
significance of a foul odor of the, 357.
thin watery, the significance of, 356.
examination of the, how to conduct, 350.

Ear, function of the, tests for, 357, 358, 359.
pain in the, common cause of, 353.
differentiated from, pain of auditory canal disease, 354.
differentiated from, pain of the Eustachian Tube affections, 354.
pain of the middle ear affections, 296, 354.

Ear, Physiology of the, 351.
polypi in the, varieties of, 365.
polypus in the, diagnosis of, 365.

Eating, effect on respiration, 41.
Ecchymoses, conjunctival, 332.
Egophony, 136.
Electrical examination, constitution of, 303.
Faradic, points to be noted in, 305.
Galvanic, order of irritability of the muscles as to contraction, in, 304.
points to be noted in, 305.
strength of the machine in, 304.
terms applied in, meanings of the, 304.
the alteration theory of, 305.
usual strength of the machine used in, 304.
forms of batteries used in, 303.
precautions necessary in the application of a battery, in, 304.
Electro-diagnosis, 303.
Emaciation, what is, 239.
general conditions producing, 239.
pronounced, in children, clinical significance of, 239.

Embolism, cerebral, the
    symptomatology of, 265.
Emphysema of the lungs,
    symptoms and physical
    signs of, 172.
  the X-ray examination of, 373.
Emphysema, of the pleura, the
    X-ray examination of the, 372.
Endocardial inflammation, the
    physical signs of, 185.
Endocarditis, acute, 199.
  malignant, 199.
  the pain of, 192.
Enophthalmos, 344.
Enteritis, acute, catarrhal, 105.
  diphtheritic, 106.
  membraneous, 107.
  phlegmonous, 106.
  ulcerative, 106.
Entero-colitis, chronic, 107.
Environment, plays a part in
    diagnosis, an example, 3.
Epilepsy, coma incident to, 300.
  convulsions of the, 281, 283, 285.
  Jacksonian, 282.
  vertigo from, 355.
  differentiation with
    Meniere's disease, 355.
Episcleritis, 340.
Epistaxis, 125.
Epithelium, in the urine,
    varieties of, 214.
Epulides, 57.
Erb's Palsy, 274.
Eruption of Scarlatina,
    relationship with fever, 9.
  of Small and Chicken Pox
    differentiated, 21.
Erysipelas, diagnostic
    symptoms of, 21.

Erysipelas, the fever of, 12.
Erythrocyte, 237.
Erythromelalgia, the pain of, 296.
Esinophilia, 237.
  marked in, 238.
Ethmoidal sinus, disease of,
    the symptoms of, 127.
Eustachian canal, abnormal
    condition of the, 359.
  catarrh, 361.
  catheter, the use of, 359.
  tube, examination of, 360.
Ewald's test-breakfast, 83.
Expectoration, containing bile,
    177.
  large, 174.
  at long intervals, 181.
  muco-purulent, 181.
  offensive, 177.
  purulent, 181.
External surface, the, 239.
Exercise, effect of, on
    temperature, 6.
  influence of, on frequency
    of respiration, 41.
  on pulse frequency, 27.
Exophthalmos, 344.
Expectoration, containing bile,
    177.
  muco-purulent, conditions
    producing, 181.
  the appearance of, 181.
  mucous, 180.
  conditions having, 181.
  serous, 180.
  conditions having, 180.
Expiration, prolonged, in, 139.
External surface, symptoms and
    diseases relating to the, 239.
Extremities, lower, lymphatic
    glands of the, 251.

INDEX

Extremities, lower, multiple
Neuritic affecting the, 276.
peripheral Palsies affecting
the, 275.
upper, lymphatic glands of
the, 251.
Eye-balls, irregular movements
of the, 347.
Eye, conjugated deviation of the,
and head, clinical significance of, 347.
examination, complete, what
constitutes, 327.
movement of the, motor area
controlling the, 308.
symptoms and diseases relating
to the, 327 to 349.
nerve supply of the muscles
of the, 344.
Eyelids, chancre of the, 327.
motor disturbances of the, 328.
swelling of the, generally
accepted causes, 327.
toxic causes, 327.
Eyes, motor area controlling the
movements of the, 308.

F

Face, causes of pain in the, 295.
Facial Neuralgia, pain in, 295.
Faecal impaction, 99.
odor in the urine, 203.
Faintness, the causes of, 291.
False membrane, in the mouth, 54.
on the pharynx, 75.
Family history, usefulness in
diagnosis, 2.
Fauces, pharynx and tonsils, 67.
Feet, motor area controlling the
movement of the, 308.
pain in the, causes of, 297.

Fever, definition of, 6.
continued, 9.
concomitant symptoms of, 11.
fall of temperature without
improvement in the associated symptoms, the
indication of, 7
fresh accession of, after the
temperature has fallen
to the normal, 7.
high, definition of, 7.
intermittent, definition of, 9.
miliary, the course of, 15.
moderate, definition of, 7.
pathological factors
producing, 8.
relapsing, what is meant by, 14.
remittent, definition of, 9.
slight, definition of, 7.
suddenly appearing, without
apparent physical or other
signs of local disease,
in infants, 9.
symptoms associated with, 9, 10.
concomitant, of, 11.
nervous, of, 12.
thermic, 17.
the usual concomitant
symptoms of, 11.
to what points in the course
of, should you pay attention, 8.
Typhoid, (see Typhoid Fever.)
Yellow, the course of, 15.
the symptoms of, 23.
Fevers, activity of the pathological process related to,
in Tuberculosis, 13.
associated with the
Anaemias, 16.
associated with vaccination, 12.

Fevers, in Croupous Pneumonia, the usual mode of onset of the, 10.
 in Malta Fever, 16.
 in Measles, 12.
 in Scarlatina, characteristic symptoms of the, 20.
 especial character of the mode of onset of the, 9.
 relationship with the time of appearance of the eruption, 9.
 in Septicaemia, the temperature-curve of, 11.
 in Small Pox, 11.
 in Tuberculosis, 11.
 Malarial, general characteristics of the, 14.
 types of, to time of occurrence of the paroxysms, 22.
 varieties of, as to recurrence of the paroxysms, 14.
 of Appendicitis, 17.
 of Cerebro-spinal Meningitis, 14.
 of Cholera Infantum, characteristics of the, 17.
 of Dengue, 14.
 of Erysipelas, 12.
 of gradual onset, 11.
 of Influenza, 14.
 of Miliary Tuberculosis, 13.
 of Pyaemia, 15.
 of Septicaemia, 15.
 of Syphilis, 16.
 of the Morphia Habitues, 16.
 presenting either continued, remittent or intermittent temperature-curve, 9.
 septic, varieties of, 15.
 varieties of, divided according to their temperature-curves, 8.

Fevers, with sudden onset, 11.
Fingers, clubbed, 249.
Fissure of Rolando, 307.
 of Sylvius, 307.
 parie to occipital, 308.
Fluoroscope, 368.
Fluoroscopic image, of the spinal cord, differentiated with that of thorax, 373.
 screen, property relative to, possessed by X-ray in examining the tissues of the body, 367.
 the influence of diaphragm on, in diseases of the thorax, 371.
 shadow, diseases of the thorax decreasing the normal, 372.
 increasing the normal, 372.
 pulsaing, indicative of, 373.
Fluoroscopy, 368.
Food, influence of, in temperature, 6.
 in weight, 240.
Foot-drop, 275.
Fremitus, friction, significance of, 137, 193.
 the bronchial, significance of, 137.
 vocal, 134.
 absent, significance of, 130.
 changes in the, 134.
 intense in, 135.
 significance of suppressed, 137.
Friction sound, pleural, 145.
Friedrich's ataxia, 273.
Frontal lobes, lesions of the, the symptoms of, 309.
 sinus, symptoms of involvements of the, 127.

Furuncles, usual location of the, 365.

G

Gait, ataxic, 261.
in-coordination of, in cerebellar disease, 262.
of Hemiplegia, 261.
of Paraplegia, 261.
of spastic Paraplegia, 261.
the Waddling, 261.
Gall-Bladder and Bile-Ducts, diseases of the, 117.
Gall-stone colic, the situation of the pain in, 103.
Gangrene, pulmonary, 166.
Gastralgia, pain of, 89.
Gastric affections, characterized by pain, 89.
analysis, a complete, what constitute, 93.
Cancer, Haematemesis of, 87.
pain of, 87.
symptoms and signs of, 96.
Catarrh, acute, the symptoms and signs of, 94.
chronic, the symptoms and signs of, 94.
contents, obtaining by expression, 83.
the chemical reaction of, 93.
the diminished total acidity, of, 93.
the increased total acidity of, 94.
the method for obtaining, 93.
the Microscopical examination of the, 87.
the presence of Lactic Acid in, the disease suggested by, 84.
Gastric contents, the significance of increased Hydrochloric Acid in, 83.
the test for Hydrochloric Acid in, 83.
the total acidity of the, the method for determining, 84.
the total Hydrochloric Acid of the, the method for determining, 84.
crises, 89.
disorders classed under motor disorders, 91.
classed under pathological process, 91.
classed under perverted functions, 91.
classed under secretory disturbance, 91.
the general divisions of, 80.
the landmarks for diagnosis of the, 80.
to what points attention should be paid in examination of the, 91.
motility, the, increased, 84.
tympany, increased in what conditions, 92.
the diminution of the area of, the causes of, 83.
the increase of the area of, the causes of, 83.
ulcers, the pain of the, 89
the symptoms and signs of, 95.
vertigo, 356.
Gastritis, the acute toxic, the symptoms and signs of, 94.
the phlegmonous, the symptoms and signs of, 96.
Gastroptosis, the symptoms and signs of, 96.

General Paralysis of the
  Insane, coma, incident to, 203.
Gingivitis, 56.
Girdle sensation, 291.
Glands, tumors in the, 253.
Glottis, the oedema of the, the
  symptoms of, 158.
Glycosuria, 212.
  association of pancreatic
    diseases with, 121.
  a test for, 212.
  the clinical significance of, 212.
  the fermentation test for, 212.
Goitre, diagnosis of, 254.
Gono-cocci, the method of
  staining for, 216.
Gout, diagnosis of, 246.
Graefe's Sign, 327.
Growing pains, of children, 297.
Gums, appearance of the, during
  dentition, 57.
  blue line along the edge of the,
    the clinical significance of, 51.
  blueness of the, 51.
  bluish-red discolorisation of
    the, 51.
  in lead-poisoning, 56.
  in Scurvy, 56.
  in Syphilitic ulcerations, 58.
  conditions of the, in
    Mercurial poisoning, 56.
  condition to take note, in
    observation, 56.
  localized swelling of the, 57.
  pallor of the, the clinical
    significance of, 51.
  receding of the, from teeth, 56, 57.
  sordes on the, 56.
  swelling and sponginess of the,
    with salivation, indicative
      of, 52.

Gums, the, 56.
  thick-brown crusts on the,
    the composition of, 52.
  indicative of, 52.
  tumors in the, 57.
Gustatory sense, test for, 65.

H

Habit, plays a part in diagnosis,
  an example, 3.
  in influence of, in weight, 240.
Habit-spasm, 282.
  as referred to the eye, 329.
Haematemesis, causes of, 87.
  definition of, 87.
  of the cancer of the stomach, 87.
  of the cirrhosis of the liver, 87.
  of the renal disease, 87.
  the constitutional diseases
    which may give rise to, 87.
Haematohidrosis, 25.
Haematuria, 206.
  a chemical test for, 206.
  suggestion by a, exited by
    slight injury, 207.
  the appearance of the urine
    in renal, 210.
  the best test for, 206.
  the color of the urine, how
    affected by reason of the
    source of haemorrhage
      in, 207.
  the conditions of bladder
    causing, 207.
  the conditions of kidneys
    producing, 211.
Haemoglobin percentage of
  the blood, 234.
  low, 236.
Haemometer, Dare's, description,
  of, 226.

INDEX

Haemometer, Fielschier's, 234.
Haemophilia, symptoms and
    haemic changes in, 229.
Haemoptysis, 174.
  a suddenly appearing, the
    quantity of blood being
    large, 175.
  conditions characterized by
    pulmonary congestion
    productive of, 174.
  conditions which may
    produce, 174.
  differentiation with
    Haematemesis, 175.
  with haemorrhage from the
    mouth and throat, 177.
  diseases of the blood associat-
    ed with, 175.
  lesions of the Tuberculosis
    productive of, 174.
  repeated attacks of, over an
    extended period, what
    is suggested by, 175.
  the usual symptoms of, 175.
Haemorrhage, from the
    bowels, 19.
  from the mouth, 177.
  differentiated from
    Haemoptysis, 177.
  from he oesophagus, causes
    of, 81.
  from the pharynx, 70.
  causes of, 75.
  from the throat, differentiated
    from Haemoptysis, 177.
  from the rectum, 112.
  intestinal, 19, 100.
  in Typhoid Fever, 19.
  into the pancreas, 122.
Hand, in Paralysis Agitans, 249.
Hay fever, the symptoms of, 126.

Head, motor area controlling the
    movements of the, 308.
Headache, brain disease in which
    it is most prominent, 277.
  due to errors of refraction, 329.
  Malarial, the special features
    of the, 278.
  rheumatic, the special features
    of the, 278.
  Syphilitic, the special features
    of the, 278.
Headaches, circulatory, the
    varieties of, 277.
  condition of the eyes specially
    liable to lead to, 279.
  congestive and anaemic,
    differentiation between, 278.
  from diseases of the female
    sexual organs, the usual
    situation of the, 279.
  neuropathic, 279.
  organic, diseases in which
    they occur, 277.
  rules governing the relation
    between the seat of pain,
    and site of the lesion,
    in, 277.
  the characteristics of, 277.
  reflex, the organs which may
    produce, 279.
  some of the toxic causes of, 278.
Hearing, centres for, 316.
  impairment of the, recent
    and moderate, not associat-
    ed with pain, what is
    suggested by, 353.
  sudden, what is suggested
    by, 352.
Rinne's test, for, 358, 359.
tests for, 358, 359.
Weber's Test, for, 358.

Heart, auscultation of the, 189.
  complications of the, in
            Typhoid fever, 18.
  dilatation of the, 192.
  disease, accompanied by
            sudden death, 197.
  associated with a slow
            pulse, 29.
  depending upon the sclerosed
            vessel of the, 39.
  symptoms which lead you to
            suspect, a, 184.
  diseases of the, associated with
            pain, 177.
  production of cough, in, 180.
  the reason for enlarged
            tongue in, 59.
  vertigo from, 354.
  which may interfere with
            respiration, 42.
  fluoroscopic image of the,
            differentiated with that of
            spinal cord, 373.
  other shadows blending with
            that of, 373.
  hypertrophy of the, what is, 185.
  some of its causes, 185.
  muscle, fatty degeneration of
            the, symptoms and
            diagnosis of, 198.
  palpitation of the, 196.
  some of its causes, 196.
  percussion of the, 187.
  the reasons for 187.
  rupture of the, the pain in, 196.
  sounds, adventitious, essential
            details in, 194.
  as heard at the apex, 189.
  changes in the, consequent
            upon a diseased muscle, 185.

Heart-sounds, changes they
  undergo, during dilatation,
            192.
  murmurs, 190.
  the decreased intensity of
            the, 189.
  the first, cause of, 185.
  the increased intensity of
            the, 189.
  the normal, in listening to,
      to what points attention
      should be paid, 186.
  the second, the cause of, 186.
  the, 184.
  the left border of the, 189.
  the right border of the, 189.
  the two areas, 188.
  the upper border of the, in
            the median line, 188.
  valvular, areas of the, 186, 187.
  aortic, 187.
  mitral, 186.
  pulmonary, 187.
  tricuspid, 187.
  X-ray examination of
            the, 373, 374.
Heat, effect of atmospheric,
            on vascular tension, 34.
  sense, examination of the, 288.
  the centre for, 320.
  -stroke, the phenomena of, 17.
Height, average relation
            between weight and, 239.
Hemaralopia, 338.
Hemi-anaesthesia, 283.
Hemianopsia, 311.
  the usual status of, 312.
Hemi-hyperaesthesia, 291.
Hemiplegia, complete, the
            symptoms of, 263.

Hemiplegia, the portion of the nervous system diseased in, 276
the gait of, 261.
what is, 260.
Hiccough, 44.
diseases and conditions accompanied by hiccough, 45.
Hippus, 342.
History of preceding diseases, in diagnosis, an example, 3.
Hodgkin's disease, 252.
Hydroa, 48.
the clinical significance of, 48.
Hydrochloric Acid, diminished or absent in what diseases, 84.
in what conditions, 85.
free, the quantitative test for, 85.
increased, in gastric contents, the significance, of, 83.
increased, in what conditions, 85.
the stomach-bucket test for, 93.
the test for, in gastric contents, 85.
total, in gastric contents, the determination of, 84.
Hydronephrosis, diagnosis of, 219.
Hydrophobia, spasm of the pharynx in, 74.
Hydrothorax, 170.
Hyperaesthesia, general, occurs in what conditions, 290.
of the pharynx, 76.
Hyperchlorhydria, 326.
Hyperidrosis, 24.
conditions suggested by, 25.
Hyperosmia, 128.
Hyperpyrexia, definition of, 7.
Hypertrophy, false, 243.
true, 243.

Hysteria, differentiation with Epilepsy, 284.
stigmata of, 286.
the features of the coma in, 302.
the convulsions, of, 284.
the delirium in, 302.
vertigo from, 355.
Hysterical respiration, 44.
spasm of the pharynx, 74.
Hysteroid convulsions, 282.
conditions characterized by, 283.

I

Icterus. (See Jaundice.)
Incontinence of urine, due to local weakness, 217.
due to reflex irritations, 217.
due to spinal affections, 217.
due to unusual strain upon the vesical sphincter, 217.
due to urinary causes, 217.
Increased arterial tension, the causes of, 32.
vascular tension, examples of, 32.
Infantile indigestion, the fever of, 16.
Inflammation, endo-cardial, 185.
pericardial, 185.
Influenza, bacillus of, in the sputum, 183.
fever of, 14.
Inspection, how performed, 130.
in kidney diseases, 218.
of the intestines, what may be learnt from, 329.

Inspection, of the oesophagus, 81.
of the stomach, 91.
what information may be had from, 130.
what is, 130.
Inspiration, shortened in, 139.
Insufficiency, 191.
Intermittent-fever, definition of, 9.
Intestinal Cancer, 108, 109.
causes of abdominal pain, 100.
colic, the pain of, 103.
hæmorrhage, the cause of, 100.
the location of, 100.
indigestion, the pain of, 100.
neuroses, 109.
non-, causes of abdominal pains, 102.
obstruction, the symptoms of, 99.
the pathological conditions giving rise to, 98.
perforation, as suggested from the temperature curve, 12.
the symptoms of, 20.
symptom dependent upon constitutional disturbance, 110.
tract, some symptoms of, 90.
Intestines, altered function of the a symptom dependent upon, 90.
examination of the, methods used, 97.
inspection of the, what may be learnt from, 97.
the, 97.
Intra-ocular tension, determination of the, 340.
Iris, symptoms of diseases in the, 340.
Iritis, appearance and course of, 340.
causes of, 341.

Irritability of the bladder,
increased, the causes of, 216.
simple diminished, 306.

J

Jaundice, the discoloration of, 255.
the pulse associated with, 29.
the varieties of, 255.
Joint lesions, diseases giving rise to, 245.
of Rachitis, 248.

K

Keratitis, interstitial, 339.
scrofulous, 339.
Kidney, action of the, the true criterion of the, 200.
amyloid 221.
disease, some general symptoms of, 218.
some of the causes of, 218.
diseases, what may be learnt by inspection, in, 218.
what may be learnt by palpation, in, 218.
floating, the diagnostic features of, 219.
Tuberculosis of the, the cardinal symptoms of, 222.
Kidneys, abscess of the, 219.
active congestion of the, 220.
diseases of the, which may produce Haematuria, 211.
which may produce Pyuria, 205.
palpation of the, the method of, 223.
position of the, 218.
the, 218.

INDEX

Knee-jerk, abolished, 259.
   increased, the clinical
      significance of, 259.
   method of eliciting, 258.
     with the patient in bed, 258.
Koplik's spots, 50, 52.
Kyphosis, 242.

L

Lactic Acid, Arnold's test for, 85.
   Kelling's test for, 85.
   tests for, 85.
   the presence of, in gastric
     contents, the disease
      suggested by, 84.
   the significance of, in gastric
      contents, 86.
   Uffelman's test for, 85.
Lagophthalmus, 329.
Laryngeal, disease, characteristic
     of the sputum from, 155.
   dyspnœa, the causes of, 155.
   image, 148.
   vertigo, 356.
Lryngismus stridulus, the
     symptoms of, 158.
Laryngitis, catarrhal, acute,
     symptoms and clinical
      course of, 155.
   chronic, symptoms and
     clinical course of, 155.
   membranous, symptoms and
     clinical course of, 157.
   oedematous, symptoms
     of, 158, 159.
   phlegmonous, acute, symptoms
     and clinical course of, 156.
   sicca, symptoms and clinical
     course of, 156.
   Tubercular, symptoms and
     clinical coure of, 157.

Larynx, affections of the
     cartilages of the, 149.
   of the mucous membrane of
     the, 148.
   of the muscles of the, 149.
   of the nerves of the, 149.
   of the vocal cords of the, 149.
   a localized Anaemia of the, 149.
   differentiation of the Tubercu-
     lar and Syphilitic ulcera-
      tions of the, 157.
   examination of the, the
     method of, 147.
   points for determination,
     in, 148.
   foreign bodies in the, the
     normal location of, 153.
   malignant growths of the, the
     common forms of, 152.
   pain in the, 154.
   structural alteration of the, 150.
   the causes of swelling in the
   mucous membrane of the, 149.
   ulcerations of the, 150.
     Lupoid, 151.
     malignant, 152.
     Syphilitic, 150, 151, 152.
     Tubercular, 150, 151, 152.
   vocal cords of the, affections
     of the, 149.
   Paralysis of the, 153.
   position and motion of the, 153.
Lead-poisoning, a cause of
     abdominal pain, 104.
   appearance of the gums in, 56.
   diagnosis of the colic in, 104.
Leg-pains, 297.
Legs, motor area controling the
     movement of the, 308.
Leucocytes, in lymphatic
     Leukaemia, 237.

Leucocytes, in spleno-medullary
    Leukaemia, 236.
  in symptomatic Anaemia, 236.
  the varieties of, 227.
Leucocytosis, some pathological
  conditions attended with, 230.
  the Physiological causes of, 237.
  what is, 236.
Leucopenia, 238.
Leukaemia, lymphatic, the forms
    of leucocytes in, 237.
  pseudo, 229.
  spleno-medullary, the forms of
    leucocytes in, 236.
  symptoms and haemic changes
    of, 227.
Linear cicatrices, 49.
Lingual tonsil, abscess of the, 65.
  disorders of the, 65.
  the, 65.
  vacicose veins of the, 66.
Linked beats, 29, 97.
Lips, alteration, in the colour
    of the, 47.
  blueness of the, the clinical
    significance of, 47.
  chancre of the, the appearance
    of, 49.
  examination of the, points to
    pay attention, 47.
  fissures on the, of infants,
    suggestive of, 49.
  pallor of the, the clinical
    significance of, 47.
Paralysis of the, suggestive of, 48.
  unilateral, of the suggestive
    of, 48.
  restlessness or twitching of the
    suggestive of, 48.
  swelling of the, suggestive of, 48.

Lips, thickness abnormal, of the,
    significance of, 48.
  congenital, of the,
    suggestives of, 48.
  thinness, abnormal, of the,
    suggestives of, 48.
  acquired, of the,
    suggestive of, 48.
  tremor of the, the clinical
    significance of, 48.
Liver, a fremitus over the, the
    conditions suggested by, 115.
  auscultation of the, informa-
    tions obtained from, 114.
  cirrhosis of the, haematemesis
    in, 87.
  dipping of the, dangerous in, 115.
  the method of examination
    by, 116.
  diseases, condition of the
    tongue in, 59.
  displacement of the, causes
    of, 117.
  differentiation with alteration
    in size, 117.
  dullness, apparent increase of,
    conditions giving rise to, 117.
  diminished conditions
    suggested by, 110.
  effect of pulmonary
    Emphysema on, 117.
  enlargement, circumscribed, the
    diseases characterized by, 114.
  differentiation between
    downward displacement.
    and, 115.
  beween the prominence from
    right-sided pleural effusion,
    and, 115.
  general, diseases characterized
    by, 117.

INDEX

Liver, enlargements, painful, 114.
  painless, 114.
  increased hardness of the, the conditions suggested by, 126.
  inspection of the, information obained from, 115.
  localized oedema over the, the significance of, 116.
  pain, usual character of the, in diseases of the, 114.
  palpation of the, information obtained from, 115.
  percussion outlines of the, normal, 116.
  physical methods for examination of the, 115.
  swellings, round, smooth, over the, fluctuating on palpation, diseases suuggested by, 116.
  the, 114.
Lobar Pneumonia, (See Pneumonia, Lobar.)
Lobes, frontal, lesion of the, 309.
  occipital the most important function of, 308.
  prefrontal, functions of the, 314.
  temporo-sphenoidal, lesions of the, 309.
Loco Motor Ataxia,
  symptomatology of, 269.
Lordosis, 243.
Lung diseases, causing interference in respiration, 42.
Lungs, abscess of the, 165.
  air-vesicles of the, collapse of, 165.
  cavity in the, the X-ray examination of the, 372.
  congestion of the, symptoms and physical signs of the, 164, 165.

Lungs, congestion of, active, 165.
  passive, 165.
  the X-ray examination of the, 372.
  consolidation of the, the X-ray examination of the, 372.
  Emphysema of the, the X-ray examination of the, 373.
  gangrene of the, 165.
  œdema of the, 165.
  the, 174.
  the X-ray examination of the, 372.
Lungs, Trachea and Bronchi, 174.
  Lymphatic glands, enlargements of the, 250.
  Syphilitic, 252.
  distribution of the, of head and neck, 250, 251.
  of the lower extremity, 251.
  of the upper extremity, 251.
  localized swellings of the, 250.
Lysis, 8.

M

Marcroglossia, 59.
Malarial attack, the stages of, 22.
  fevers, characteristics of, 14.
  types of, to time of occurrence, 22.
  varieties of, 14.
  headaches, 278.
  parasites, aestivo-autumnal, 232.
  different, 230.
  general forms of, 230.
  quartan, 232.
  tertian, 230.
Malta fever, characteristics of, 15.

Mania delirium in, 303.
Mastoid disease, symptoms and diagnosis of, 365.
Mastoid proecss, inflammation of the, 354.
Measles, mouth lesion in, 50, 52.
symptoms of, 21.
temperature-curve of, 12.
Medulla oblongata, centres lying in the, 320.
Megaloblast, 237.
the clinical significance of, 237.
Memories, centres for, 316.
Meniere's disease, 354.
differentiation with epileptic vertigo, 355.
Meningitis, cerebro-spinal, the diagnostic symptoms of, 22.
the temperature-curve of, 14.
spinal, symptoms and diagnosis of, 269.
Mensuration, 132.
Metallic tinkling, occurs in, 141.
Meteorism, the causes of, 105.
Micturition, difficult, causes of, 217.
painful causes of, 216.
Mitral area, 186.
regurgitation, murmurs of the, 191.
sphygmographic evidence of, 38.
stenosis, murmurs of the, 191.
systolic murmurs, the endocardial causes of, 194.
Monoanaesthesia, 283.
Monoplegia, 260.
nervouus system involved in, 276.
Morphia habitutes, the characteristics of the fever of, 16.
Morton's disease, 297.

Motion, portion of the cord governing, 320.
Motor aphasia, 310.
area controlling the movements of the arm, 308.
of the feet and legs, 308.
of the trunk, 308.
area of the cortex, 303.
the lesions of the, 309.
disturbance of the eyelids, 328.
neurons, lower, 319.
upper, 319.
neuroses of the stomach, 96.
point of a nerve, 205.
power, loss in, of the nervous system, determination of, 260.
of the stomach, test for, 84.
decreased, 87.
increased, 86.
tracts of the brain and spinal cord, their respective functions, 312.
direct, 312.
indirect, 312.
Mouth, 49.
alteration in the shape of, in post-nasal adenoids, 51.
Anatomical structures entering into the composition of mouth, 47.
as a site for taking temperature, 5.
cyanotic hue of the mucous membrane of the, suggestive of, 52.
dark or bluish-red hard spots in the, 49.
differentiation between thrush and deposits of milk-curds in the, 50.
examination of the, the points to pay attention, 49.

INDEX

Mouth, false membrane in the, 54.
  lesion of the, characteristic of Measles, 50.
    of Scarlatina, 50.
    of Variola, 50.
  pallor, undue, of the, 49.
  pathological lesions of the, 47.
  redness, patchy, of the, 52.
    undue, of the. 49.
      diseases suggestive of, 52.
      without ulceration, 53.
  symptoms of Scurvy, 51.
  Syphilitic ulcerations of the, 50.
  tumors, in the, 54.
  ulceration of the, simple, 53.
  white platches, raised, looking like milk-curds, in the, 49.
  yellowish discoloration of the, suggestive of, 52.
  yellowish-white spots, small, breaking down to form ulcers, suggestive of, 53.
Multipolar cells, function of the, 324.
Mumps, the symptoms of, 254.
Murmur, aortic systolic, a, causes of, 194.
  endocardial, 191.
  meaning of the term as applied to heart-sounds, 190.
  mitral systolic, a, the endocardial causes of, 194.
  pericardial, 191.
  differentiation from endocardial murmur, 191.
  to determine the origin of a given, in the cardiac region, 190.
Murmurs, 190.
  associated with lesions affecting the aortic valve, 184.
Murmurs, functional, description of one of the so-called, 195.
  of mitral regurgitation, 191.
    stenosis, 191.
  regurgitant, 192.
  stenotic, 192.
    differentiation with the regurgitant, 192.
  to distinguish the character of 190.
  varieties of, as to quality, 190.
    as to mechanism of the valves, 190.
  as to time, 190.
Muscles, inflammatory swellings of the, the appearance of, 244.
  with bilateral representation, 309.
Muscular atrophy, arthritic, 272.
  juveniles, the symptoms and diagnosis of, 271.
  progressive, spinal, 267.
  equilibrium of the eye, tests for, 348.
  insufficiency of the eye, 347.
  sensibility, examination of the, 288.
Mydriasis, 342.
Myelitis, acute, 273.
Myocarditis, 198.
Myosis, 342.
  conditions producing, 343.
Myxoedema, tongue in, 59.

N

Nasal discharge, profuse, infectious diseases characterized by, 125.
  purulent, condition producing, 125.
  unilateral purulent, in adults, suggestive of, 125.

Nasal discharge, unilateral
purulent, in children, 126.
disease, pain in the causes of, 129.
relationship to certain neuroses 129.
with menstruation, 128.
obstruction, appearance of the face in, 124.
causes of, 129.
conditions capable of producing, 126.
some evil effects of, 124.
symptoms, of the constitutional disease, 129.
Neck, enlargements and tumors in the, 253.
Nephritis, acute, 220.
chronic, 210.
chronic interstitial, 221.
parenchymatous, 220.
with most marked albuminuria, 210.
Nephrolithiasis, 222.
Nephroptosis, 223.
Nervous affections, peripheral, capable of producing anaesthesia, 288.
chills, 24.
symptoms of, Typhoid Fever, 20.
system, 258.
Neuralgia, facial, 295.
intercostal, 176.
the diagnostic features of, 176.
the pain of, 292.
Neurasthenia, vertigo from, 355.
Neuritis, Arsenic, 274.
brachial, the pain of, 292.
Influenzial, 290.
multiple, affecting the lower extremities, 276.

Neuritis, multiple,
symptoms and diagnosis of, 276.
the common forms of Paralysis in, 326
optic, 338.
appearance of, 338.
causes of, 338.
clinical significance of, 338.
prognostic significance of, 339.
pain of, 292.
post-Alcoholic, 289.
post-lead, 274.
post-Typhoid, 274.
simple, diagnosis of, 289.
Neurons, motor, lower, 319.
upper, 319.
Neuroses, intestinal, 109.
Noma, 49.
Normoblasts, 237.
Nose, diseases of the, having profuse serous discharge, 125.
hypertrophy of the turbinated bodies of the, true and false, differentiation of, 128.
method of examination of the, 124.
the, 124.
turbinated enlargement of the, due to engorgement, differentiated with that due to tissue-formation, 125.
ulceration of the, 126.
Numbness, causes of, 292.
Nyctalopia, 338.
Nystagmus, 347.

O

Obesity, causes of, 240.
evil-effects of, 241.

INDEX

Occupation, the influence of, in diagnosis, an example, 3.
Oesphageal, abscess, 80.
  cancer, 80.
  obstruction, caused by Aneurysm of the aorta, 81.
    gland-disease causing, 81.
  tube or sound, contra-indication to the use of, 80.
    manner of passing the, 80.
    points to note when passing 80.
Oesophagus, 79.
  Anatomy of the, 79.
  Auscultation of the, 81.
  haemorrhage from, 81.
  inspection of the, 81.
  measurement of the, 79.
  method of examination of the, 80.
  organic obstruction of the, 80.
  pain in diseases of the, 80.
  palpation of the, 81.
  Paralysis of the, 81.
  subjective symptonms referred to the, 81.
Offensive breath, 66.
Oliguria, 200.
Ophthalmo-scopic examination, 349.
Opisthotonos, 286.
Optic chiasm, lesions of the, giving rise to symptoms, 311.
  nerve, atrophy of the, 343.
  Neuritis, 338.
    appearance of, 338.
    causes of, 338.
    clinical significance of, 338.
    prognostic significance of, 339.
Orthopnoea, diseases accompanied by, 46.
Otitis, media, catarrhal, 361.
  chronic, 362.
  suppurative, 363.

Otitis Media, suppurative, chronic, 363.
Oxalate of the crystals in the urine, the microscopic appearance of, 204.

P

Pain, abdominal (see abdominal pain).
  causes of, 292.
  centre for sensibility to, 320.
  epigastric, 89.
  from facial Neuralgia, 295.
  increased by motion, 295.
  at night, 295.
  in Acute Aortitis, 195.
  in Acute Enteritis, 101.
  in Aneurysm of the aorta, 195.
  in Angina Pectoris, 196.
  in Appendicitis, 101.
  in Brachial Neuritis, 296.
  in Cholera Morbus, 102.
  in diseases of the blood-vessels, 177.
    of the chest, 176.
    of the heart, 177.
  in diseases of the liver, 114.
  in diseases of the middle ears, 296.
  in diseases of the spinal cord, 293.
  in duodenal ulcer, 101.
  in Dysentery, 102.
  in Endocarditis, 196.
  in Erythromelagia, 296.
  in Gall-stone colic, 103.
  in Gastralgia, 89.
  in gastric affections, 89.
  in gastric Cancer, 87.
  in gastric Crises, 89.
  in gastric ulcers, 89.

Pain, in Hernia, 101.
in intestinal colic, 103.
in intestinal indigestion, 100.
in larynx, symptomatic of, 154.
in lead colic, 101.
in Pericarditis, 195.
in Phlegmasia alba Dolens, 297.
in rupture of the heart, 196.
in the face, 295.
in the chest, causes of, 176.
diseases producing, 176.
in the pharynx, 72.
in the rectum, 112.
in Tic Douloureux, 296.
of renal calculus, 224.
renal, causes of, 104, 219.
sense, 288.
sensibility to, the centre of, in the spinal cord, 320.
Pains, dull, causes of, 294.
epigastric, 89.
facial, 295.
gouty, 294.
gnawing, 295.
growing, 297.
Hysterical, 294.
increased by motion, 295.
in the back (see Backache.)
in the feet, 297.
of Neuralgia, 292.
of Neuritis, 292.
of spinal-cord diseases, 293.
from Hysteria, 294.
from reflex condition, 293.
from toxic causes, 293.
general forms of, 326.
paroxysmal causes of, 294.
radiating, 295.
reflex, 293.

Pains, rheumatic, 294.
sharp, causes of, 294.
shifting, 295.
Palate, Paralysis of the, 69.
conditions producing, 74.
deformity of the, 73.
soft, perforation of the, 73.
Palpation, 131.
of the abdomen, 97.
of the kidneys, 223.
of the liver, 115.
of the oesophagus, 81.
of the stomach, 82.
points to pay attention in, 82.
value of it on examination, 91.
qualities of sounds to use, in, 135.
Palpitation, 196.
some causes of, 196.
Palsy, differentiation of cerebral and spinal, 273.
Erb's, 274.
peripheral, affecting the lower extremities, 275.
ocular, the causes of, 344.
the symptoms of, 344.
Pancreas, Anatomy of the, 121.
cancer of the, 123.
haemorrhage into the, 122.
Pancreatic calculi, 122.
cysts, 123.
diseases, symptoms of the, 121.
association of Glycosuria with, 122.
secretion deficient, symptoms resulting from, 121.
Pancreatitis, acute, 122.
chronic interstital, 122.
Paraesthesiae, 283.
of the pharynx, 76
Paralyses, cerebral, 262, 263.

INDEX

Paralyses, cerebral, from laceration of the brain, 264.
ocular, 345, 346.
of slow onset, 263.
spinal, associated with muscular atrophy, 266.
associated with pain in the extremities, 266.
not associated with atrophy or severe pains, 267.
of rapid onset, 266.
of slow onset, 267.
of the vocal cords, 153.

Paralysis, 260.
acute ascending, 268.
agitans, tremor of the, 280.
hand of, 249.
as to location of lesions, 262.
bulbar, parts paralyzed in, 69.
cerebral, caused by lesions of slow onset, 263.
caused by lesions of sudden onset, 262.
from brain disease, general form of, 326.
from cerebral haemorrhage, 263.
from injury, 277.
general, of the insane, the coma of, 300.
glosso-labio-laryngeal, 10.
in Multiple Neuritis, general form of, 326.
of sudden onset, the significance of, 281.
of the accommodation, 343.
of the anterior crural nerve. 275.
of the arms, 275.
of the circumflex nerve, 275.
of the diaphragm, 42.
of the eyelids, 329.

Paralysis, of the fourth nerve of the eye, 346.
of the lips, 48.
unilateral, 48.
of the lower extremities, 275.
of the musculo-spiral nerve, 275.
of the oesophagus, 81.
of the palate, 69.
conditions producing, 74.
of the pharynx, the clinical manifestation of, 74.
conditions producing, 69.
of the sixth nerve, 346.
of the superior rectus, of the eye, 346.
of the inferior rectus, 346.
of interior rectus of the eye, 346.
of the third nerve of the eye, 345.
of the tongue, 61.
bilateral, 61.
unilateral, 61.
post-diphtheritic, 79.
progressive bulbar, 271.
pseudo hypertrophic, 271.
spinal, 266, 267.
general form of, 326.

Paranaesthesia, 283.

Paraplegia, 260.
ataxic, gait of, 260.
symptoms of, 270.
gait of, 260.
portion of the nervous system affected, 276.
spastic, gait of, 261.
symptoms of, 270.

Parasite, aestivo-autumnal, special features of the, 232.
malarial, the general forms of, 230.

Parasite, Malarial, types of fevers poduced by the, 230.
quartan, 232.
differentiation with the tertian parasites, 232.
tertian, 230, 231, 232.
Parosmia, 128.
Paroxysmal, tachycardia, 28.
Pectoriloquy, 136.
Peptone, a test for, 86.
Percussion, 131.
in examination of the chest, 131.
position of the patient, in, 135.
of the stomach, 92.
sounds, duration, intensity and pitch of, 135
Percussion sounds, the duration of, 135.
the intensity of, 135.
the pitch of, 135.
Perforation of the tympanic membrane, 361.
of the soft palate 73.
Pericardial inflammation, the physical signs of, 185'
Pericarditis, 199.
pain in, 195.
Pharyngeal catarrh, atrophic, 78.
disease, relationship with an aural disease, 366.
haemorrhage, causes of, 75.
lesions giving rise to, 70.
Pharyngitis, catarrhal, 78.
follicular 79.
gangrenous, 77.
gouty, 76.
herpetic, 77.
phlegmonous, 77.

Pharyngitis, rheumatic, 77.
Syphilitic, 78.
Tubercular, 77.
Pharynx, abnormally roomy, in 69,
alteration in the shape of, 71.
anaesthesia of the, 76.
capacity of the, increased in, 73.
capillary pulsations in the 71.
change in color in the mucous membrane of the, 71.
cyanosed hue of the, 71.
dryness of the, 72.
examination of the, 70.
exudation of mucus, in the, 74.
of pus, in the, 74.
false membrane in the, 70.
appearance of, 75.
follicular ulcerations of the, 70.
hyperaesthesia of the, 76.
malignant ulcerations of the, 75.
method of examination of the, 70.
points to be noted in, 71.
pain in the, in conditions, 72.
pallor of the, clinical significance of, 71.
paraesthesia of the, 76.
Paralysis of the, symptomatic of, 69.
production of mucus in the, increased, 70.
pus in the, 70.
spasm of the, observed in, 70.
Hysterical, 74.
in Hydrophobia, 74.
swelling of the, 67.
localised, 68.
Syphilitic ulceration of the, 75.

INDEX

Pharynx, Tubercular ulceration
    of the, 75.
  ulcerations of the, follicular, 70.
    malignant, 75.
    syphilitic, 75.
    tubercular, 75.
  yellowish hue of the, indicative
    of, 71.
Phlebitis, 39.
  causes of, 39.
  suppurative, symptoms of, 39.
  symptoms of, 39.
  varieties of, 39.
Phlegmasia Alba Dolens, pain
    in, 297.
Phlyctenules, 331.
Phosphates, tripple, in the urine,
  microscopic appearance of, 204.
Phthisis, acute pneumonic,
    symptoms and physical
    signs of, 167.
Physical diagnosis, 30.
  methods in use, for, 31.
  what constitutes a, 2.
  signs, the representation of, 2.
Pica, 88.
Pile-bearing inch, Anatomy
    of the, 112.
Pinguecula, 334.
Pleurisy, acute dry, symptoms
  and physical signs of, 164.
  with effusion, symptoms and
    physical signs of, 163.
Pneumonia, Broncho, symptoms
  and physical signs of, 163.
  catarrhal (see Broncho.)
  Chronic interstitial, symptoms
    and physical signs of, 171.
  circumstances when cough is
    absent in, 180.

Pneumonia, croupous, mode of
    onset of the fever in, 10.
  the symptoms and physical
    signs of, first stage, 161.
  second stage, 161.
  third and fourth stage, 162.
  Lobar, (**See** Croupous).
  temperature, high, the relative
    prognostic value of, in 7.
  X-ray examination of, 372.
  shadows growing darker in,
    significance of, 372.
  usual position of the
    shadows in the, 372.
Pneumonic Phthisis, acute, 167.
Pneumothorax, X-ray examination
    of, 372.
Poikilo-cytosis, 237.
  clinical significance of, 237.
Polio-myelitis Anterior, acute, 267.
  chronic, 276.
Polypi, in the ear, 365.
  varieties of, 365.
Polygraph, 35.
Polyuria, 200.
Pons varoli, lesions of the, giving
  rise to symptoms, 310.
Posture, influence of, on pulse
    frequency, 27.
Propetone, 86.
Pruritus Ani, 113.
Pterygium, 333.
Ptosis, morning, cause of, 329.
Pulmonary area, 187.
  congestion, 164.
  active, 165.
  Haemoptysis in, 174.
  passive, 165.
  fibrosis, 171.
  gangrene, 166.

Pulmonary oedema, 165.
  second sound, the accentuation of, 186.
Pulsations, venous, 39.
  how to detect, 40.
  pathological, 39.
  Physiological, 39.
  symptoms of, 39.
  the side in which, is most prominent, 40.
  systolic, in jugular veins, indication of, 40.
Pulse, examination of the, 26.
  by hand, 26.
  by instrument, 26.
  method for determining the tension of, 32.
  method for recording information, 26.
  points to pay attention in, 26.
  precaution to avoid errors in, 26.
  dicrotic, 33.
  prominent feature in, 34.
  frequency, for every degree rise of temperature, 27.
  influence of age, in, 27.
  influence of exercise, in, 27.
  influence of pain, in, 28.
  influence of posture, in, 27.
  influence of sex, in, 27.
  influence of temperature in, 27.
  safe limit of, in Typhoid Fever, 29.
Pulse, in Jaundice, 29.
  in Uraemia, condition of, 29.
  intermittent, the, 30.
  irregular, conditions causing, 31.
  causes of, 31.
  of aortic insufficiency, 33.

Pulse, of aortic stenosis, 33.
  of Miliary Tuberculosis, 29.
  the feature of, 31.
  radial, the delay of, 35.
  slow, disease of the heart associated with, 29.
  poisons causing, 29.
  value of, in Diphtheria, 29.
  the, 26.
  -tracing, 35.
  apsymmetry of, 36.
  component parts of a, 35.
  unilateral disturbance of the, the causes of, 35.
  water hammer, 33.
Pulsus allorhythmia, 30.
  alternans, 30.
  bigeminus, 30.
  et alternans, 30.
  paradoxus, 31.
  trigeminus, 30.
Pupils, Argyll-Robertson, 341.
  consensual reaction of the, 342.
  refusal to contract during blindness, suggestive of, 342.
Purpura, symptoms and blood-changes of, 230.
Pus in the secretion from bowels, 107.
Pyaemia, fevers of, 15.
Pyelitis, cardinal symptoms of, 221.
Pylorus, Cancer of the, the situation of the palpable tumor in, 82.
Pyorrhoea alveolaris, 56.
Pyrosis, 89.
Pyuria, 204.
  dseases of bladder producing, 206.
  intermitetent, 205.
  origination of, in, 205.

Pyuria, tests for determining, 206.
  value of chemical reaction in diagnosis, 205.
  vesical, 205.

Q

Questioning the patient, one practical way of, 1.

R

Rachitis, joint lesions of, 248.
Radiograph, 367.
Radiography, 369.
  comparison of the observations of, with those of fluoroscopy, 371.
  principles underlying, 368.
Rales, crepitant, 142.
  division of, 141.
  dry, conditions represented by, 141.
  varieies of, 141.
  moist, conditions represented by, 141.
  sub-crepitant, 142.
Ranula, 54.
Records, necessity of keeping accurate and systematic, 1.
  of physical conditions, 3.
Rectal examination, particulars of the, 110.
  points for determination, 111.
  preparation of the patients for, 111.
  pain, causes of the, 112.
Rectum, abscess of the, 113.
  balooning of the 113.
  bleeding from the, 112.
  cancer of the 112.
  digital examination of the, 111.

Rectum, digital examination, points to take note in, 112.
  fissure of the, 113.
  instrumental examination of the, 112.
  portion of the spinal cord controlling the, 320.
  stricture of the, 113.
  the, 110.
Reflex, abdominal, the method of eliciting, 259.
  cremaster, the method of eliciting, 259.
  epigastric, the method of eliciting, 259.
  gluteal, the method of eliciting, 259
  superficial, abolished in, 260.
Reflexes, superficial and deep, 262.
Refraction, errors in, cause of headache, 329.
Regurgitation, aortic, 184.
  sphygmographic evidence of, 38.
  mitral, the murmurs of, 191.
  sphygmographic, 38.
Renal calculus, the pain of 224.
  the situation of the pain in, 104.
  enlargements, conditions capable of producing, 223.
  special features of, 223.
  varieties of, 219.
  pain, the causes of, 219.
Resonance, vocal, diminished, 137.
  increased, 137, 140.
  suppressed, 137.
Respiration, 41.
  affections of the cranial nerve for interference in, 42.
  amphoric, 136.
  Cheyne-Stokes, 43.

Respiration, Cheyne-Stokes,
    clinical significance of, 46.
    diseases and conditions
        accompanied by, 46.
  deficient, 43.
  effect of cold air on, 41.
    of eating on, 41.
    of exercise on, 41.
    of rarefied air on, 41.
    of sleep on, 41.
  factors necessary for proper
        performance of, 42.
  frequency of, normal 41.
  Physiological variations of
        the, 41.
  Hysterical, 44.
  interference in, by affections
        of the cranial nerve, 42.
    by diseases of the heart, 42.
    by disorders of the blood, 42.
    by obstruction of the air-
        passages, 43.
    the nervous causes of, 42.
    the pleural causes of, 43.
    the pulmonic causes of, 42.
  interrupted, in conditions, 140.
  points to take note in
        observation of, 41.
  sighing, 44.
  yawning, 44.
Respiratory sings, 138.
  of beginning consolidation, 145.
  of complete consolidation, 145.
  of slight consolidation, 145.
Respiratory sound, bronchial, 143.
  broncho-vesicular, 144.
  cavernous, 144.
  diminished in, 143.
  increased in, 142.
  interrupted or cog-wheel, 144.
  prolonged, 144.

Respiratory sound, suppressed,
        143.
  symptoms of the Typhoid
        Fever, 20.
Retention of urine, the causes
        of, 216.
Retina, functional disturbances
        of, 337.
Retinitis, 336.
  albuminuria, 336.
    prognostic value of, in
      interstitial Nephritis, 336.
  diabetic, 337.
  leukaemic, 337.
Rheumatic Pharyngitis, 77.
Rheumatism, acute inflammatory,
        diagnosis of, 245.
  chronic articular, diagnosis
        of, 246.
  of the abdominal walls, 105.
Rigidity, muscular, 98.
  spinal cord affections
        associated with, 288.
Rigidities, occur in, 287.
Rigors, 23.
  greatest diagnostic value of, 23.
  in continued fever is
        suggestive of, 24.
  Pathological causes of, 23.
  Physiological causes of, 23.
  symptoms associated with, 23.
Rose-spots in Typhoid fever, 18.

S

Saliva, 66.
  acid reaction of the, 66.
  composition of, 66.
Salivery flow, diminished in, 66.
  increased, in, 66.
Salivation, the drugs producing,
        66.

INDEX

Scarlatina, character of the mode of onset of the fever, in, 9.
    mouth in, 50.
    relation of the fever of, with the appearance of the eruption, 9.
    significance of smoky urine in, 203.
Scarlet fever, characteristic symptoms of, 20.
    complications met with, in, 20.
Sclerosis, amytrophic lateral, 268.
    disseminated, 270.
    tremors of, 280.
Scoliosis, 243.
Scurvy, blood-changes in, 229.
    mouth symptoms of, 51.
    the gums in, 56.
Secretory neuroses of the stomach, 97.
Sensation, "bearing down", 291.
    cold and chilly, 291.
    girdle, 291.
    of faintness, 291.
    of numbness, 292.
    of tingling 292.
    portion of the cord governing, 319.
Sense, muscular, centres of, 320.
    tests for, 288.
    pain, tests for, 288.
    gustatory, tests for, 65.
    heat sense, centres of, 320.
    tactile, tests for, 288.
    temperature, tests for, 288.
Sensory, Aphasia, 310.
    neuroses of the stomach, 96.
    tracts of the brain, 313.
    tracts of the spinal cord, 313.
Septicaemia, fevers of, 15.
    temperature curves of, 11, 13.

Septic fevers, varieties of, 15.
Septum, perforation of the, causes of, 128.
Sex, influence of, in diagnosis, an example, 3.
Sighing, 44.
Sign, definition of the term, 2.
Signs, physical, the representation of the, 2.
Sinus, ethmoidal, involvements of the, 127.
    frontal, involvements of the, 127.
Skin, changes in the, in Arsenical Poisoning, 256.
    discoloration of the, in Jaundice, 255.
    Pathological, 234.
    pallor of the, indication afforded by, 255.
    pigmentation of the, diseases which cause a, 256.
    Syphilitic, 257.
Small-pox, (*see* Variola)
Smell, centres for, 316.
Sordes, 52.
Spasm, 281.
    clonic, 281.
    habit, 282.
    of the pharynx, 70, 74.
    in Hydrophobia, 74.
    hysterical, 74.
    of the tongue, occurs in, 62.
    tonic, 281.
Spasms, local, instances of, 285.
    found in conditions, 285.
Special senses, centres of the, 315.
Sphygmograph, 35.
    method of application of the 35.
    method of preparing smoked films for the 35.
    tracing by the 35.

Sphygmograph, tracing, aortic
notch of the, 37.
information given by, 35.
the component parts of a, 35.
summit wave of the, 36.
tidal wave of the, 37.
Sphygmographic evidence of
aortic regurgitation, 38.
of aortic stenosis, 37.
of combined regurgitation and
stenosis, 38.
of mitral regurgitation, 38.
of mitral stenosis, 38.
of the arterial tension,
high, 37.
of the arterial tension, low, 37.
Spinal Cord, cervical section of
the, the functions of, 320.
circulation of the, 323.
disease of the, the common
form of Paralysis, in, 326.
the depressive and destructive
symptoms of, 326.
the irritative symtoms of, 326.
the pain in, 293.
dorsal section of the, the
functions of, 321.
fluoroscopic image of the,
differentiated with that
of heart, 373.
general Anatomy of the, 318.
general functions of the, 324.
grey matter of the, 318.
functions of the, 325.
lower end of the, lesions of, 322.
lumbar section of the,
functions of, 321.
motor neurons of the, lower, 319.
motor neurons of the, upper, 319.
tracts of the, 312.

Spinal cord, multipolar cells of
the functions of, 324.
pain of, from reflex
conditions, 293.
from Hysteria, 294.
from toxic causes, 293.
portion of the, controlling
bladder, 320.
controlling the rectum, 320.
governing motion, 320.
governing sensation, 319.
sensory tracts of the, 313.
softening of the, from
Thrombosis, 274.
special centres in the,
functions of, 324.
the centre for heat sense, 320.
the centre for muscle
sense, 320.
the centres in the upper
enlarged portion of the, 320.
white matter of the, 318.
the functions of, 325.
Spinal localization, 318.
Splanchnoptosis, 110.
Spleen, displacements of the,
causes of, 120.
enlargements of the,
conditions producing, 120.
physical methods for
examining of, 120.
situation of the, 120.
the condition of, in Typhoid
Fever, 15.
Splenic percussion dullness,
the normal limits of 120.

INDEX

Sputum, black, 174.
  Charcot-Leyden crystals in the, the appearance of, 182.
  collection of, for microscopic examination, 176.
  elastic fibres in the, 176.
  fibrinous coagula in the, the appearance of, 182.
  Influenza bacilli in the, the appearance of, 183.
  method of preparation of, for examination, 177.
  of laryngeal disease, characteristic of, 155.
  Pneumo-coccus in the, the appearance of, 182.
  Frankel's, in the, 183.
  Friedlander's, in the, 183.
  purulent, the appearance of, 181.
  rust-colored, 177.
  spirals in the, the appearance of, 182.
  tubercular bacilli in the, the examination of, 177.
Squint, concomitant, 345.
  convergent, 345.
Stenosis, 191.
  aortic, 184.
  mitral, the sphygmographic evidence of, 38.
  murmurs of, 191.
  the pulse of, 33.
  the sphygmographic evidence of, 37.
Stellwag's Sign, 328.
Stomach, absorptive power of the, the determination of, 86.
  Anatomy of the, 90.
  ausculation of the, how performed, 92.
Stomach, auscultation of the, value of, in examination, 92.
  -bucket, 93.
  cancer of the 96.
  contents of the, (*see* Gastic contents.).
  dilatation of the, 95.
  dimension of the, 90.
  diseases of the, classed under motor disorders, 91.
  classed under Pathological processes, 91.
  classed under perverted functions, 91.
  classed under secretory disturbances, 91.
  general divisions of the, 90.
  landmarks for diagnosis in, 90
  in which free Hydrochloric Acid is diminished or absent, 84.
  in which free Lactic Acid is present, 84.
  points to pay attention, when examining, 91.
  what may be learnt from inspection of, 91.
  increased resistance of the, when palpating, 82.
  method of inflating the, for inspection and palpation, 82.
  method of palpating the, 82.
  points to pay attention in, 82.
  motor power of the, diminished in conditions, 87.
  increased in conditions, 86
  tests for determining the, 84.
  neuroses of the, 96.
  motor, 96.
  secretory, 97.

Stomach, palpation of the, how performed, 91.
   value of, in examination, 91.
   percussion of the, how performed, 92.
   value of, in examination, 92.
   -tube, contra-indication of the use of, 83.
Stomatitis, 53.
   apthous, 54.
   small yellowish-white spots in, 53.
   when frequently observed, 52.
   catarrhal, 54.
   undue redness of the mouth in, 53.
   gangrenous, 49, 55.
   Mercurial, 55.
   mycotic, 49, 55.
   ulcerative, 55.
   swelling and sponginess of the gums in, 53.
Stool, black, 104.
   clay-colored, 104.
   effect of retention of faeces on the color of, 107.
   fatty, 105.
   formed, 104.
   mucous, 104.
   normal, 104.
   pus in the, 104.
Stupor, 296.
Subjects of enquiry, the principal in medical cases, 1.
Sub-normal temperature, a morning, with an evening rise is indicative of, 24.
   constitutional diseases associated with, 24.
   nervous conditions producing, 24.

Subnormal temperature, Pathological state associated with, 24.
   the, 24.
   what constitutes a, 24.
Sunstroke, 17.
   coma incident to, 301.
Sweat, 24.
Symblepharon, 334.
Symptom, definition of the term, 2.
   objective, 130.
   subjective, 130.
Syphilis, blood-vessels usually attacked, in, 34.
   fevers of, 16.
   lymphatic enlargements, in, 252.
Syphilitic pigmentation of the skin, 257.
   teeth, 58.
Syringomyelia, 272.

T

Tachycardia, 28.
   conditions producing, 28.
   general conditions associated with, 28.
   paroxysmal, conditons producing, 28.
Tactile sense, examination of, 288.
Taste, centre for, 316.
   perverted, 65.
Teeth, caries of the, conditions favoring, 58.
   deformities met with in the, 58.
   grinding of the, the significance of, 58.
   receding of the gums from the, causes of, 57.
   Syphilitic, characteristies of the, 58.
Teething in children, 57.
Temperature, 4.

INDEX

Temperature, accurate way for determining bodily, 4
-curve of cerebro-spinal Meningitis, 14.
of Measles, 12.
of Septicaemia, 11.
resemblance with Tuberculosis, 13.
of Small Pox, 11.
of Typhoid Fever, typical, 10.
departures from, 10.
fall of, sudden, in Typhoid Fever, 10.
influence of age on, 6.
of exercise on, 6.
of food on, 6.
of seat of local diseases, 4.
of time of day on, 6.
Physiological, 5.
normal, cold and chilly sensation in, 291.
observation of, with thermometer, how long to be kept in situ, 4.
in cases where rectum or vagina is used, 5.
in cases where taking by mouth is inadmissible, 5.
means for recording, 6.
places available for, 4.
precautions to be adopted,
when taking by the axilla, 5.
when taking by the mouth, 5.
when taking by the rectum, 5.
when taking by the vagina, 5.
Physiological influences causing variance in the, 5.

Temperature, relative differences of, taken by mouth, axilla and rectum, 5.
sense, examination of, 288.
symptoms, of Tuberculosis, 11.
Temperature, sub-normal, 24.
cold and chilly sensation in, 291.
constitutional diseases associated with, 24.
nervous conditions having, 24.
pathological states associated with, 24.
the morning, with evening rise, suggestive of, 24.
Thalamus Opticus, functions of the, 317.
Thermic fever, 17.
Thermometer, observation of temperature with, 4.
how long to be kept in situ, in, 4.
necessary factors for accuracy of the, 4.
places available for, 4.
the age of the, affecting its reading, 4.
the seat of local diseases affecting the reading of, 4.
Thoracic Aneurysm, shadows of the, in X-ray examination of the, 371.
Thorax, (*see* Chest).
Thirst, marked, clinical significannce of, 88.
Thrill, (See Cardiac thrills).
Throat, anaesthesia of the, causes of, 290.
haemorrhage from the, differentiated with Haemoptysis, 177.
variations in the color of the, 71.

Thrombosis, cerebral, 265.
   softening of the cord, from 274.
Thrush, differentiated with
               milk-curds, 50.
   the lesion of, 40.
Thyroid glands enlargements,
               of the, 253.
Tinkling, metallic, 141.
Tinnitus Aurium, 353.
   the causes of, 353.
Tongue, 58.
   appearance of the, in
               Aneamia, 59.
   atrophy of the muscles of the,
      the lesions or diseases
               producing, 59.
   black, drugs staining the, 60.
   blackish spots on the, clinical
             significance of, 60.
   blueness of the, clinical
             significance of, 60.
   coated, 62.
   coatings of the, 62.
   conditions of the, in liver
               diseases, 59.
   cyanosed, 62.
   cyanosed hue of the, clinical
            significance of, 60.
   denuded dry, 62.
   diminution in the size of the,
              causes of, 59.
   dryness, abnormal, Pathological
        conditions producing, 61.
   dryness of the, Physiological
             causes of, 60.
   prognostic significance of, 61.
   encrusted dry, 62.
   dry and brown, significance
               of the, 62.
   enlarged causes of, 58.

Tongue, enlarged, in heart dis-
      eases, the reasons for, 59.
   in Myxoedema, the reason
              for, 59.
   observed in conditions, 59.
   examination of the, points to
            pay attention, 58.
   fissures of the, significance
             of, 63, 64.
   furred, 62.
   furrowed, 64.
   moisture in the, the absence
             of, the value of, 63.
   the presence of, the value
             of, 63.
   orange-yellow, the substance
            staining the, 60.
   pallor of the, clinical
             significance of 59.
   Paralysis, bilateral of the 61.
   of the, occurs in, 61.
      as a sequel of an
           infectious disease, 61.
   unilateral, of the, 61.
   plastered, clinical significance
             of, 63.
   protrusion of the, slowly, 61.
   with abnormal readiness, 61.
   purplish spots on the, clinical
            significance of, 60.
   red, dark (merging almost to
      black), conditions producing,
              60.
   reddish, later becoming bluish
       to black sub-cutaneous
       blotches on the, 60.
   redness, abnormal, the diseases
      and conditions producing, 60.
   red, raw and denuded, clinical
            significance of, 60.
   shaggy, 62.

INDEX

Tongue, spasm of the, occurs
    in, 62.
  stippled, 62.
  plus coated, 62.
  strawberry, 62.
  swelling, enormous, the
    disease suggested by, 58.
  great, of half the, the
    diseased suggested by, 59.
  tremor of the, clinical
    significance of, 61.
  ulceration of the, common
    forms of, 63.
  dyspeptic, 65.
  Syphilitic, 64.
Tubercular, 64.
  yellow, the substance staining
    the, 60.
Tonsillar hypertrophy, true and
  false, differentiation of, 73.
Tonsillitis, catarrhal,
    appearance of the, 68.
  definition of, 73.
  follicular, differentiation with
    Diphtheria, 69.
  objective conditions observed
    in, 68.
  herpetic, definition of, 73.
  objective conditions observed
    in, 68.
  suppurative, definition of, 73.
  objective appearances of
    the, 68.
Tonsils, enlarged, post-nasal
    space observed in, 68.
  enlargement of the, causes
    of, 68.
  swelling of the, conditions
    producing, 68.
  the, 67.

Tonsil, the lingual, (See Lingual
    Tonsil).
Trachea, bronchi and lungs,
Tracheal tugging, 193.
Trachoma, 331.
Tremor, Alcoholic, 280.
  asthenic, definition of, 279.
  observed in, 279.
  definition of, 279.
  of disseminated sclerosis, 280.
  of the lips, the significance of,
    48.
  of the Paralysis Agitans, 280.
  of the tongue, the clinical
    significance of, 61.
  tobacco, 280.
  toxic causes of, 281
Tricuspid area, 187.
Trunk, motor area controlling
    the movements of the, 308.
Tubercle bacilli in the sputum,
    examination of, 177.
  in the urine, method of
    staining for, 215.
Tuberculoses, activity of the
    Pathological process
    suggested by fevers in, 13.
  characterized by complete
    absence of fever, 14.
  great variety of ranges,
    high Remittent fever, 13.
Tuberculosis, acute, miliary,
  differentiation of the fevers
    in, with Typhoid Fever, 13.
  the fevers of, 13.
  the pulse of, 29.
  the features of the, 31.
  Fibro-caseous, the symptoms
    and physical signs of, 168.
  Fibroid, the symptoms and
    physical signs of, 170.

Tuberculosis, Fibroid, lesions of the, producing Haemaptysis, 147.
relationship with Dactylitis, 249.
temperature symptoms of, 11.
the varieties of, 22.
the X-ray examination of, 371.
Tumor of the Pylorus, 82.
Tumors, about the neck, 253.
cerebral, coma incident to, 299
fluctuating, 242.
lateral, 242
of the glands, 253.
of the gums, 57.
of the mouth, 54.
pelvic, 241.
wandering, 242.
Turbinated bodies, 128.
Tympanites, the causes of, 105.
Tympanic membrane, normal, appearance of the, 359.
points to be noted in examination of the, 360.
Tympanum, abnormalities of, 360.
chronic suppurative disease of the, 360.
Tympany, gastric, 83.
Typhoid Fever, complication of the heart in, 18.
crusts, thick brown, on the gums, in, 52.
differentiation of the fever of, with that of Tuberculosis, 13.
enlargement of the spleen in, 18.
haemorrhage from bowel in, the diagnosis of, 19.
high fever, persistent, in, value of, 7.
intestinal perforation, suggestion from the temperature-curve of, 12.

Typhoid Fever, intestinal perforation, the symptoms, of, 20.
prodromal symptoms suggestive of, 18.
prognosis of, 20.
pulse-frequency in, the safe limits of, 29.
pulse in, 13, 34.
rose-spots in, 18.
sudden fall of temperature, in, 10.
temperature curve of, typical, 10
departure from, 10..
temperature, high, the relative prognostic value of, in, 7.
the abdominal symptoms of, 19.
the gastro-intestinal symptoms of, 19.
the nervous symptoms of, 20.
the respiratory symptoms of, 20.
the second week of, 18.
urinary examination in, the value of in diagnosis, 19.
Widal reaction of, 232.

U

Ulceration of the cornea, 335.
of the gums, syphilitic, 57.
of the larynx, lupoid, 131.
malignant, 152.
Syphilitic, 150.
Tubercular, 150.
of the mouth, 53.
Syphilitic, 50.
of the nose, 125, 126.
of the pharynx, follicular, 70.
malignant, 75.
Syphilitic, 75.
Tubercular, 75.

INDEX

Ulceration of the stomach,
(*See* Gastric ulcers).
of the tongue, common forms of, 63.
dyspeptic, 65.
Syphilitic, 64.
Tubercular, 64.
Uraemia, the coma incident to, 301.
the pulse in, 29.
Urination, decreased, the Pathological causes of, 200.
difficult, causes of, 216.
increased, the Pathological causes of, 200.
painful, causes of, 216.
Urine, acidity of, the, increased, the causes of, 209.
albumin in the, two tests for determination of, 209.
the heat and acid tests for, 209.
the Picric Acid tests for, 209.
alkalinity of the, causes of, 209.
Ammoniacal, 203.
analysis of the, points to pay attention in, 202.
what constitute a complete, 202.
appearance of the in renal Haematuria, 210.
bile in the, clinical significance of, 211.
test for, 211.
black, conditions producing, 202.
blood in the, best test ordinarily for, 206.
chemical test for, 206.
blue, causes of, 201.
casts in the, 214.
pseudo- in the urine, 215.
waxy, 204.

Urine, Chemical reaction of the, method for determining the, 208.
normal, 209.
Chlorides in the, when absent, 213.
cloudiness of the, appearing on cooling, 203.
disappearing on addition of an acid, 203.
in freshly-passed, the significance of, 207.
not changed by alkalis or acids, 203.
cloudy, causes of, 201.
clearing on application of heat, what is suggested by, 202.
on the addition of an acid, 202.
color of the, affected by source of haemorrhage in Haematemesis, 207.
normal, 201.
concentrated, produced by, 202.
cylinders in the, 215.
daily quantity of, normal, in adults, 200.
in children, 200.
deposit, white, in the, suggestive of, 209.
earthworm-like clots in the urine, suggestive of, 207.
epithelium in the, varieties of, 214.
faecal odor in the, 203.
greenish-yellow, conditions producing, 202.
incontinence of the, local weaknesses causing, 217.
reflex irritation causing, 217.

Urine, incontinence of the,
    spinal affections causing, 217.
    the urinary causes of, 217.
    unusual strain on the vesical sphincter causing, 217.
microscopic examination of the, preparation of a specimen for 213.
the method of staining for Gono-cocci for, 216.
the method of staining for tubercle bacilli for, 215.
milky, causes of, 203.
Oxalate of lime in the, microscopic appearance of, 204.
pale, abnormal, diseases producing, 215.
causes of, 201.
clinical significance of, 214.
of high specific gravity, 202.
Physiological variations in quantity, of, 200.
pus in the, Chemical tests of, 204.
flakes of, clinical significance of, 205.
of vesical or renal origin, value in Chemical reaction, 205.
quantity of, normal, daily, in adults, 200.
    in infants, 200.
    Physiological variations in, 200.
retention of, causes of, 216.
smoky, the significance of, in Scarlatina, 203.
specific gravity, normal of the, 207.

Urine specific gravity of, allowance for temperature, when freshly passed, 208.
precautions to avoid inaccuracies in determining the, 207.
sugar in the, test for, 212.
sugary odor in the, 203.
sweat odor in the, 203.
tripple Phosphates in the, the microscopic appearance, 204.
urea in the, decreased, in conditions, 212.
    increased, causes of, 211.
    the method for determining the percentage of, 211.
Uric Acid crystals in the, microscopic appearance of, 212.
urinary solids in the, the method of estimation of, 208.
    the proportion of the, with urea, 208.
waxy casts in the, 204.
white deposit, abundant, in the, suggestive of, 209.
whitish, what is suggested by, 202.
yellowish-green and milky, what is suggested by, 202.
pale, causes of, 201.
Uvula, oedema of the, the clinical signifiance of, 69.

V

Vaccination, the character of the fever associated with, 12.
Varicella, the eruptions of, differentiated from those of Small Pox, 21.

INDEX

Varicose veins of the lingual tonsils, 66.
Variola, the eruptions of, differentiated from those of Chicken Pox, 21.
 the febrile curve of, 11.
 the mouth lesion of, 50.
 the principal diagnostic features of, 21.
Venous pulsations, 39.
Vertigo from cardiac diseases, 355.
 from disturbance in a special sense, 356.
 from Epilepsy, 355.
 from Hysteria, 355.
 from Meniere's disease, 355.
 from Neurasthenia, 355.
 from organic disease of the brain, 355.
 from toxic conditions, 356.
 of ear disease, 354.
 peripheral, 356.
Vision, centres for 315.
Visual field, test for, 348.
 memories, centres for, 310.
Vocal cords, affections of the, 149.
 normal position and motion of the, 153.
 Paralysis of the, 153.
 fremitus, absent, the significance of, 138.
 changes in the, in palpating the chest, 134.
 the side of the chest, in which it is far intense, 135.
 suppressed, the significance of, 137.
resonance, diminished and suppressed in, 137.
 increased, found in, 137.
signs, 138.

Vocal signs, loud and most important, 139.
Vomiting, cerebral, characteristics of the, 87.
 of blood, (*See* Haematemesis.)
 Uraemic, characteristics of, 88.

W

Water-hammer pulse, 33.
Waxy casts, 204.
Weber's test for, auditory functions, 358.
Weight, average relation between height and, 239.
 influence of age on, 239.
 of climate on, 239.
 of food and drink on, 239.
 of habit on, 239.
 Physiological factors of, 238.
Whisper, bronchial, increased in, 137.
 cavernous, conditions represented by, 137.
Whispering Bronchophony, 136.
Whooping cough, the cardinal symptoms of, 183.
Widal reaction, 232.
 method for preparing the blood for, 233.
 the clinical value of, 233.
Winged scapula, the lesion producing, 275.
Wrist-drop, double, the clinical significance of, 275.

X

X-ray, diagnosis, 367.
 discovery of, 367.
 drawbacks of the surgical and medical clinicians, 375.

X-ray, examination, adjustment of the tubes to secure high or tubes to secure high or low vacuum, 369.

affections of the thorax in which employed, 371.

influence of the diaphragm in, 371.

consolidation shadow in, suggestive of, 372.

diseases of the brain in which it assists materially to diagnose, 370.

dressing of the patient in, 369.

effects on the shadows, by congestion and consolidation of the lungs, 372.

in intra-spinal disease, why of no service, 371.

in which the normal fluoroscopic shadow is increased, 372.

necessity of a dark-room in, 367.

enlightening the patient about the nature of the, beforehand, 367.

of Emphysema of the lungs, 372.

of the pleura, 372.
of Pneumonia 372.
of Pneumothorax, 372.
of Tuberculosis, 372.
of the chest, 372.
of the lungs, 372.

X-ray examination, of the oesophagus, mechanical aid used for, 374.

of the stomach, mechanical aid used for, 374.

position of the patient in, 368.

of the shadows in Pneumonia, 372.

shadows of the heart, in, 374.

of the thoracic Aneurysm, 374.

the shadow growing darker at the base during convalescence of Pneumonia, in, suggestive of, 372.

the value of, in diagnosis, 370.

forms of apparatus chiefly used in, 367.

fundamental principles of the, in its application to medical and surgical diagnosis, 370.

-picture. evidence in interpreting of, 371.

-plates, 370.

the contribution of, to medicine and surgery, 375.

the value of, to the medical diagnostician, 367.

Y

Yawning, 44.
Yellow Fever, symptoms suggesting, 23.
the course of, 15.

THE END.